*Perspectives in Cardiovascular Psychophysiology*

T.M.

# *Perspectives in*
# CARDIOVASCULAR
# PSYCHOPHYSIOLOGY

*Edited by*

JOHN T. CACIOPPO
*The University of Iowa*

*and*

RICHARD E. PETTY
*The University of Missouri, Columbia*

THE GUILFORD PRESS
*New York*
*London*

LIBRARY OF CONGRESS CATALOGING IN PUBLICATION DATA

Main entry under title:

Perspectives in cardiovascular psychophysiology.

  Includes bibliographies and indexes.
  1. Cardiovascular system—Diseases—Psychosomatic aspects. 2. Cardiovascular system.
I. Cacioppo, John T. II. Petty, Richard E. [DNLM: 1. Cardiovascular system—Physiology.
2. Psychophysiology. WG 101 F652]
RC 669.P47     616.1'08     81-6766
ISBN 0-89862-613-7          AACR2

*To our spouses*
BARBARA L. CACIOPPO AND VIRGINIA L. PETTY

# Contributors

CHRIS BERKA, BA, Department of Neurosciences, University of California, San Diego, California

JOHN T. CACIOPPO, PhD, Department of Psychology, The University of Iowa, Iowa City, Iowa

DAVID DANFORTH, MA, Department of Psychology, Boston University; and Department of Biobehavioral Science, University Hospital, Boston, Massachusetts

JAMES E. DAVIA, MD, Walter Reed Army Medical Center and Department of Medicine, Uniformed Services University School of Medicine, Bethesda, Maryland

BERNARD T. ENGEL, PhD, Laboratory of Behavioral Sciences, National Institute on Aging, Gerontology Research Center, Baltimore City Hospital, Baltimore, Maryland

DON C. FOWLES, PhD, Department of Psychology, The University of Iowa, Iowa City, Iowa

DAVID C. GLASS, PhD, Graduate Center, City University of New York, New York, New York

JAMES HASSETT, PhD, Department of Psychology, Boston University, Boston, Massachusetts

LARRY D. JAMNER, PhD, Department of Psychology, State University of New York at Stony Brook, Stony Brook, New York

DAVID S. KRANTZ, PhD, Department of Medical Psychology, Uniformed Services University School of Medicine, Bethesda, Maryland

PHILIP M. McCABE, PhD, Department of Psychology, University of Illinois, Champaign–Urbana, Illinois

JAMES H. McCROSKERY, PhD, Department of Psychology, State University of New York, Oswego, New York

PAUL A. OBRIST, PhD, Department of Psychiatry, University of North Carolina, Chapel Hill, North Carolina

ALEKSANDER PERSKI, PhD, Laboratory of Behavioral Sciences, National Institute on Aging, Gerontology Research Center, Baltimore City Hospital, Baltimore, Maryland

RICHARD E. PETTY, PhD, Department of Psychology, The University of Missouri, Columbia, Missouri

STEPHEN W. PORGES, PhD, Department of Psychology, University of Illinois, Champaign–Urbana, Illinois

JOHN L. REEVES II, PhD, Department of Anesthesiology, University of California, Los Angeles, California

CURT A. SANDMAN, PhD, Departments of Psychiatry and Psychobiology, University of California Irvine Medical Center, Orange, California; and Fairview Hospital, Costa Mesa, California

MARC A. SCHAEFFER, BA, Department of Medical Psychology, Uniformed Services University School of Medicine, Bethesda, Maryland

GARY E. SCHWARTZ, PhD, Department of Psychology, Yale University, New Haven, Connecticut

DAVID SHAPIRO, PhD, Department of Psychiatry and Biobehavioral Sciences, University of California, Los Angeles, California

BERNARD TURSKY, PhD, Laboratory for Behavioral Research, Department of Political Science, State University of New York at Stony Brook, Stony Brook, New York

BARBARA B. WALKER, PhD, Ann Arbor VA Medical Center, University of Michigan, Ann Arbor, Michigan

BRANDON G. YONGUE, MA, Department of Psychology, University of Illinois, Champaign–Urbana, Illinois

# *Preface*

At a time when much of the research in psychophysiology is on the human brain, we have chosen to focus on the frontiers in cardiovascular psychophysiology. This perspective is selected not to discount the importance of other research, but rather to serve as a starting point from which the functions of the brain and bodily systems can be investigated. There are several advantages to this focus. First, the instrumentation and techniques for measuring cardiovascular variables are becoming increasingly agreed upon and economical. Second, there is a long history of research in this area that has yielded a large data base from which sophisticated behavioral hypotheses can be derived and tested. Third, the application of current theory in cardiovascular psychophysiology has generated a number of procedures that show promise in the areas of clinical psychology and behavioral medicine.

Furthermore, using as a starting point the long line of research that has derived from the field of cardiovascular psychophysiology recognizes the complex interactions between the central and peripheral nervous systems. The cardiovascular system contributes so importantly to the life-maintaining function of the organism that, from an evolutionary viewpoint, it is obvious why the reliable operation of the cardiovascular system and the system's responsiveness to environmental demands are tied so closely (albeit complexly) to physiological functioning generally and behavior. It should not be surprising, then, that dynamic changes in cardiovascular functioning can be initiated by a number of control systems and can emerge as altered heart rate, stroke volume, vascular resistance, and so forth. Interestingly, these dynamic changes can alter specific parameters within cardiovascular functioning (e.g., transiently accelerated heart rate, for instance, may affect blood pessure but not stroke volume or vascular resistance; vascular resistance may change primarily within one area of the circulatory route), yet interact with functions of other organs and physiological systems (e.g., via baroreceptor reflexes).

Accordingly, a focus on cardiovascular psychophysiology can be expected to yield a variety of viewpoints. The reader can anticipate disagreements among our contributors regarding the behavioral significance of changes in cardiovascular functioning and regarding the mechanisms underlying the observed effects. The variety of views offered by the contributors not only provides students with an up-to-date treatment of the history, methods, theory, and applications of cardiovascular psychophysiology, but also should stimulate discussion and study of a number of important issues emerging from this field.

We have sought to maintain a level of readability throughout the book that is steady and accessible to the advanced undergraduate or graduate student who has had at least one advanced course in psychology. To the extent that we were successful in this effort, we owe our thanks to the contributors.

We are indebted to a large number of people and groups. First of all, we are grateful to the special research support provided us by our universities (University Faculty Scholar Award, Old Gold Fellowship), the National Science Foundation (BNS 78-18667 and BNS 80-23589), and the National Institutes of Health (BRS-U.I. G603). Their generous support enabled us to develop and complete this project with a minimum of delays.

Working with the contributors has been a pleasure, and for their efforts and understanding we are sincerely thankful. Gary E. Schwartz, Paul A. Obrist, and Don C. Fowles were particularly encouraging and helpful in the early stages of the project. We also acknowledge a debt to earlier works on cardiovascular psychophysiology from which we learned so much, but especially the work by the Laceys and the 1974 tome on this subject by Obrist, Black, Brener, and DiCara. Seymour Weingarten, editor-in-chief at The Guilford Press, has been unusually facilitative, and we thank him sincerely. Our students (especially Leo Quintanar, Charlotte Lowell, Mary K. Braccio, and John P. Holbrook) and our secretaries (Gertrude Nath and Sue Staub) also made valuable contributions to the book. Finally our families (Barbara, Lynn, Cyrus, Mary Katherine, Edmund, Jo Ann, Susan, Dominick, Bob, Renee, Arlene, Jane, and Tom) have made our work environments conducive and extraordinarily pleasant.

J.T.C.
R.E.P.

# Contents

*Perspectives in Cardiovascular Psychophysiology*

# Editors' Overview

The present book draws together some of the most current work representing a cross-section of approaches to the study of cardiovascular psychophysiology in particular (e.g., heart rate, blood pressure, and cardiac lability) and psychophysiology in general (e.g., interactions with electrocortical activity, and respiration). Research in the field of cardiovascular psychophysiology has a long tradition of being germinal for other areas of investigation, and the contributions to this book will likely continue this tradition.

The book begins with a brief overview of the cardiovascular system. In the first chapter, Hassett and Danforth outline the history of cardiovascular psychophysiology and briefly discuss cardiac physiology. Tursky and Jamner in the second chapter delve deeper into cardiac physiology and provide a benchmark review of the techniques for measuring, quantifying, analyzing, and interpreting cardiovascular functioning.

The chapters that follow deal explicitly with the psychological and behavioral significance of the cardiovascular responses of interest to psychophysiologists. In 1899 Angell and Thompson noted an empirical pairing of specific kinds of tasks and cardiovascular responses. Chester

Darrow (1929) refined this early analysis by determining that "sensory," "ideational," and "disturbing ideational" stimuli led to a slowing, slight speeding, and significant speeding of heart rate, respectively. These effects remained unexplained for about 30 years while investigators focused on physiological "arousal" and behavioral organization. During the 1950s, psychophysiologists, but most notably the Laceys, elaborated upon the earlier observations of stimulus–response stereotypy and directional fractionation. A host of principles of psychophysiology soon emerged (see Sternbach, 1966).

Currently, there is a consensus that cardiac activity does not covary invariantly with other measures of arousal, and increasingly common is the distinction by investigators of reportable arousal, the intensity of a response or syndrome of responses, and behavioral excitation (see Chapters 3–5). The contribution focused most explicitly on physiological arousal and behavior is the third chapter, by Fowles, who proposes a sophisticated model based on Gray's theory of motivation and behavior.

Another theme that has emerged in cardiovascular psychophysiology is that cardiac changes are related in complex ways to information processing and affect. The fourth chapter, by Shapiro and Reeves; the fifth chapter, by Cacioppo and Petty; and the sixth chapter, by Sandman, Walker, and Berka, advance variations on this theme. Shapiro and Reeves demonstrate, for instance, that altering the cardiovascular component of a person's reaction to a stressful stimulus (e.g., a cold-pressor test) modifies reports of its painfulness. Cacioppo and Petty review the social psychological research on physiological responses and attitude change. Cacioppo and Petty argue that the psychological and behavioral significance of cardiovascular responses must be interpreted not only within the context of other physiological responses, but also within the context of an individual's reportable state. The significance of a given cardiovascular response can be influenced by factors such as whether or not the response was detected, and if detected, whether it was detected interoceptively or exteroceptively. Sandman, Walker, and Berka review their work on cardiac activity, perception, and the average evoked potential (AEP). Though their early studies were in accord with the Laceys' hypotheses regarding sensory intake–rejection, their data on heart rate and AEPs suggest that the underlying mechanism may be considerably more complex than originally anticipated.

A third focus can be characterized by an emphasis on explicating the physiological mechanisms underlying cardiovascular responses. Porges,

McCabe, and Yongue, for instance, review the physiological evidence relating fluctuations in heart rate to respiratory activity. They indicate that the amplitude of the respiratory sinus arrhythmia (RSA) is related to vagal tone and can be used to index fetal neuropathology and fetal well-being during birth. Obrist, in the next chapter, traces his productive program of research from its origins when investigating the sensorimotor concomitants of heart rate responses to its present focus on hypertension. Interestingly, Obrist argues that the major contributions to be garnered from cardiovascular psychophysiology pertain to issues in behavioral medicine (e.g., the development and treatment of hypertension) rather than to the study of more traditional, theoretical constructs in psychology.

The clinical applications of work in the field of cardiovascular psychophysiology are the thrust of Chapter 9, by Perski, Engel, and McCroskery; and Chapter 10, by Krantz, Glass, Schaeffer, and Davia. In Chapter 9 the authors describe their work on the modification of cardiovascular responses using operant conditioning procedures. Their research, which also highlights a number of important issues in clinical biofeedback, holds promise in improving patients' recovery from ischemic episodes. The chapter by Krantz et al. contains a review of data relating Type A behavior to coronary heart disease. They provide interesting evidence that this relationship may be mediated by long-term alterations of cardiovascular functioning resulting from the behavior and physiological responsivity of Type A individuals.

The epilogue chapter by Schwartz details the many different mechanisms that can operate to produce any given "cardiovascular response." Schwartz describes the principles of general systems theory and specifies the implications of this theory for thinking about and research in cardiovascular psychophysiology. This chapter, which also serves as an interesting commentary on the preceding chapters, underscores the importance of a systems, or multivariate, approach to the study of cardiovascular psychophysiology in particular and psychophysiology in general.

## REFERENCES

Angell, J. R., & Thompson, H. B. A study of the relations between certain organic processes and consciousness. *Psychological Review*, 1899, *6*, 32–69.
Darrow, C. W. Differences in the physiological reactions to sensory and ideational stimuli. *Psychological Bulletin*, 1929, *26*, 185–201.
Sternbach, R. A. *Principles of psychophysiology*. New York: Academic Press, 1966.

# 1

# An Introduction
# to the Cardiovascular System

JAMES HASSETT
DAVID DANFORTH

## EARLY VIEWS OF THE CARDIOVASCULAR SYSTEM

The importance of the heart and the circulatory system was recognized even by primitive man. The cave drawings of Neolithic hunters often included a symbol of the heart within the breast of their prey. Scholars disagree about whether these drawings suggest a belief in the magical powers of the heart or were simply meant to teach other hunters to aim for this bull's-eye.

When ancient Egyptian priests prepared a body for mummification, they wrapped the heart in linens and left it in place in the body. Less important organs such as the stomach and brain were removed and thrown away. In the eyes of some commentators, this custom suggests that the Egyptians viewed the heart as the seat of the soul. There is no reason to believe, however, that the Egyptians had any understanding of

James Hassett. Department of Psychology, Boston University, Boston Massachusetts.

David Danforth. Department of Psychology, Boston University; and Department of Biobehavioral Science, University Hospital, Boston, Massachusetts.

the circulation of the blood, nor of the cardiovascular diseases to which so many of them succumbed.

The honor of being the first psychophysiologist may belong to Erasistratos, an Alexandrian physician three centuries before Christ. Erasistratos was called on to treat Antiochus, the son of one of Alexander the Great's most powerful generals, for a strange and debilitating disease. Strongly believing in mind–body holism and finding no somatic problem, Erasistratos concluded that the young prince suffered from mental strain. The ancient Greek biographer Plutarch offered the following account of the physician's method (quoted in Mesulam & Perry, 1972):

> Wishing to discover who was the object of his passion . . . he would spend day after day in the young man's chamber, and if any of the beauties of the court came in, male or female, he would study the countenance of Antiochus. . . . when anyone else came in Antiochus showed no change, but whenever Stratonice (his step-mother) came to see him as she often did . . . those telltale signs of which Sappho sings were all there in him—stammering speech, fiery flashes, darkened vision, sudden sweats, irregular palpitations of the heart, and finally . . . helplessness, stupor, and pallor. (p. 547)

Based on these physiological observations, Erasistratos concluded that his patient suffered from love sickness. The Greek physician Galen later made a similar diagnosis on another patient by observing changes in her pulse rate.

The *Mo Ching*, or Chinese Pulse Treatise, was written in the 3rd century A.D. and contained descriptions of various pulse signs and their implications. For example, "a pulse like the pecking of a bird or water dripping on a roof means death in four days." The Chinese stressed the idea that the pulse can be used to diagnose disease or emotional turmoil.

Greek physicians traditionally believed that the arteries contained only air. But Galen, a physician who lived about a century and a half after Christ, argued that the blood did not diffuse through the body "like water in unbaked pottery," as Aristotle maintained, but rather flowed through the arteries and veins. His conclusions were based on dissections of lower animals, and his gory observations as physician to the gladiatorial school in Pergamon. However, Galen erroneously believed that the blood ebbed and flowed through the vessels like the ocean tide, and that only the veins delivered blood to the organs.

The facts and fictions of Galen's view of the cardiovascular system dominated science until the Renaissance. Leonardo da Vinci was the first to correctly draw the heart as having four rather than three chambers. Less serious misconceptions were corrected by other anatomists. But the most radical advances came from the work of William Harvey, the court physician to King James I of England. A contemporary of Newton and Shakespeare, Harvey was a fellow of the Royal College of Physicians, an institution which fined its lecturers for any criticism of Galen's teachings. Nevertheless, Harvey tried to solve the puzzle of cardiovascular function by observation and experiment, rather than limiting himself to studying the writings of earlier experts.

Harvey measured the pumping action of the heart and discovered that it was far greater than anyone had ever imagined. In 1628 he wrote in *De Mortu Cordis*:

> At last I perceived that the veins should be quite empty, and the arteries on the other side be burst with too much blood, unless the blood did pass back again some way out of the veins into the arteries and return into the right ventricle of the heart. . . . I began to bethink myself if it might not have a circular motion. (Willis, 1847/1965, p. 58)

Interestingly, Lehrer (1979) notes that Harvey reached this conclusion on the basis of several erroneous calculations:

> He derived his results by measuring the volume of the left ventricle in one cadaver, then multiplying this figure by the pulse rate. But in the first place, he measured the volume incorrectly, and then he made an enormous error by using a pulse rate of 33 beats per minute, about half the actual average rate. The final figure he obtained for cardiac output is less than one thirty-sixth of the lowest value accepted today. Nonetheless, Harvey had proved his point, because even by his calculations the output of the heart in thirty minutes far exceeded the total weight of blood in the body. (p. 9)

Apparently, the Royal College of Physicians was not an institution in which researchers published or perished. Harvey performed repeated experiments and published the results 12 years after first reaching his dramatic conclusion. Although the theory that the blood circulates through the body led to a storm of controversy, Harvey gave little reply, preferring to let his painstakingly derived facts speak for themselves. He lived to see the acceptance of his theories mark the beginning of a new era of experimental physiology. Using a crude microscope in 1661, Malpighi discovered the capillaries, the "missing link" which transported blood from the arteries to the veins.

Arterial blood pressure was measured for the first time in 1733. Much to the dismay of the British Anti-Vivisectionist Society, Reverend Stephen Hales attached a vertical glass tube to a major artery in a horse. The blood rose to a height of 8¼ feet. Since that time far less drastic procedures have been developed for measuring blood pressure. In 1896 the Italian physician Riva-Rocci invented the mercury sphygmomanometer, the precursor to the familiar blood pressure cuff now used in medical settings.

## THE BEGINNING OF THE MODERN ERA

In 1899 James Angell and Helen Thompson published a paper entitled "A Study of the Relations between Certain Organic Processes and Consciousness." According to their review of the literature, an Italian physiologist named Angelo Mosso performed the first study of cardiovascular psychophysiology in 1881 when he demonstrated that psychic activity increased the flow of blood to the brain and decreased blood flow to the periphery.

Inspired by the theories of emotion proposed by Wilhelm Wundt and William James, other 19th-century researchers soon turned to the question of how the cardiovascular system responds to affective stimuli. Most of these early studies relied on plethysmographic measures of blood flow. The Greek root "plethysmos" means enlargement. When blood flows to most parts of the body, the influx of liquid makes that body part swell. A plethysmograph measures this change in volume, which waxes and wanes with each beat of the heart.

For example, blood flow was often measured by immersing the hand in a container filled with liquid and sealed with a stretchable diaphragm. As blood flowed into the hand and its volume increased, a small amount of liquid was displaced, causing the diaphragm to be stretched. This movement often activated a mechanical system of levers and pulleys which ultimately moved a stylus over a slowly revolving drum, and thus provided a permanent record of blood flow changes.

The Angell and Thompson (1899) study was partially designed to see whether a device like this could distinguish physiologically between agreeable and disagreeable sensations and emotions. It could not. Angell and Thompson found instead that almost every stimulus led to vasoconstriction. They were able to show, however, that mild stimuli (such as an unexpected knock on the door) decreased blood flow less than more dramatic stimuli (such as thinking suddenly of a friend's illness).

Through the 1920s psychophysiological researchers continued to rely on the plethysmograph to measure physiological responses to emotion. Surprisingly few experimented with the new technologies of electrocardiography (ECG) for measuring heart rate or various cuff methods for measuring blood pressure. Instead, many of the early studies of the psychophysiology of blood pressure grew out of the work of the Italian criminologist Cesare Lombroso. Lombroso had suggested that blood pressure measurements during a criminal interrogation could reveal whether or not a suspect was telling the truth. This claim laid the foundations for the lie detection business, which unfortunately developed a life of its own outside the mainstream of psychophysiological research.

In 1929 Chester Darrow published a monumental study of the physiological effects of different classes of stimuli. His subjects were 70 coworkers at the Illinois Institute for Juvenile Research. Darrow measured respiration, electrodermal activity, and plethysmographic changes in the finger. He also measured blood pressure from a cuff on each person's ankle, designed to be more comfortable and less affected by artifact than the ordinary arrangement.

Dr. Darrow chose over 100 stimuli to elicit a wide range of reactions. After the experiment was over each subject classified the stimuli. These ratings were combined with others from neutral observers to form three categories. Twenty "sensory" stimuli included hearing a shout, a finger snap, and a gun fire, as well as being slapped in the face and having the hair pulled. Fifty-three "indifferent ideational" stimuli included hearing the words "apple," "boot," and "tree," and answering the question "Do you like cheese?" The 41 "disturbing ideational" stimuli were more emotionally charged. They included the words "constipation" and "masturbation," looking at pictures of men and women in their underwear, and answering the questions "Ever contemplate suicide?" and "Afraid I'll find out something?"

What Darrow found out was that he could indeed distinguish these categories physiologically. He found that sensory stimuli were "relatively more effective in increasing cardiac activity as indicated by blood pressure or pulse rate" (Darrow, 1929, p. 300). He also found that the responses to disturbing ideational stimuli tended to be larger than those to the indifferent group.

In historical terms, this study is important because Darrow was one of the first to find systematic classes of stimuli which produced physiologically distinct responses. But, as we shall see later, his work had little influence until John and Beatrice Lacey uncovered a similar distinction nearly three decades later.

## CONTEMPORARY VIEWS

It is now widely accepted in medical practice that stress and tension are often associated with increases in cardiovascular function.

With the aid of portable measuring devices, observations have been made of increased heart rate (HR) and/or blood pressure (BP) in many stressful real-life situations. Indeed, the use of such portable machines has often been crucial for diagnosis of heart problems that cannot be seen in the relative tranquility of the doctor's office. Gunn, Wolf, Block, and Person (1972), for example, tell of one patient whose abnormally high heart rate (paroxysmal atrial tachycardia, to be exact) appeared only in measurements during a contract bridge tournament, with his wife as his partner. Some years later this same patient had a heart attack and died during a similar bridge tournament. Other situations in which cardiovascular increases have been seen include driving a car, donating blood, being interviewed by a psychiatrist, preparing for a ski jump, landing a plane on an aircraft carrier, and working in a brokerage house while the stock market is open (Gunn et al., 1972).

Increases in cardiovascular function are also observed, of course, during the muscular strain associated with physical activity. One of the more interesting examples of this phenomenon was in Masters and Johnson's (1966) studies of sexual activity. For women, at least, the increase in HR appears to be related to the intensity of the orgasmic experience.

Studies of sexual activity also point to the importance of local changes in blood flow. Genital erection is largely controlled by increased blood flow to the penis and clitoris. The "sex flush" frequently observed during sexual excitement is also a product of increased blood flow to the skin. The innocent blush of embarrassment is nothing more than a dilation of facial arteries leading to increased circulation and a warming of the skin.

Despite Darrow's insights, early psychophysiological researchers often used measurements of the cardiovascular system as indices of arousal. For example, one series of studies showed higher HRs and BPs right before class examinations (Brown & Van Gelder, 1938). A. E. Nissen (1928) found BP increases in two patients sitting in the dental chair when their dentist walked into the room. Landis (1926) induced three of his colleagues to undergo a 2-day fast without sleeping. The subjects were then given the strongest electrical shock they would stand for as long as they would permit it. The physiological reactions to the shock included marked sweating, gasping, nausea—and BP increases.

The concept of overall activation in the cardiovascular system is a reasonable first approximation. But the concept of patterning of cardiovascular responses in different states was the next step.

In a classic study in 1953, Albert Ax directly confronted the issue of whether one emotion could be distinguished from another on the basis of its physiological concomitants. He measured the cardiovascular, electrodermal, respiratory, and muscle systems, while an "incompetent technician" deceptively produced feelings of anger and fear. Each emotion produced its own physiological pattern. The major cardiovascular finding was that diastolic blood pressure increases and heart rate decreases were more common for anger than fear. Overall, the fear pattern appeared related to the chemical action of the hormone adrenaline (epinephrine); the anger pattern was more closely related to noradrenaline (norepinephrine) action. In a recent extension of this study, Weerts and Roberts (1976) found similar patterns of physiological response when people simply imagined being in situations that made them angry or fearful.

The next major advances in the understanding of cardiovascular function grew out of the work of John and Beatrice Lacey at the Fels Research Institute. In 1959 Lacey attacked simplistic concepts of global arousal and substituted the idea of "directional fractionation": that different fractions of the total somatic response pattern may respond in opposite directions. He went on to argue that cardiovascular increases *cause* decreases in brain function.

In the earliest studies Lacey (1959) demonstrated that, for most people, a task like solving a mental arithmetic problem led to a classical arousal reaction in which both HR and skin conductance increased. The same people, when they listened to a series of tones, showed HR decreases along with skin conductance increases—thus, an example of "directional fractionation." As more tasks were discovered to show similar patterns, Lacey, Kagan, Lacey, and Moss (1963) went on to argue that "environmental intake" (attention to external events) led to phasic HR decreases. Still later Lacey (1967) emphasized the presumed basis of this observation: HR and BP increases increased baroreceptor (pressure-sensitive receptors in the aortic arch and carotid sinus) firing, which provided feedback to the brain and decreased its activity.

A number of critics attacked this view, most notably Paul Obrist and his colleagues at the University of North Carolina Medical School.

The Obrist, Webb, Sutterer, and Howard (1970) theory of cardiac-somatic coupling stresses more commonsense notions of cardiovascular function—namely, the heart beats faster to supply more blood to the tissues that need it. In an impressive series of studies on humans and lower animals, HR and electomyogram (EMG) activity have covaried directly. That is, when muscle tension increased (thus increasing muscular demands for $O_2$ and nutrients), HR also increased; when EMG decreased, so did HR. HR and EMG are seen in this view as concomitant changes produced by the same central nervous system mechanism. It is not that one causes the other; rather, the body is built in such a way that the two ordinarily change together.

Thus, the HR decrease observed when a person attends to the surrounding world is merely an indication, for Obrist, that our individual is sitting quietly. Cardiovascular increases seen in mental arithmetic are a sign that a person tenses his/her muscles when he/she tries to solve a problem.

Some of the research generated by this controversy is described elsewhere in this volume; much of our current understanding of the psychophysiology of the cardiovascular system can be traced to this source.

## ANATOMY AND PHYSIOLOGY

The heart is a muscular pump, the strongest and most efficient muscle in the body. It weighs a little less than a pound (between 250 and 400 g in the normal adult) and pumps the average human's 6 quarts of blood through the entire circulatory system in just over 1 min. Assuming an average heart rate of about 70 beats per minute, the heart beats over 100 thousand times a day, or more than 2.5 billion times in a life of 70 years. It pumps about 1800 gallons of blood a day, for a lifetime total of 46 billion gallons.

The heart rests in the pericardium, a cone-shaped sac of protective tissue which is situated slightly to the left of center in the thoracic cavity. On either side of the heart are the lungs; in the front it is protected by the sternum.

There are three layers of heart tissue. The outermost, the epicardium, contains the coronary vessels, which deliver the heart's own blood supply, and the cardiac autonomic nerves. The inner walls of the heart chambers are lined with the cells of the endocardium, which are so smooth that they offer little resistance to blood flow within the heart. Between these two layers lies the myocardium; it is composed of layers of muscle tissue wrapped in a spiral fashion not unlike a turban. When cardiac muscle contracts, it resembles the sliding and folding of a Chinese fan. This allows the chambers of the heart to forcefully contract and expand without unduly displacing the heart within the pericardium.

The heart is divided by impermeable membranes, or septa, into four chambers. The left and right atria act as reservoirs or receptacles for incoming blood. The left and right ventricles provide the main pumping power.

In a functional sense, there are two hearts and two circulatory systems. With any luck at all, blood does not pass directly from the right to the left side of the heart or vice versa. Instead, the left and right ventricles act as two pumps operating in series and firing simultaneously. In the systemic circulatory system, blood rich with oxygen is passed out of the heart from the left ventricle, through the arterial system to target organs, where nutrients are removed and wastes are added, then through the veins and back into the right atrium. The pulmonary system is concerned with passing the now oxygen-deficient blood through the lungs. Blood is pumped through the right ventricle, through the pulmonary artery (the only artery in the body that carries oxygen-deficient blood), through the capillary system of the lungs, where wastes are removed and oxygen replaced, and back out the pulmonary vein to the left atrium.

A one-way flow through the entire system is ensured by the many unidirectional valves in the arteries and veins, and (most crucially) by the four major valves in the heart. The mitral and tricuspid valves allow blood to pass from the left and right atria to the left and right ventricles,

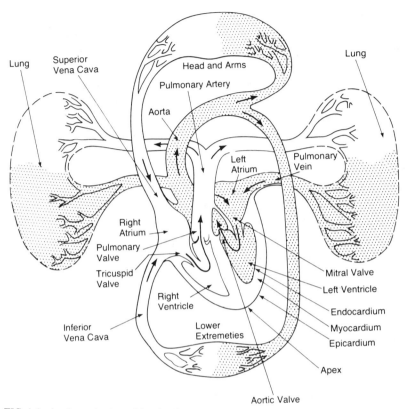

FIG. 1-1. A schematic view of the circulatory process. See text for details. From *A Primer of Psychophysiology*, by James Hassett. Copyright 1978 by W. H. Freeman. Reprinted by permission.

respectively. They are also known as the atrioventricular, or inlet, valves. The two outlet valves, the aortic and the pulmonary, control the ejection of blood to the systemic circulation and the lungs, respectively, upon contraction of the ventricles. The opening and shutting of these valves make the familiar "lub–dup" sound of the heart beating in the chest. The "lub" sound corresponds to the sudden closure of the atrioventricular valves accompanied by a contraction of the thick muscular walls of the arteries. "Dup" is the sound of the sharp closure of the aortic and pulmonary valves. When these sounds are abnormal, one is said to have a heart murmur, which usually indicates that the valves are not closing properly. Such faults, particularly in the atrioventricular pair, may result from infection such as rheumatic fever or from congenital defects. These deficiencies may lead to fatigue and fainting from reduced cardiac output, particularly when an individual is under stress (cf. Gazes, 1975).

The course of circulation may be thought of as a continuous, non-intersecting figure eight. When the heart is in its resting phase, or diastole, the oxygenated pulmonary venous blood (the only oxygen-rich venous blood in the body) returning from the lungs enters the left atrium through the four pulmonary veins. It then passes through the mitral valves, upon atrial contraction, down into the left ventricle: This is the larger and stronger of the ventricles, since its cylindrical contractions must pump blood for the longest distance. When the ventricles contract, in the systolic phase, blood is thrust out of the left ventricle into the aorta. From there, it branches out to the systemic circuit, consisting of the cerebral, muscular, renal, and splanchic (liver and spleen) networks.

At the cellular level, blood is deoxygenated in the capillary bed; there it also picks up $CO_2$ and cellular waste products. At this point, it enters the venous half of the circuit. Upon arriving back at the heart, the "used" blood enters the right atrium at diastole through the inferior and superior venae cavae. Upon atrial contraction, once again this blood passes through the tricuspid valve and is ejected at systole from the right ventricle into the two pulmonary arteries which carry it to the lungs for "recycling." While the systemic circulation is a "high-resistance circuit" with a large pressure difference between the arteries and veins, the blood flow through the lungs normally encounters little resistance.

The blood is spread into a very thin layer in the dense alveolar capillary network in the lungs. The total surface area of this network is about the size of a tennis court. The blood is spread until it is only about 10 millionths of a meter thick; thus $O_2$ and other atmospheric gases are easily exchanged for $CO_2$ in the blood. This entire process of moving through the alveolar capillary bed and exchanging gases takes only about 1 sec. But effective oxygenation depends on the condition of one's alveoli. Respiratory disorders may collapse some alveoli. In effect, this sends venous blood back to the heart, making the heart work harder and stressing the entire system. Thus, it is easy to see why respiratory and cardiovascular disorders such as coronary disease and hypertension are integrally related to such risk factors as cigarette smoking and inadequate exercise.

Although in some respects the heart is a self-regulating organ, it remains under the control of both the autonomic and central nervous systems. Sympathetic nervous system impulses increase heart activity (a "pressor effect" resulting from the release of adrenaline), while parasympathetic nervous system messages decrease it. Electrical impulses from the hypothalamus and parts of the brainstem can have either pressor or depressor effects on heart rate and related output.

It is now clear that portions of the cerebral cortex which are involved in either motor behavior or in emotion have a strong influence on the activity of the heart. Psychophysiologists who hope to clarify the relationships between psychological events and cardiovascular function are particularly interested in these interactions.

The regular beating of the heart is controlled by a complex series of electrical events. A high-density network of muscle cells called Purkinje fibers constitutes the "hard wiring" of the circuit. These cells run through the myocardium and have a distinct action potential which allows contraction of the heart muscle in a rapid, coordinated pattern. When the electrical impulses which cause the heart to contract are not properly coordinated, parts of the muscle will contract and relax too haphazardly— as, for example, in fibrillation.

The sinoatrial (SA) node is the electrical pacemaker which coordinates the contractions of the heart. The SA node consists of a group of specialized muscle cells surrounded by a mass of autonomic nerve endings. It is located high on the wall of the right atrium near the entrance of the superior vena cava.

Once the SA node fires, a wave of excitation quickly spreads to the right and left atria, causing them to contract, and the atrioventricular valves to open. A second center of electrical firing, the atrioventricular (AV) node, is located near the bottom of the right atrium, where the rapid-conduction Purkinje network begins. At this point, muscle fibers are gathered into a conducting cable called the "bundle of His" which carries impulses from the atria to the ventricles at a speed of about 400 or 500 cm/sec. In the wall between the two ventricles, the bundle of His divides into two branches which reach down through each ventricle and cause ventricular contraction.

The electrocardiogram (ECG) is a recording of the electrical events associated with the muscular contraction of the heart. Since these electrical events are so massive compared to other body potentials, the ECG can be recorded with electrodes placed far from the heart. Typically, electrodes are placed on the right forearm, the left forearm, and the calf of the left leg. The ECG may be recorded from any pair of these electrodes.

These placements were specified by Einthoven in 1903 when he discovered the ECG, and they are commonly known as "Einthoven's triangle." In a clinical diagnostic setting, the ECG may be recorded from as many as 12 different pairs of leads—half on the chest and the other half on the limbs. Each pair of leads detects a potential electrical difference across the sides of the heart, and each gives subtly different information about both the placement of the heart in the chest and the actual mechanisms of its beating.

As a wave of excitation passes through the heart, depolarization of the myocardial fibers occurs, resulting in the recording of an electrical potential (see Figure 1-2). The first portion of the ECG wave is called the P wave and results from the depolarization of the atria at the onset of atrial contraction. Next follows what is commonly referred to as the QRS complex, as the ventricular myocardium depolarizes from the inside outward. The final T wave signifies the recovery, or the repolarization, of the ventricles. An isoelectric interval, when no electrical activity occurs, indicates diastole between the T wave and the following P wave.

Clinically, the ECG recording may reveal the existence of many different cardiac defects. In part, this is because the rate at which depolar-

FIG. 1-2. ECG waveform and electrical events in the heart. See text for details. From *A Primer of Psychophysiology*, by James Hassett. Copyright 1978 by W. H. Freeman. Reprinted by permission.

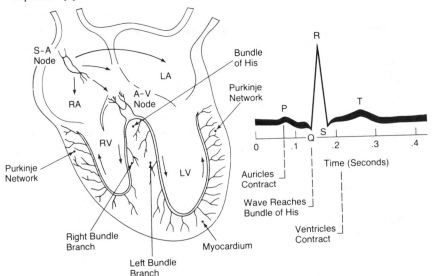

ization is supposed to occur in different sections of the heart is a known constant. For example, conduction from the bundle of His leading to complete depolarization of the ventricles should take no more than .12 sec in an adult male. If the measure of the QRS complex takes longer than .12 sec, it is fair to assume that either the left or right branch of the bundle is damaged.

## CONCLUSION

This brief orientation is intended to place cardiovascular psychophysiology in historical perspective, and to provide a basic understanding of key anatomical and physiological principles. The next chapter describes the measurement of the most widely studied aspects of cardiovascular function such as heart rate, blood pressure, and photoplethysmography. However, it is worth noting here that recent technological advances promise to increase our understanding of the complex adjustments and responses of the cardiovascular system still further. New refinements in impedance cardiology permit the measurement of stroke volume from electrodes on the surface of the body (Miller & Horvath, 1978). A somewhat more invasive procedure (which at first involved injection of a radioactive chemical into the carotid artery and later relied on gas inhalation) allows psychophysiologists to measure localized changes in blood flow in the brain as a person performs a variety of tasks (Risberg & Ingvar, 1973).

Technological advances like these, and the conceptual advances which are described throughout this book, make this an exciting period for cardiovascular psychophysiologists. A close reading of this material will make it clear just how far we have come since Galen diagnosed love sickness on the basis of fluctuations of the pulse. But it will also illustrate the awesome complexity of the cardiovascular system and remind all of us just how far we still have to go.

## ACKNOWLEDGMENT

Portions of this chapter were adapted from *A Primer of Psychophysiology*, by James Hassett. Copyright 1978 by W. H. Freeman. Used with permission.

# REFERENCES

Angell, J. R., & Thompson, H. B. A study of the relations between certain organic processes and consciousness. *Psychological Review*, 1899, *6*, 32–69.

Ax, A. F. The physiological differentiation between anger and fear in humans. *Psychosomatic Medicine*, 1953, *15*, 433–442.

Brown, C. H., & Van Gelder, D. Emotional reactions before examinations: I. Physiological changes. *Journal of Psychology*, 1938, *5*, 1–9.

Darrow, C. W. Electrical and circulatory responses to brief sensory and ideational stimuli. *Journal of Experimental Psychology*, 1929, *12*, 267–300.

Gazes, P. C. *Clinical cardiology: A bedside approach*. Chicago: Year Book Medical Publishers, 1975.

Gunn, C. G., Wolf, S., Block, R. T., & Person, R. J. Psychophysiology of the cardiovascular system. In N. S. Greenfield & R. A. Sternbach (Eds.), *Handbook of psychophysiology*. New York: Holt, Rinehart, & Winston, 1972.

Lacey, J. I. Psychophysiological approaches to the evaluation of the psychotherapeutic process and outcome. In E. A. Rubinstein & M. B. Parloff (Eds.), *Research in psychotherapy*. Washington, D. C.: American Psychological Assocation, 1959.

Lacey, J. I. Somatic response patterning and stress: Some revisions of activation theory. In M. H. Apley & R. Trumbull (Eds.), *Psychological stress*. New York: Appleton-Century-Crofts, 1967.

Lacey, J. I., Kagan, J., Lacey, B. C., & Moss, H. A. The visceral level: Situational determinants and behavioral correlates of autonomic response patterns. In P. H. Knapp (Ed.), *Expression of the emotions in man*. New York: International Universities Press, 1963.

Landis, C. Studies of emotional reactions: V. Severe emotional upset. *Journal of Comparative Psychology*, 1926, *6*, 221–242.

Lehrer, S. *Explorers of the body*. New York: Doubleday, 1979.

Masters, W., & Johnson, V. *Human sexual response*. Boston: Little, Brown, 1966.

Mesulam, M., & Perry, J. The diagnosis of love-sickness: Experimental psychophysiology without the polygraph. *Psychophysiology*, 1972, *9*, 546–551.

Miller, J. C., & Horvath, S. M. Impedance cardiography. *Psychophysiology*, 1978, *15*, 80–91.

Nissen, A. E. *Influence of emotions upon systolic blood pressure*. Unpublished master's thesis, Columbia University, 1928.

Obrist, P. A., Webb, R. A., Sutterer, J. R., & Howard, J. L. The cardiosomatic relationship: Some reformulations. *Psychophysiology*, 1970, *6*, 569–587.

Risberg, J., & Ingvar, D. H. Patterns of activation in the gray matter of the dominant hemisphere during memorizing and reasoning. *Brain*, 1973, *96*, 737–756.

Weerts, T. C., & Roberts, R. The physiological effects of imagining anger-provoking and fear-provoking scenes. *Psychophysiology*, 1976, *13*, 124.

Willis, R. *The works of William Harvey, M.D.: Translated from the Latin with a life of the author*. New York: Johnson Reprint Corp., 1965. (Originally published in London by Sydenhan Society, 1847.)

# 2

## Measurement of Cardiovascular Functioning

BERNARD TURSKY
LARRY D. JAMNER

## INTRODUCTION

The development of cardiovascular instrumentation in both clinical medicine and psychophysiology advanced rapidly as the need for more accurate measures of cardiovascular functioning increased. Much of the present development of instrumentation to record heart rate, blood pressure, and blood volume resulted from a symbiotic relationship between the psychophysiologist and the bioinstrumentation engineer (Tursky, in press). In this relationship the cardiovascular psychophysiologist's research needs were translated into the development of transducers, signal processors, and recording instruments by the engineer, and the improved instrumentation made it possible for psychophysiologists to increase their research productivity. In recent years this relationship has been extended to include the computer specialist, whose development of digital hardware (microprocessor systems) and software (computer programs to detect artifact,

Bernard Tursky. Laboratory for Behavioral Research, Department of Political Science, State University of New York at Stony Brook, Stony Brook, New York.

Larry D. Jamner. Department of Psychology, State University of New York at Stony Brook, Stony Brook, New York.

control-sampling rates, and experimental events) has made it possible for the cardiovascular psychophysiologists to increase their research capability and to improve the accuracy and validity of their measurements of cardiovascular events.

Most hemodynamic functions (blood pressure, blood flow, and blood volume) and some cardiodynamic functions (contractile force and cardiac output) can be most accurately determined by the use of invasive measurement techniques. It is, therefore, reasonable to postulate that the accurate recording of cardiovascular activity may pose greater problems for the research psychophysiologist than the clinician. The clinical investigator, usually a physician or a psychophysiologist working in a hospital setting with patients whose medical condition warrants the use of invasive recording methods for diagnostic or monitoring purposes, can utilize these direct methods to record many of the individual's cardiovascular functions. The nonmedical research psychophysiologist, limited both by professional ethics and the possible stressful effects of the use of invasive recording techniques, must be satisfied with cardiovascular measures derived from the use of noninvasive indicators of heart function and blood pressure, flow, and volume.

Although the research goals and clinical objectives may often differ between the psychophysiologist and the clinical investigator, the instrumentation and measures developed for one can be adapted for use by the other. Indeed, many of the measures employed in psychophysiological research were developed from, or can be validated by, the information obtained from the more direct invasive clinical measures. For example, a pressure-sensitive transducer directly coupled to an artery by an indwelling catheter produces an accurate measurement of systolic and diastolic blood pressure for each heart cycle. The use of a sphygmomanometer can provide only a maximum of a single relative reading of systolic and diastolic blood pressure every 30 sec. This indirect measure has the advantage of being noninvasive, but it is also inferential since the pressure information is inferred from arterial events detected at the skin surface that are caused by a systematic alteration in applied cuff pressure. This intermittent blood pressure measurement technique is useful for research and clinical purposes only because the relationship between the sphygmomanometer measure and the directly obtained invasive arterial pressure measures has been demonstrated to be correlated by empirical observations (Tursky, 1974).

The inferential relationship between direct and indirect measures indicates that a number of specific criteria should be utilized in evaluating current instrumentation and methodology in cardiovascular psychophysiology. All laboratory instrumentation should be carefully evaluated for stability, fidelity, range sensitivity, and signal-to-noise ratio (Cobbald, 1974; Ferris, 1978; Geddes & Baker, 1968), and all indirect cardiovascular measures should be evaluated for:

1. Accuracy—measured by the relationship between the indirectly obtained measure and its direct standard. A functional or statistically valid relationship between these measures should be established.
2. Specificity—Does the instrument measure only the variable of interest?
3. Reactivity—How does the recording procedure affect the measure of interest?
4. Reproducibility—What is the test-retest reliability of the dependent variable?

The investigator's ability to make statements concerning the functioning of the cardiovascular system must reflect his/her capability for measuring its basic physical properties. The types and accuracy of the measurements employed depend in part upon the investigator's understanding of the cardiovascular system and his/her knowledge of the possible effects of physical or psychological stimulation on the system. Various chapters in this text and other sources (such as Abel & McCutcheon, 1979; Guyton, 1976) are recommended for an in-depth analysis of cardiovascular physiology and an understanding of the system's reaction to environmental and psychological manipulation.

This chapter attempts to examine the measurement techniques utilized in the study of cardiodynamics (characteristics of heart activity) and hemodynamics (characteristics of blood circulation). The techniques of obtaining accurate measurements and the methodologies utilized in their interpretations are discussed.

## THE MEASUREMENT OF CARDIODYNAMICS

Cardiac activity generates signals in several energy forms, and each of these signals can be quantified by a specific measurement technique. Table 2-1 lists four major cardiac energy modalities and their primary measurement techniques.

TABLE 2-1. Cardiac Energy Modalities

| Form of energy | Measurement technique |
|---|---|
| Electrical | Electrocardiography (ECG) |
| Mechanical | Ballistocardiograph, cardiac output |
| Auditory (heart sounds) | Phonocardiography |
| Chemical | Biochemical analysis |

The researcher's choice of signal and measurement technique is dependent upon the experimental and information requirements of each study. The need for a physical response capability by the subject, the ease of recording, and the accuracy of interpretation of the obtained record may govern the choice of signal and measurement technique. The response characteristics, advantages, and disadvantages of each energy form and measurement modality are discussed in the following pages.

ELECTROCARDIOGRAPHY

## Etiology of Cardiac Biopotentials

The heart is equipped with a special excitatory and conductive system which results in a spontaneous self-generation of action potentials. These potentials spread in a controlled manner throughout the cardiac muscle mass in such a way as to cause the synchronous contractions of the atria and ventricles. In the normally functioning heart, the action potential which triggers each cardiac cycle originates in a specialized group of nerve fibers called the sinoatrial (SA) node. Due to a higher permeability to sodium ions (relative to other cardiac fibers) the SA node self-excites at a rate of approximately 80 times per minute (Guyton, 1976). This action potential propagates throughout the atrial synctum, resulting in the atrial systole (contraction). As the action potential progresses to the atrioventricular (AV) node, transmission is delayed by approximately one-tenth of a second to allow for adequate filling of the ventricles. Following the activation of the AV node, the signal is transmitted along the AV bundle (also called the "bundle of His"), through the Purkinje fibers, and finally throughout the ventricular synctum. Because the body is a good volume conductor, fluctuations in myocardial potentials can be recorded at the surface of the body. These potentials are referred to as electrocardiograms, or ECGs. When measured at the body surface, the ECG voltage ranges from .5 to 2 mV, with a frequency bandwidth of .1 to 250 Hz. The components of the ECG (see Figure 2-1) are directly related to the events of the cardiac cycle. The P wave is produced by atrial depolarization; the QRS complex, by ventricular depolarization; and the ST segment and the T wave, by ventricular repolarization.

## Historical Development of the ECG Recording

According to Geddes and Baker (1968), the electrical activity associated with cardiac events was discovered by Kolliker and Mueller in 1856. In their procedure, they utilized the beating ventricle of a frog's heart to initiate contractions in an isolated muscle fiber. The first accurate representations of the R- and T-wave components of ventricular functioning were obtained by Burdon-Sanderson and Page in 1878 (Geddes & Baker, 1968). Continuous measurement of cardiac activity was first achieved by

FIG. 2-1. (A) Dynograph record of normal Lead II electrocardiogram. R-R represents the interbeat interval, and the P to T waves identify the sequential electrical events of the cardiac cycle. P—depolarization of the atrial muscle, Q,R,S—depolarization of the ventricular myocardium, T—repolarization of the ventricles. (B) Beat-to-beat tachometer recording. Note 60–120 bpm calibration and 30 bpm change in heart rate in three-beat interval.

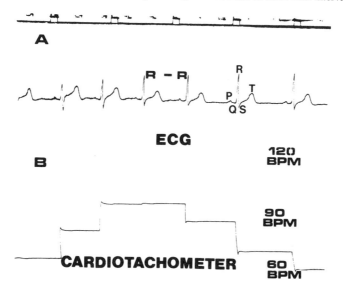

use of the capillary electrometer, an instrument consisting of a mercury–sulfuric acid interface within a capillary tube. Current generated by a group of cells was transmitted through a connecting electrode and thus effected a change in the mercury meniscus. Photographic techniques were utilized to produce permanent records of these variations in the meniscus. Measurements obtained by this method were prone to stimulus artifacts, and were insensitive to rapid changes. However, this crude recording device led to the development of the string galvanometer, an instrument which was capable of higher-frequency recording. This recording instrument was invented in 1903 by Einthoven, who is credited with the development of clinical electrocardiography (Geddes & Baker, 1968). The present-day galvanometer, though many times more sophisticated and sensitive than Einthoven's original model, is still the primary ECG recording instrument. The invention of the direct-writing electrocardiograph in the 1940s standardized the apparatus used in the recording of ECGs. This equipment has remained essentially the same over the years except for improvements in the sensitivity and frequency response of the amplifiers, and the reduction of noise in the recording instruments.

## Electrocardiography in Current Psychophysiology

The ECG signal is primarily recorded for the clinical assessment of cardiac functioning, and this information is considered to be a major source of information of the cardiac health of each patient. Through the use of electrocardiographic and vectorcardiographic techniques, cardiologists are able to isolate specific regions of malfunctioning in the heart organ itself. The psychophysiologist's major interest in the ECG is not the diagnosis of cardiac well-being, but rather the utilization of this signal as a measure of autonomic nervous system activity.

The measures of interest for the psychophysiologist that can be produced from the ECG are heart period (HP), defined as the R-R interval (see Figure 2-1), and heart rate (HR), which is the frequency of heart action. HP and HR have been extensively employed in psychophysiology as dependent measures in the study of emotions such as anger (Ax, 1953; Hokanson & Burgess, 1964), depression (Dawson, Schell, & Catania, 1977), anxiety (Hodges & Spielberger, 1966; Reeves, Shapiro, & Cobb, 1979), fear (Ax, 1953; Lang, Melamed, & Hart, 1970), reaction time (Jennings & Wood, 1977; Light & Obrist, 1980), pain (Engel, 1959; Tursky & Greenblatt, 1967), relaxation (Grings & Schandler, 1977; Paul,

1969), attention (Tursky, Schwartz, & Crider, 1970), classical conditioning (Furedy, 1979; Obrist, 1968), and operant conditioning (Cacioppo, Sandman, & Walker, 1978); and as an independent measure in reaction time tasks (Lacey & Lacey, 1974) and as a measure of learned autonomic nervous system (ANS) control (Engel, 1972).

*Electrodes and Electrode Placement*

Several types of surface electrodes have been utilized in the recording of the ECG signal. The most common is the plate electrode. Usually made of nickel, copper and zinc alloys, or nickel-plated steel, these electrodes range in size from 1 to 4 square inches. They are usually applied to the limbs or chest by the use of perforated straps. Suction bulb electrodes (Roth, 1933-1934) are often used to record clinical ECGs from the chest because they can be easily moved from one location to another. The need for constant monitoring of the cardiac functions of patients in hospital intensive care units has resulted in the design of several types of disposable ECG electrodes made up of a metal, metal foil, or metalic mesh contact bonded to an adhesive collar (Geddes & Baker, 1968). The one-time use of these disposable electrodes ensures no transmission of skin ailments from one patient to another. To reduce noise and drift potentials in the recording of physiological signals (O'Connell & Tursky, 1960), the biopotential electrode was developed. These electrodes consist of a silver–silver chloride disk or sponge recessed into a plastic cup with a rim flange that permits the easy attachment of the electrode by use of an adhesive collar; continuing low-impedance contact with the skin is accomplished through the sodium chloride electrolyte that fills the cup. Application of any surface electrode requires that the skin be thoroughly cleansed with warm water or alcohol, and that an electrolyte paste or solution be briskly rubbed into the skin surface to penetrate the nonactive stratum corneum layer of the epidermis, thus reducing the electrode skin impedance to provide adequate electrical contact with the underlying tissue.

The large ECG electrical potential reduces the need for critical placement of the ECG electrodes for psychophysiological recording. The sequence of electrical events occurring during the cardiac cycle can be recorded by measuring the potential difference between any two sites across the surface of the body. Three standard configurations of electrode placement, known as the "Einthoven triangle" system (see Figure 2-2), are commonly used: the Lead I configuration, in which electrodes are attached

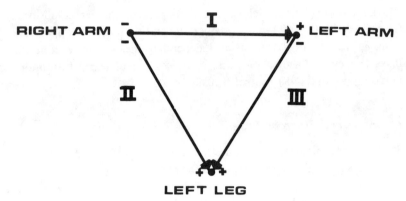

FIG. 2-2. Einthoven triangle electrocardiogram electrode configuration. Maximum electrical energy produced by Lead II electrode placements.

to each of the upper arms; the Lead II configuration, in which electrodes are attached to the right upper arm and the left lower leg; and the Lead III configuration, in which the electrodes are attached to the upper left arm and the lower left leg. Each lead placement produces a distinctive ECG wave configuration. The Lead II configuration provides the largest-magnitude signal (Schneiderman, Dauth, & VanDercar, 1974). This enhanced reproduction of the R wave is often used by psychophysiologists to initiate stimulus events and as a biological clock for sampling other physiological measures (Elmore & Tursky, 1981).

Cardiotachometry

Heart rate (HR) is usually described in terms of the number of heart cycles or beats that have occurred in 1 min. Beats per minute (bpm) can be obtained for any period of time by counting the number of heart cycles (R waves) that have occurred in the period of time of interest and converting to bpm by the use of a simple mathematical transformation.

$$HR\,(bpm) = \frac{Number\ of\ cardiac\ cycles \times 60}{Time\ (sec)}$$

Although simple, this process cannot provide information about HR on a beat-to-beat basis unless the time between two adjacent R waves can be accurately measured. Early beat-to-beat rate information was arrived at by recording the ECG at an extremely fast paper speed so that the R-R interval could be accurately measured. To reduce the manual measurement time, special-purpose calipers were designed to read out in HR when the legs of the calipers bridged two adjacent R waves. Electronic circuits developed in the 1950s provided the necessary instrumentation to accurately measure beat-to-beat interval or beat-to-beat HR. There are two basic types of cardiotachometers which provide the necessary signal processing to record rate or time on either an averaging or interbeat basis. The averaging cardiotachometer electronically determines the average HR by counting cardiac cycles during a specified period of time. Figure 2-3 presents a block diagram of the circuitry used in this process. The preamplified ECG signal is coupled through a 10- to 50-Hz bandpass filter that represses low-frequency noise and baseline drift, and reduces high-frequency artifact due to movement and muscle potentials. This filter passes the frequencies (25–35 Hz) primarily associated with the QRS complex (Neuman, 1978) to a threshold detector. The most frequently used threshold detector circuit is the Schmitt trigger, an electronic switch that operates when the signal amplitude exceeds some predetermined level. However, the use of this circuit for ECG detection may create several problems. If the P, R, or T peaks of the ECG are of relatively equal amplitude, double triggering may produce erroneously rapid averaged HR values. It is also possible that the Schmitt trigger, because of its preset and constant operating voltage level, will be sensitive to variations

FIG. 2-3. Block diagrams of averaging and beat-to-beat cardiotachometers.

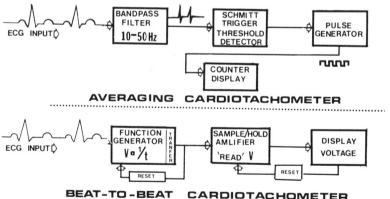

in R-wave amplitude due to respiration or movement artifacts and miss some heart beats, thus producing erroneous indications of HR slowing. An alternative circuit described by Shimizu (1978) operates as a phase-related peak detector which can identify phase-related points in the ECG signal, irrespective of amplitude. The output of either of these detection circuits can be used to trigger a pulse generator. As HR increases, so does the frequency of pulses from the pulse generator, which in turn results in an increase in the output voltage from the circuit, thus producing an equilibrium voltage related to the average of several cardiac cycles.

The beat-to-beat cardiotachometer determines rate by calculating the reciprocal of the R-R interval for each heart cycle and presenting it as the rate for that particular interval. Mathematically this can be represented as $HR = (1/T)(60)$. As shown in Figure 2-3, the beat-to-beat cardiotachometer operates in two stages. The amplified and filtered R wave triggers a function generator which produces a hyperbolically decreasing voltage across time. This voltage is fed to a sample-and-hold amplifier which samples the voltage produced prior to the current R-R interval, holds it through that R-R interval, and produces a meter or vertical pen deflection proportional to the change in HR.

If one were more concerned with HR trends, the averaging cardiotachometer is sufficient and perhaps desirable (see later section on methodological considerations). However, the beat-to-beat cardiotachometer, because its output reflects alterations in rate from one QRS complex to the next, is capable of providing information concerning the variance in HR across beats. Various designs for cardiotachometers can be found in the literature (Fitchenbaum, 1976; Taylor & Mandelberg, 1975).

## Heart Period Data Collection

Heart period (HP) is the measure of time in milliseconds between successive heart beats. Several instruments have been developed to measure and record R-R intervals. Brown (1972) designed an event per unit time (EPUT) meter; cardiotachometers are available that can express HP variability on a continuing-time basis. The output voltage from these instruments provides an analog graphic (paper) or magnetic (tape) record. Shimizu (1978) has described a digital cardiac period meter capable of parallel output modes: One is digital for data analysis, and the other is analog for data inspection; both records are proportional to HPs (R-R intervals).

Methodological Considerations in Cardiac Measurement Selection

Both HR and HP are derived from the relationship between time and the ECG signal. HP, or interbeat interval (IBI), is the time interval between R waves, and beat-to-beat HR is measured as the reciprocal of HP. The nonlinear relationship between HR and HP (Jennings, Stringfellow, & Graham, 1974; Khachaturian, Keer, Kruger, & Schacter, 1972) may introduce errors into obtained means, variances, and skewness of frequency distributions (Khachaturian *et al.*, 1972). Thus a consistent increase in the R-R interval does not necessarily result in a consistent decrease in HR. Thorne, Engel, and Holmblad (1976) reported that the IBI transformation into bpm results in bpm rates exceeding true rates, since shorter R-R intervals are weighted excessively. They also reported that this derived rate from a cardiotachometer is greater than true HR when HR is decreasing monotonically, such as in reaction time tasks; and that cardiotachometer rates provide less than true HR information when HR is increasing monotonically, as in the onset of electric shock stimulation. Several investigators (Heslegrave, Ogilvie, & Furedy, 1979; Jennings *et al.*, 1974; Khachaturian *et al.*, 1972; Thorne *et al.*, 1976) have concluded that the differences between IBI and bpm distributions become increasingly important and tend to favor IBI measurement as one approaches extreme HR values, as in infant research. Others disagree with this premise (Graham, 1978a; Richards, 1980) and point out that HR meets the assumptions of normalcy of distribution and homogeneity of variances better than does HP.

HR, unlike most psychophysiological measures, has an inherent time component, and when phasic changes in cardiac activity are examined, it is traditional to compute rates or periods based upon either successive beats (cardiac time) or successive seconds (real time). Graham (1978b) has suggested that, although rate and period have been described in terms of both cardiac and real time, only rates, calculated over real-time units (seconds), and periods, calculated over cardiac time units (beats), yield an unbiased average representative of the total data. In terms of deciding upon which time unit is appropriate, Graham (1978b) suggested per second units, since they have the advantage of facilitating the coordination of cardiac activity with stimulus events. Conversely, the cardiac unit of analysis can provide a biological clock against which other cardiac events can best be evaluated. This may be of particular value in the design of biofeedback studies (Elmore & Tursky, 1981).

Evoked cardiac changes have also been examined in terms of their variability. Kahneman, Tursky, Shapiro, and Crider (1969); Porges (1969); Tursky, Shapiro, and Schwartz (1972); and Walter and Porges (1976) have suggested that attention-demanding tasks that require some degree of information processing produce a stabilization of HR; that is, there is a decrease in HR variability. Heslegrave, Ogilvie, and Furedy (1979) have suggested that variance may not be an optimal measure of HR variability, and that the results of studies that utilize the variance statistic to assess baseline–treatment differences may be invalid due to nonrandom trends in HR. It is this nonrandomness of the cardiac response that violates one of the assumptions of the variance statistic. They suggest the use of the successive difference mean square statistic (Bennett & Franklin, 1954), which minimizes the effects of gradual nonrandom trends.

One of the most critical issues that affects the analysis of HR data is the Law of Initial Values (LIV). This law states that HR level at any particular moment is in part due to baseline HR level. When HR level is high, the acceleratory response is more restricted than when the level is low, and the deceleratory response is less restricted at high than at low levels. Thus the question that the investigator must be able to determine is what proportion of poststimulus variance is systematic and what portion can be explained by the prestimulus level.

A further consideration in evaluating HR data involves individual differences in the range of responses. That is, a change of 20 bpm for two subjects cannot be said to be indicative of the same degree of autonomic activity. A number of statistical transformations (i.e., log, square root, and $z$-score) have been utilized to overcome these variance and range problems in the analysis of HR response and level information. An innovative procedure proposed by Lykken (1972) is the range correction transformation, which reduces error variance due to individual range differences for tonic HR levels.

## Computer/Microprocessor Support Systems

Technological advances in computer engineering have produced computer systems that are extremely useful in the recording and analysis of cardio-vascular information. These instruments range from laboratory-assembled microprocessor systems (Welford, 1962) designed specifically for the psychophysiology laboratory, to the more general commercial laboratory digital computer system designed to process both analog and digital laboratory data. In either case, at moderate cost one can obtain a system that can sample up to 16 channels of physiological or behavioral data at any desired rate. The use of this equipment reduces the data-processing and analysis time from weeks to hours. The on-line capabilities of these systems permit the dynamic control of experimental variables and the formation of intricate binary and continuous feedback displays for use in biofeedback studies (Elmore & Tursky, 1981; Lang & Twentyman, 1976). In these computer systems the amplified analog physiological information is sampled at an appropriate rate by an analog-to-digital (A/D) converter. This information is massaged through the use of appropriate computer programs and then stored in some form of computer memory (tape, disk, floppy disk, or cassette) for future analysis.

The complexity and utility of computer software may vary with the computer equipment being utilized. Many laboratory computer systems can be programmed in easily learned BASIC, but this relatively slow-responding language severely limits the processing of rapid HR information. Programming in FORTRAN, a more complex computer language, tends to reduce this problem. A number of packaged programs are available to carry out a variety of operations on cardiac data. Wilson (1974) has described his CARDIVAR program written in FORTRAN IV, which can appraise and analyze the dynamic properties of polyphasic cardiac responses via analysis of variance and trend analysis. Abel and McCutcheon (1979) have described a number of BASIC programs which can compute mean blood pressure, HR, maximum $dP/dt$, and blood volume from an analog input.

Physiological Considerations

An important consideration for the psychophysiologist is the necessity to separate HR responses related to experimental manipulation from alterations in HR due to the natural physiological and physical factors that systematically affect this measure.

The investigator should bear in mind that the cardiac activity is to a large extent internally autoregulated and is also complexly interrelated with other components of the vascular and somatic systems. The primary function of the cardiovascular system is metabolic; oxygen and nutrients must be delivered to the cells, and metabolic byproducts and carbon dioxide must be removed. Hence, the variable most likely to manifest alterations in the activity of the cardiovascular system is the metabolic requirements of the organism. An increase in metabolic requirements results in dilation of the arterioles and capillaries due to a relaxation of vasomotor tone, thus causing a decrease in peripheral resistance. If there were no homeostatic regulation in the cardiovascular system, a large drop in mean arterial pressure would result. However, baroreceptic, chemoreceptic, thalamic, and homeometric feedback mechanisms all serve to bring about increases in the output of the heart (i.e., increases in HR and stroke volume), thus maintaining homeostatis. Obrist *et al.* (Obrist, 1968; Obrist, Webb, & Sutterer, 1969; Obrist, Webb, Sutterer, & Howard, 1970) have expounded the concept of the cardiac–somatic relationship, which takes into account the metabolically relevant relationship between cardiac activity and somatic processes. Briefly, their research indicates that increases in HR are associated with increases in somatic activities, that cardiac decelerations are concomitant to diminished electromyographic EMG activity, and that manipulations which modify the magnitude or direction of the somatic system have a similar effect upon the cardiac system. This work suggests that measurements of cardiac activity should be accompanied by somatic measurements such as EMG to evaluate and account for the effects of somatic mediation.

HR also varies systematically with respiration (Brener, 1967; Schneiderman *et al.*, 1974). "Sinus arrythmia" is the term used to describe the systematic cardiac acceleration during inspiration and cardiac deceleration during expiration (Guyton, 1976). Sroufe (1971) found that depth and rate of respiration differentially affect HR and HR variability: Increased respiration rate reduces HR variability, while decreased respiration rate increases HR variability; and increased respiration depth increases HR level and HR variability, while decreased respiration depth (shallow breathing) has the effect of decreasing HR level and variability. As in the case of cardiac–somatic coupling, the investigator should consider the use of breathing controls such as respiratory pacing (Clemens & Shattock, 1979) or paced respiration via a respirator (Schneiderman *et al.*, 1974). Other factors with which HR varies systematically are ambient room temperature (Thauer, 1965) and carbon dioxide concentration.

Although it may appear that HR is hopelessly confounded with respiration and somatic activities, there are investigators who hold contrary opinions. For example, some degree of HR control has been demonstrated when respiration is experimentally controlled (Brener & Hothersall, 1967; Sroufe, 1969). A number of investigators have taken issue with Obrist's conclusions (Lacey & Lacey, 1974). One argument against the notion of cardiac–somatic coupling is that HR is not the sole indicator of the metabolic requirements of the organism. Lacey and Lacey stated: "The metabolically relevant variable is cardiac output, not heart rate. Heart rate is only one factor in the determination of cardiac output, and the two are imperfectly correlated" (1974, p. 563).

## PHONOCARDIOGRAPHY

### Development

Phonocardiography (PCG) is the recording of the sounds and vibrations of the heart due to the opening and closing of the cardiac valves and the turbulance of the blood in the filling and emptying of the heart chambers. Auscultatory evaluation of heart sounds has been utilized by physicians as a diagnostic tool since the beginnings of medical practice. Though heart sounds can be identified by placing the ear directly on the chest wall, the development of the stethoscope made it possible to detect, identify, and diagnose sounds related to individual cardiac events. Aberrations of the lub–dub sound of the healthy heart serve as a warning to physicians to investigate the possibility of a cardiac problem.

Electrical recording of heart sounds began in 1894 when Einthoven and Geluk used a carbon granule microphone connected to a capillary electrometer to record these auditory events (Geddes & Baker, 1968). Today, the piezoelectric transducer (crystal microphone) and the high-fidelity dynamic microphone are the transducers most commonly employed in the detection and recording of heart sounds and pulse waves. Heart sound and pulse wave microphones may be coupled to the skin by means of an air-filled tube, or a transducer may be applied directly to the skin surface.

### Physiological Mechanisms

Four heart sounds have been identified and associated with electrical and mechanical cardiac events. $S_1$ reflects the oscillations and vibrations resulting from the closing of the AV valves and the consequent opening of the similunar valves (due to the ventricular systole). $S_2$ is a low-frequency vibration resulting from the deceleration and flow reversal of the blood in the aorta and the snapping shut of the semilunar valves due to this backflow. This event corresponds to the incisural notch observed in pressure pulse wave recording.

$S_3$ is a small-amplitude, low-frequency vibration associated with vibrations of the relaxed ventricular muscle walls as a result of sudden termination of the rapid-filling phase. $S_4$, also referred to as the atrial sound, represents vibrations as a result of the atrial systole. $S_4$ is usually inaudible but may be recorded by the PCG.

## Response Characteristics/Recording Techniques

Sound energies produced by cardiac events are greatly attenuated by the acoustical properties of the body, particularly in compressible tissues such as the lungs (Peura, 1978). The least attenuation occurs at several sites on the chest where lung thickness is minimal (see Burton, 1972). Due to the sound-damping qualities of the body, heart sounds have extremely small amplitudes, with a frequency spectrum of .1 to 2000 Hz. Adequate reproduction of heart sounds requires that the recording system have a frequency response of 25 to 2000 Hz. For the reproduction of pulse waves, the recording system must have a frequency response bandwidth of .1 to 100 Hz. The piezoelectric (crystal) microphone is capable of frequency responses as low as .17 Hz (Cobbold, 1974), with an upper limit of about 2000 Hz (Webster, 1978), thus making it ideal for the recording of both heart sounds and pulse waves. However, the dynamic microphone, while suitable for most PCG purposes, cannot be used in the detection of pulse waves because of its inadequate low-frequency response.

## PCG Applications in Psychophysiology

The PCG is primarily utilized by physicians as a supplement to the use of the stethoscope in evaluating the cardiac health of the patient. The major problem with PCG as a primary diagnostic tool is the difference between the behavior of the human ear and the responses of conventional microphones, amplifiers, and recorders. The human ear is a nonlinear sound transducer, and it is difficult to produce a PCG record that accurately mimics this nonlinearity. Attempts have been made to modify the electronic audio systems to duplicate this auditory response (McKusick, Webb, Humphries, & Reid, 1955). There has been increasing interest among psychophysiologists in measures that employ heart sound production as a reference point (Newlin & Levenson, 1979; Obrist, Light,

McCubbin, Hutcheson, & Hoffer, 1979; Weiss, Delbo, Reichek, & Engelman, 1980). Measures such as systolic time intervals and preejection period (PEP) are gaining attention among psychophysiologists interested in cardiodynamic evaluation. The interest in these measures may place the PCG in a more prominent role in the psychophysiology laboratory.

CARDIAC OUTPUT

Cardiac output (CO) is a measure of the amount of blood in liters per minute that the heart pumps. Cardiac output has also been expressed in terms of cardiac index (CI), which is CO per square meter of body surface area (BSA).

Figure 2-4 illustrates the complex interaction between the physiological mechanisms that regulate cardiac output and arterial pressure.

Measurement of cardiac output or of its components (e.g., contractile force) has not received very much attention in psychophysiological research. This may in part be due to the relative ease of obtaining other electrophysiological information concerning cardiac activity and the elusiveness of an unobtrusive, accurate measure of the physical aspects of

FIG. 2-4. Block diagram of physiological mechanisms that contribute to the regulation of cardiac output and arterial blood pressure.

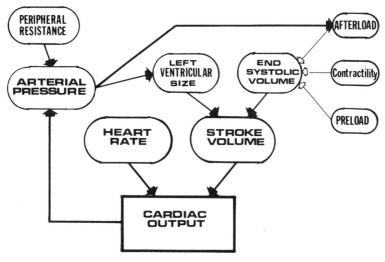

cardiac functioning. Obrist, Gaebelein, and Langer (1975) pointed out that the significance of cardiac output as a parameter in psychophysiological research is of increasing importance because of the usefulness of this parameter in investigations regarding hypertension and metabolic homeostatis. In attempts to separate the relative contributions of the sympathetic and parasympathetic nervous systems to cardiodynamics, a component of cardiac output, contractile force, has been associated with increased sympathetic activity, whereas HR is assumed to be largely controlled by vagal activation or inhibition (Obrist, Howard, Lawler, Sutterer, Smithson, & Martin, 1972).

## Invasive Measures

The methods used to accurately measure CO require procedures which range from the sampling of blood and the injection of dye, to the surgical implantation of transducers. While these invasive procedures are not suitable for most psychophysiological research, several of the measures generated by this procedure have been established as the standard clinical determinants of CO. Since the noninvasive methods of determining CO used in the experimental psychophysiology laboratory rely upon these measures for their validation and quantification, it is necessary to present a brief description of these invasive techniques and measures.

### The Fick Principle

The Fick method is used to measure CO and is represented by the equation

$$CO\,(liters/min) = \frac{O_2 \text{ consumption (ml/min)}}{arterial - venous\ O_2\ content\ difference\,(ml/liter)}$$

The amount of oxygen ($O_2$) consumed by the subject can be derived from the volume of air expired over a 3-min period and comparing the $O_2$ concentration of that sample to the concentration in inspired air (predetermined atmospheric concentration). The arterial $-$ venous $O_2$ concentrations can be determined from blood samples from central arterial and venous systems. Given that a fixed amount of $O_2$ requires a fixed flow to circulate it, total flow or CO can be derived.

*Indicator Dilution Methods*

The indicator dilution method involves the injection of a known quantity of a dye such as methylene blue or indocyanine green into a systemic vein on the right side of the heart. Following this injection, a time–concentration curve is obtained from blood sampled at a constant rate from the brachial or femoral artery. Dividing the area of the resultant curve by the total time across which the curve was plotted provides the mean concentration of indicator. CO can then be derived from the relationship

$$CO = \frac{I \times 60}{C_m \times t}$$

where I is the amount of dye injected (in mg), $C_m$ is the mean concentration of dye (in mg/liter), and t is the total curve duration (in sec). For a thorough review of indicator methodology see Guyton, Jones, and Coleman (1973).

*Flowmeters*

There are a number of electromechanical transducers which utilize blood flow to rotate magnets mounted on frictionless bearings (Potter Electro-turbinometer), or raise a ball or float until the downward force due to the weight of the ball is equal to the lifting force produced by the flow (Shipley & Wilson, 1951), or cause the pendulum in a pendulum flowmeter to deviate from its resting position. The most frequently used flowmeters are the perivascular electronic electroflowmeters and electroflow probes which surround the intact vessel.

Noninvasive Measures of Cardiac Output

Noninvasive measurement procedures may be inferential and susceptible to measurement error since they are one step removed from the hemodynamic event of interest. However, these disadvantages must be weighed against the possible problems of danger, trauma, and reactivity that may accompany invasive techniques. Specifically, the procedures and restraints imposed upon the subject with the use of invasive methods may affect the physiological system being measured. Some noninvasive techniques, such as ballistocardiography, have been in use for approximately 100 years (Starr, 1965). Others, such as rate of pressure change (dP/dt), are just recently receiving attention and critical evaluation in psychophysiology (Heslegrave & Furedy, 1980). Although the validity of these noninvasive measures is still conjectural, Obrist and Light (1980) are optimistic about the ultimate utility of these procedures in cardiovascular psychophysiology.

*Ballistocardiography*

Ballistocardiography (BCG) is based upon Newton's Third Law, which states that for every action there is an equal and opposite reaction. BCG measures cardiac output by means of recoil forces. With each systole, blood is ejected through the aorta. This explosive event results in the recoil of the body. Cardiac output can then be calculated from a measurable physical reaction to this recoil.

There are two basic types of ballistocardiographic methods. In the older method, high-frequency BCG, the subject is restrained and force is measured by displacement of a supporting spring. In ultra-low-frequency BCG, the subject is free to move and force is calculated from his/her mass and the measured acceleration. Typically, in obtaining a BCG the subject lies on a light, frictionless table which is either suspended from the ceiling or supported from below on an air cushion. The movements of this ballistotable, resulting from body movements produced by cardiac activity, are transduced into electrical energy by means of either mechanoelectronic tubes (Geddes & Baker, 1968) or a compound transducer in which movement of the table is converted into a varying light intensity (Ferris, 1978).

Dock and Taubman (1949) recorded body movements without the use of a ballistotable by devising a photoelectric transducer which was attached to the shins of the subject. Cardiac-induced body movements alter the transmission of light to these photoelectric detectors, thus producing a variable electrical output proportional to movement.

One factor which reduces the accuracy of the BCG in representing cardiac functioning is the fact that the ejected blood dissipates its forces in many directions, due to the anatomy, variations in compliance of the circulatory system, and body mass. Thus, the forces measured from a BCG do not represent the total force of cardiac output.

Though BCG has not been employed extensively as a dependent measure in psychophysiology, several studies have been conducted that utilize BCG as a measure of cardiodynamic change (Ax, 1953; Schacter, 1957). (For a comprehensive essay on BCG, see Starr, 1965.)

*Impedance Cardiography*

Impedance change techniques for detecting alterations in physiological events have been used to reflect changes in respiration, blood flow, contractions of cardiac muscle, or any event that exhibits a change in dimension, dielectrics, or conductivity of the thorax (Geddes & Baker, 1968). The principle behind impedance cardiography is that when a high-frequency (20 to 200 kHz) constant-current electrical signal is applied across the thoracic cavity, the impedance of the signal measured between two electrodes will vary as a function of the volume of the contained region. Impedance (Z), measured in ohms, decreases as volume increases.

Bipolar (Atzler, 1933, 1935) and tetrapolar (Nyboer, 1950) configurations of electrodes attached to the arms (Mann, 1953), both sides of the thorax (Atzler, 1933), and around the neck and the chest at diaphragm level (Miller & Horvath, 1978) have been employed. Although bipolar electrode placements have been frequently used, the tetrapolar configuration is considered superior since it delivers a more uniform current distribution across the electrodes (Geddes & Baker, 1968). Kubicek, From, Patterson, Witsoe, Castenda, Lilleki, and Ersek (1970) have suggested an electrode configuration of aluminum film 1 mil thick by 63 mm long deposited on 1-inch-wide mylar tape. They also suggested that current flow is most uniform when the two recording electrodes are placed at least 3 cm from the excitation electrodes. Figure 2-5 is a diagram of a representative tetrapolar electrode placement; observed changes in impedance should reflect cardiac activity. Impedance cardiography is subject to a number of limitations. For example, any change in the thorax (related to blood flow), the expansion or contraction of the lungs, or an increase in fluids may alter the conductance of the thorax and thus may contribute to the measured impedance change. Due to the possible contamination of these variables and the inferential nature of the signal, it is difficult to calibrate impedance measures in physiological terms. Kubicek *et al.* (1970) and Kinnen, Kubicek, and Patterson (1964), using the tetrapolar configuration, have attempted to validate the impedance cardiogram as an indirect method of measuring stroke volume (SV) in human subjects. These efforts have produced SV values that fall within 20% of those obtained with the more direct Fick method. Miller and Horvath (1978)

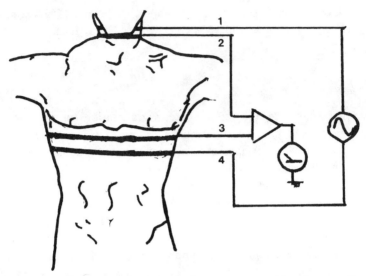

FIG. 2-5. Representative tetrapolar electrode placements to record impedance cardiogram. Electrodes 1 and 4 are connected to high-frequency signal source. Change in impedance is recorded across electrodes 2 and 3.

concluded that impedance cardiography can provide a fairly reliable intrasubject index of relative changes in SV and CO if impedance change measurements ($\Delta Z$) are made at the same phase of each respiratory cycle. Interpretation of the obtained measurements is further complicated by the fact that observed thoracic impedance changes are also affected by systolic discharge from both right and left ventricles. Research with dogs (Denniston, Maher, Reeves, Cruz, Cymerman, & Grover, 1976) suggests that the right ventricle contributes approximately 20% of the total pulsatile impedance amplitude. Thus any statement concerning the true value of CO or SV derived from impedance cardiography must be made with caution. Although at present impedance cardiography remains an uncalibrated indirect measure, it does reflect cardiac events and can, therefore, be useful as a noninvasive measure in evaluating relative changes in cardiac activity.

*Contractile Force as Measured by dP/dt*

Contractile force, which is an indicator of the strength of the contraction of the heart, has been suggested as the measurement of choice in assessing the $\beta$-adrenergic (sympathetic) contribution to cardiac activity (Lawler &

Obrist, 1974). Anatomical research indicates that while the SA node (the group of fibers responsible for determining HR) and the two atria are well supplied with both parasympathetic and sympathetic innervation (Guyton, 1976), HR is more representative of vagal (parasympathetic) influences, and the ventricles are mainly innervated by the sympathetic nervous system (Guyton, 1976). Obrist *et al.* (1972), employing an aversive classical conditioning paradigm and pharmacological manipulation with dogs as subjects found that cardiac contractile changes more clearly reflected sympathetic influences than did changes in HR. Obrist, Lawler, Howard, Smithson, Martin, and Manning (1974), using human subjects in a stressful reaction-time paradigm, demonstrated that while HR changes were dependent upon level of somatic activity (cardiac–somatic coupling), changes in contractility were independent of somatic activity, an instance of cardiac–somatic uncoupling. Thus an investigator interested in a "purer" measure of sympathetic influences on cardiac activity, relatively uninfluenced by parasympathetic innervation or somatic mediation, might consider the measurement of contractile force. Precise measurements of contractile force can be obtained by a number of invasive techniques, such as the implantation of strain gauges in the ventricular wall or the introduction of a pressure manometer catheter into the left ventricle. However, these difficult procedures can be utilized only with experimental animals. A noninvasive method of assessing contractile force that holds promise for the psychophysiologist is a measure of the maximum rate of change of ventricular pressure (dP) with respect to a change in time (dt). $dP/dt$ is a measure of the first derivative or the slope of the pulse pressure wave for each cardiac cycle. Obrist *et al.* (1972) examined aortic $dP/dt$ in dogs using a pressure-sensitive manometer catheter. A specially designed circuit calculated the first derivative (slope) of that waveform, and an output voltage proportional to the point of a maximum rate of change was obtained for each cardiac cycle. Thus ventricular performance could be determined on a beat-to-beat basis.

Obrist *et al.* (1974) compared the use of photoplethysmographic techniques, the vibrocardiogram (VCG), and a microphonic recording of the carotid artery pulse wave. The carotid pulse wave was detected using a low-frequency microphone placed over the region of the left carotid artery, where the pulse wave is most easily recorded. The microphone was held in place with an adhesive electrode collar, covered with a section of foam rubber to eliminate extraneous noise, and held in place using an elastic bandage. In addition, a neck collar was utilized to minimize movement artifacts. Their results suggest that the slope of the carotid pulse wave recorded by the microphone produced a superior index of contractility. Pulse waves obtained with photoplethysmography seemed to reflect changes in vasomotor tone as opposed to contractile influences, while the VCG produced variable, nonviable signals.

Although carotid dP/dt (measured in mm Hg/sec) may provide a reasonable noninvasive index of contractile force, there are a number of inherent difficulties associated with this particular technique (see Heslegrave & Furedy, 1980; Obrist & Light, 1980). Movement of any type, including swallowing, causes variations in microphone–skin contact pressure, which result in artifacts and variations in the amplitude of the pressure pulse (Obrist *et al.*, 1974).

Rate of change of pressure measurement is a function not only of myocardial excitation but also of other cardiovascular parameters (see Figure 2-4). The rate at which the ventricle can eject its contents is greatly affected by the resistance it will meet from aortic pressure levels (diastolic blood pressure, DBP). The greater the DBP, the lower the dP/dt. This artifact is known as the afterload factor. Preload factors such as left-ventricle end volume (LVEV) also affect dP/dt, since more blood filling the ventricles results in greater distention of the cardiac muscle fibers and has the effect of increasing the force of the contractions (Frank–Starling mechanism). Light and Obrist (1980) have suggested that regardless of how the indirect measures of carotid dP/dt are quantified, calibration is impossible, thus limiting the investigator's ability to make between-subject comparisons.

Recently, myocardial performance has also been evaluated by the measurement of pulse transit time (PTT) (Obrist *et al.*, 1979). This measure was found to be highly influenced by $\beta$-adrenergic manipulations on the myocardium; PTT was found to be significantly correlated with carotid dP/dt and HR. Later in this chapter, PTT measurement and methodology will be examined in detail as an indirect measure of arterial blood pressure.

*Cardiac Activity and Systolic Time Intervals*

Another noninvasive measurement of cardiac functioning is the evaluation of various systolic time intervals (STIs). The STIs used are those of electromechanical systole (Q-$S_2$), left-ventricular ejection time (LVET), and preejection period (PEP). Q-$S_2$ is the interval commencing at the start of the ventricular depolarization (the Q wave of the ECG) until the detection of the high-frequency heart sounds associated with the closing of the semilunar valves ($S_2$). LVET is the interval from the beginning of the ascending limb of the arterial pulse wave to the dichrotic notch, and the preejection period (PEP) is derived by subtracting LVET from $Q$-$S_2$ [$PEP = (Q\text{-}S_2) - LVET$] (see Figure 2-6). The calculated PEP therefore represents all electrical and mechanical cardiac events prior to ejection.

STI measures, commonly used in cardiology, are now being investigated in psychophysiological studies. Obrist *et al.* (1979) have suggested

FIG. 2-6. Temporal relationships between the ECG, the peripheral pulse wave, and the phonocardiogram (heart sounds). These event and time relationships determine several systolic time intervals (STIs): (A) electromechanical systole (Q to $S_2$); (B) left-ventricular ejection time (LVET); (C) preejection period (PEP).

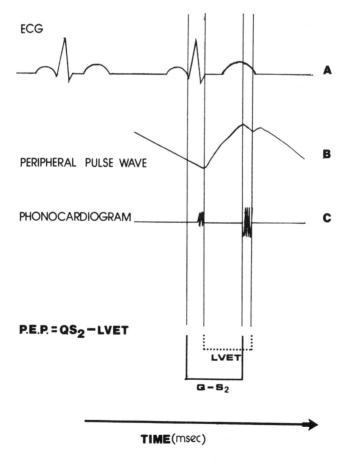

ECG

PERIPHERAL PULSE WAVE

PHONOCARDIOGRAM

A

B

C

P.E.P.=$QS_2$−LVET

LVET

Q−$S_2$

TIME(msec)

that observed changes in PTT partially reflect changes in PEP. Newlin and Levinson (1979) have provided evidence that PEP may be a better index of cardiac contractility than either carotid dP/dt or PTT.

The measurement of STIs requires that the temporal aspects of the ECG Q wave, a peripheral pressure pulse wave, and a PCG signal be simultaneously recorded and evaluated with respect to each other. The Q-S$_2$ interval is determined by the detection of the ECG Q wave by conventional ECG methods described earlier, and the employment of PCG techniques to make the critical assessment of the second heart sound (S$_2$). LVET determination can be made from the peripheral pressure pulse wave detected by low-frequency direct-contact microphones (Obrist et al., 1979) or by photoplethysmographic techniques at a variety of locations such as the carotid artery, the finger, and the pinna of the ear. Haffty, Kotilainen, Kobayashi, Bishop, and Spodick (1977) suggested the detection of the pulse at the ear because this site provides tracings that are relatively free from movement artifacts. The PCG techniques and signal processing are discussed in more detail in a preceding section. Newlin and Levenson (1979) described the measurement of PEP by the use of digital computer techniques and provided the necessary algorithms to accomplish the measurement. STI measurements such as PEP hold a distinct advantage over other noninvasive measures of cardiac activity in that, unlike carotid dP/dt or PTT, STIs can be calibrated, thus extending the validity of these measurements across subjects. Future research in cardiovascular psychophysiology will demonstrate the increased employment of these relatively unobtrusive, calibratable, noninvasive measures of the cardiovascular system.

## THE MEASUREMENT OF HEMODYNAMICS

Hemodynamics is the study of the circulation of blood in the cardio-vascular system. Many hemodynamic factors can be studied by applying the principles of hydrodynamics (the field of study that deals with the properties of moving fluids), but the direct application of hydrodynamic principles to hemodynamics is limited by several controlling factors. The study of hydrodynamics assumes the vessels in which fluids move to be rigid and the fluid itself to be incompressible. The human circulatory system consists of a web of flexible tubing (arteries, arterioles, veins, venules, and capillaries) of varying size and degrees of distensibility and compliance. In addition, the fluid (blood) is not incompressible. These factors complicate the understanding and predictability of hemodynamic events. To date no complete hemodynamic model has been formulated; however, bearing in mind the existing limitations, it is possible to utilize some of the basic relationships and principles of hydrodynamics to provide a basis for the interpretation of hemodynamic events.

The variables of interest in the study of the movement of blood in the peripheral vasculature include pressure, rate of flow, and impedance, or resistance of flow. Using appropriate hydrodynamic measures, both pressure and flow can be directly quantified, while resistance can be indirectly derived from the relationship between flow and pressure.

BLOOD PRESSURE

Definition and Units

Blood pressure is a measure of the force that the blood exerts on the walls of the blood vessels as it flows through the circulatory system. Millimeters of displacement of a mercury column (mm Hg) has conventionally been used as the unit of measurement in most (air, water) pressure determinations. Millimeters of mercury has also become the unit of choice in the direct and indirect recording of arterial blood pressure, and the mercury manometer has been utilized as the standard instrument for blood pressure measurement (Guyton, 1976).

In the normal adult individual, blood pressure can vary from a minimum of approximately 0 mm Hg pressure in the vena cava to a maximum of $120 \pm 20$ mm Hg in the large arteries. Psychophysiologists and clinicians are primarily interested in recording the pulsatile (systolic and diastolic) pressures produced in the major arteries by the rapid discharge of a bolus of blood from the left ventricle with every beat of the heart. Figure 2-7 depicts the pulsatile pressure waveform produced by this event with each heart cycle. The ascending, or anacrotic, limb of the wave represents the rise in pressure caused by the rapid ejection of blood from the left ventricle when the semilunar valves open. The peak pressure is referred to as the systolic blood pressure. This is followed by the closure of the semilunar valves, depicted by the incisura or dicrotic notch. The slower descending (catacrotic) limb indicates the passage of the pressure

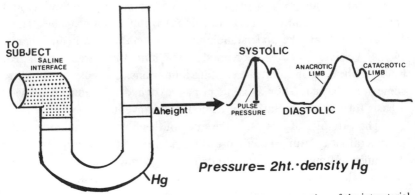

FIG. 2-7. Diagram of U-tube mercury manometer and a representation of the intraaterial pulsatile pressure waveform that is produced by each heart cycle. Major aspects of the pressure wave are identified.

wave; the lowest pressure in each heart cycle is called the diastolic pressure, and arterial blood pressure is usually reported as systolic over diastolic pressure. The difference between these pressures and the mean arterial pressure has been empirically defined as one-third the difference between systolic and diastolic plus the diastolic. It is important to emphasize that pulsatile arterial blood pressure is not constant from beat to beat and can vary by as much as 30 mm Hg in any one-minute period (Tursky, 1974).

Accurate measures of arterial blood pressure have been directly recorded on a beat-to-beat basis by coupling a cannula inserted into a major artery to a pressure-sensitive mechanical or electrical transducer. These devices convert pressure into a recordable mechanical or electrical signal. Recently, attempts have been made to develop noninvasive techniques that utilize PTT as an analogue of beat-to-beat blood pressure (Gribbin, Steptoe, & Sleight, 1976). Arterial blood pressure has also been determined indirectly on an intermittent basis by recording the amount of cuff pressure that is necessary to occlude the flow of blood in a major artery (systolic pressure) and the pressure at which the cuff no longer impedes the flow of blood in that artery (diastolic pressure). Manual and automatic counterpressure systems have been devised to indirectly record arterial blood pressure. Attempts have been made to overcome the intermittent qualities of these measures by initiating a method of tracking change in pressure on a beat-to-beat basis.

Subsequent sections of this chapter describe in detail the development and characteristics of the invasive (direct) and counterpressure (indirect) methods of recording arterial blood pressure.

## Invasive Measurement Techniques

Olmsted (1967) has described one of the first experiments related to the measurement of blood pressure; in 1711 curate Stephen Hales inserted a brass pipe into the crural artery of a restrained horse, which was then connected to a glass tube 9 feet long. Hales noted that blood rose to a level of 8 feet, 3 inches, which corresponds by present standards to a mean blood pressure of approximately 200 mm Hg. Blood pressure measurement was made more practical with the invention of the U-tube mercury manometer by Poiseuille in 1826. With one arm of the tube directly connected to an artery, pressure measurements were obtained by noting the difference in height between the two arms of the column of fluid (see Figure 2-7); pressure is equal to twice the change in height of the free arm times the density of mercury (13.6 g/cm³). The high viscosity of mercury reduces the utility of the U-tube manometer as a measure of the pulsatile intrabeat (systolic/diastolic) fluctuation in arterial blood pressure. However, this slow-responding (highly damped) system can be useful in the direct determination of mean arterial blood pressure.

There are several electrical and mechanical transducer techniques that are available for the continuous monitoring of the pulsatile arterial and venous pressures. These direct techniques often require a fluid connection between a diaphragm and a blood vessel; pressure in mm Hg is determined by measuring the displacement of the diaphragm.

There are basically three categories of electrical pressure transducers: resistive, inductive, and conductive. Each of these transducers may be applied intravascularly on a catheter tip or may be hydraulically coupled via a saline solution extravascularly. For a thorough discussion of these measures, the reader is referred to Cobbald (1974), Geddes (1970), Geddes and Baker (1968), and Webster (1978).

### Pulsatile Pressure: Resistive Transducers

In 1898 Grunbaum described the first use of an electrolytic transducer mounted on the end of a catheter (Geddes & Baker, 1968). In this device an electrode attached to the outside of a zinc-chloride-filled pressure capsule was separated from an electrode within the capsule by a thin rubber window. Pressure applied to the capsule reduced the distance between the two electrodes, thus decreasing the electrical resistance between the two electrodes. Electrolytic strain gauges have fallen into disuse because of their tendency to deteriorate due to the instability of the electrolyte. The electrolytic strain gauge has been replaced by more sensitive, less vulnerable resistance transducers which utilize a thin wire filament or a film vacuum-deposited conductive material as the resistive element. Electrical resistance is proportional to the diameter and length of the resistive element. A filament of wire in a physical configuration that can be altered by a change in pressure will produce a change in resistance proportional to the pressure change. Modern resistance strain gauge transducers use several types of bonded and unbonded wire designs (Lambert & Wood, 1947). The unbonded strain gauge (Statham P23Db) is one of the most frequently used resistance transducers because of its high sensitivity and stability. Up to four resistive elements can be connected as a wheatstone bridge to compensate for systematic artifacts due to fluctuations in temperature or extraneous movement.

Alterations in blood pressure exert a force upon the diaphragm causing it to flex, which produces a recordable output voltage from the wheatstone bridge that varies proportionally in amplitude with changes in pressure.

*Pulsatile Pressure: Inductance Transducers*

In the inductive transducer system, resistance elements and the wheatstone bridge are replaced by a system in which movement of the diaphragm causes a displaceable core to alter its position along a single, double, or triple set of transformer windings, thus producing inductance changes. The most frequently used inductive displacement transducer is the linear variable differential transformer (LVDT). Displacement of the core, as a function of pressure changes acting on the diaphragm, serves to alter the coupling between the primary and secondary windings of this differential transformer. At 1 V with an excitation frequency of 60 Hz (line frequency), the sensitivity of most commercial units (e.g., Sanborn) is in the range of 1.5 to 2 V/mm of diaphragm displacement. LVDT transformers have been developed that have a frequency response of 1000 Hz (Allard, 1962).

*Pulsatile Pressure: Conductance Transducers*

The capacitive transducer has been extensively employed in the measurement of blood pressure, replacing the cumbersome Hamilton Optical Manometer in the late 1930s (Geddes & Baker, 1968). In the capacitance method of measuring blood pressure, a stiff elastic diaphragm is exposed to the fluctuations in blood pressure. This diaphragm constitutes one plate of the capacitor; the other plate is proximal and stationary. Lilly (1942) was among the first investigators to employ the conductance transducer for the measurement of blood pressure. Commercial units (e.g., Lilly Technitrol) have a frequency response of 300 Hz and very high compliances on the order of $1 \times 10^{-20}$ ml/100 mm Hg (Abel & McCutcheon, 1979).

### Response Characteristics of the Blood Pressure Waveform

The frequency response necessary in transducers and instruments for the high-fidelity reproduction of the pressure waveform is approximately 20 Hz, assuming an HR of 120 bpm (Peura, 1978). If measurements of the first derivative of a pressure pulse are to be taken, as in dP/dt measures, then a greater bandwidth is required. The necessary frequency response can be estimated by a Fourier analysis that includes the first 10 harmonics. It is important to evaluate the frequency response of transducers since transducers with inadequate frequency responses will produce distorted waveforms. Underdampened distortion of the pulse waveform results in the amplification of high-frequency wave components, which leads to the overestimation of both systolic and diastolic blood pressure levels. Overdampened distortion results in the attenuation of the recorded systolic and diastolic levels, resulting in an underestimation of these blood pressure values (Cobbald, 1974; Krausman, 1975).

### Indirect Measurement of Blood Pressure

Invasive blood pressure measurement techniques are the only methods that can produce an accurate, continuous recording of beat-by-beat pulsatile arterial blood pressure. Ethical and stress-producing considerations make these methods unsuitable for most casual clinical blood pressure evaluations or for experimental psychophysiological investigations. The development of manual and automatic noninvasive counterpressure measurement techniques have made it possible for the clinician and the psychophysiologist to record blood pressure from the intact human on an intermittent basis. These intermittent measures have been utilized as a psychophysiological index of activation (Sternbach, 1966; Alexander, 1972), personality variables (Berger, 1964; Williams, Kimball, & Willard, 1972), sexual arousal (Hoon, Wincze, & Hoon, 1976), and emotions (Ax, 1953); and for the investigation of the detection of deception (Landis & Wiley, 1926; Podlesny & Raskin, 1978; Tháckray & Orne, 1968). These indirect measures of blood pressure may sometimes produce an unacceptable level of measurement error (Tursky, 1974; Tursky et al., 1972), or they may produce discomfort due to the frequency of occlusive inflations (Clancy, 1978; Freis & Sappington, 1968).

There has been an increased interest in the recording of arterial blood pressure due in part to heightened awareness of the relationship between hypertension and the increased risk of myocardial infarction (Stallones, 1980), the possible employment of biobehavioral techniques (e.g., biofeedback) as a part of a treatment regimen for hypertensive populations, and an interest in using blood pressure as a parameter demonstrating voluntary control of autonomic functioning. These new interests have led to investigations of the relationships between systolic and diastolic pressures and stressors (Obrist et al., 1979), coping (Manuck, Harvey, Lechleiter, & Neal, 1978), coronary-prone behavior patterns (Manuck & Garland, 1979), and relaxation (Fey & Lindholm, 1978).

Just as at the turn of the century—when a number of indices of blood pressure were developed as the need increased for a methodology to improve the measurement of blood pressure (Geddes, Hoff, & Badger, 1966)—so these new interests are contributing to the development of equipment and measurement procedures that are capable of meeting the contemporary requirements of blood pressure determination.

Several noninvasive blood pressure measurement techniques have been developed (Elder, Longacre, Welsh, & McAfee, 1977; Newlin & Levenson, 1979; Shapiro, Greenstadt, Lane, & Rubinstein, in press; Steptoe, 1976; Tursky, 1974). These techniques, coupled with the use of minicomputers, have brought the cardiovascular psychophysiologist closer to a more convenient, more continuous measure of relative arterial blood pressure.

*Sphygmomanometry: Historical Development*

The most commonly used indirect method of blood pressure determination employs the use of an occluding cuff to provide a measurable counter-pressure against the pressure of blood in the artery. These methods are all labeled "sphygmomanometric."

Sphygmomanometry is derived from the Greek word "sphygmo," meaning "to pulse" or "to throb" and the French word "manomètre" for "measuring force," and refers to the noninvasive measurement of blood pressure.

The first indirect determination of systolic pressure by use of a counterpressure was accomplished in the late 1860s by Marey (Geddes *et al.*, 1966). Employing a fluid-filled glass chamber encasing the arm of a subject, Marey observed that increasing fluid pressure resulted in blanching (increased skin pallor) of the arm. The fluid pressure at which color (blood flow) returned to the limb was labeled the "systolic level." The contemporary counterpart of this method, the "flush technique," employs the same basic principles using a pneumatic occluding cuff and the finger at the observation site.

The use of an occluding cuff in the measurement of arterial blood pressure was simultaneously introduced by Riva-Rocci in 1896 and Hill and Barnard in 1897 (Geddes *et al.*, 1966). This method employs an inflatable cuff wrapped around the upper arm to provide a controllable and measurable counterpressure to the blood pressure in the artery. A gradual reduction of cuff pressure from the occluding level to the lowest pressure level that impedes the flow of blood in the artery produces turbulence in the artery that can be detected by one of several methods: palpation of the artery, pressure oscillations in the cuff, or auscultatory changes (Korotokoff sounds) detected at the cubital fossa through the use of a stethoscope. The palpatory method is currently considered to be a highly unreliable measure of arterial blood pressure, producing systolic determinations that may be 30 mm Hg lower than concurrent intraarterial determinations (Van Bergen, Weatherhead, Treolar, Dobkin, & Buckley, 1954). This is primarily caused by the inability of palpation to detect the lowest level of turbulence as the cuff is deflated (Abel & McCutcheon, 1979).

The introduction of the occluding-cuff technique led to the refinement of the recording of pressure oscillations. Marey had observed that as the pressure of the liquid in the occluding chamber fell below the systolic level, low-level pressure oscillations were registered. With continued reductions in liquid pressure, these oscillations first increased, then decreased, and gradually disappeared. Erlanger in 1903, employing the pneumatic occluding-cuff technique of inflation above the systolic level followed by gradual deflation, graphically recorded this rise and fall of oscillations with sufficient amplitude to allow for critical evaluation of the changes in magnitude (Geddes et al., 1966). The point of increased oscillation amplitude was thought to indicate the systolic pressure as read on the mercury manometer, and the point at which oscillation amplitudes were maximal was thought to indicate the diastolic pressure (Geddes et al., 1966). Recent studies (Geddes & Newberg, 1977; Papillo, Tursky, & Friedman, 1981) indicate that maximum oscillations occur at mean arterial pressure, and that these oscillations are systematically reduced at the systolic and diastolic pressure levels.

The auscultatory technique had its genesis in Korotokoff's (1905) discovery of the various sounds associated with lessening degrees of arterial compression. Korotokoff, employing the Riva-Rocci cuff technique, reported that at some point in the release of cuff pressure, a short snapping sound was detected using a stethoscope. This first sound represented the systolic pressure. With continued reductions in cuff pressure, murmuring occurred, followed by the recurrence of more defined sounds. As cuff pressure was further reduced, all sounds disappeared completely. According to Korotokoff, this point represented the minimum, or diastolic, pressure.

These sounds have since been named "Korotokoff sounds" and are detected by a variety of sound and electronic transducers. Many of the principles that underlie modern blood pressure measurement are drawn from this history.

### Auscultatory Blood Pressure Measurement

The ascultatory method of determining systolic and diastolic blood pressure has been almost universally adopted as the clinical measure of arterial blood pressure. The procedure involves the rapid inflation of an occlusive cuff to approximately 40 mm Hg above systolic pressure (Lywood, 1967); the cuff is then deflated at a rate of 2–3 mm Hg/sec (see Figure 2-8). The cuff pressure at which pulsatile flow begins is identified

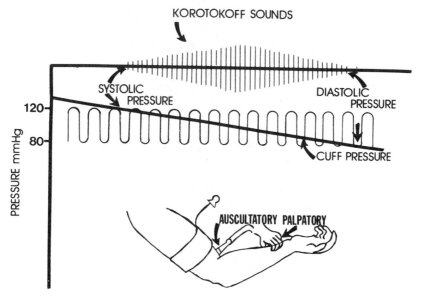

FIG. 2-8. Diagram of sphygmomanometric blood pressure record demonstrating the relationship between applied cuff pressure and Korotokoff sounds in the determination of systolic and diastolic arterial pressure. Turbulence in the artery can be detected by auscultation (stethoscope) or palpation.

as the systolic pressure, and the cuff pressure at which flow is no longer impeded is identified as the diastolic pressure.

The most frequently utilized method of identifying the systolic and diastolic blood pressure levels involves the detection of a change in the sound characteristics produced by the pulse wave passing through the constricted artery. The Korotokoff sounds go through a series of five systematic phases as a function of decreasing cuff pressure. Kirkendall, Burton, Epstein, and Freis (American Heart Association, 1967) have described the acoustic qualities of Phase I, in which clear tapping sounds of increasing intensity first appear; Phase II, during which the tapping sounds are replaced by a "swishing," murmur-like sound; Phase III, marking the return of clear thumping sounds which increase in intensity; Phase IV, a period marked by the abrupt muffling of sound which now has a soft, blowing quality; and Phase V, which represents the point at which all sounds disappear.

Detection of these sounds is accomplished with the use of an acoustic or electronic stethoscope, or by a pressure-sensitive transducer (i.e., piezoelectric crystal). The detection of Phase I indicates an equilibrium between the applied cuff pressure and peak pressure within the artery (see Figure 2-8). At that point, the cuff pressure, as measured by a mercury or aneroid manometer, is recorded as the systolic pressure. Although the beginning of Phase IV (muffled sounds) has been generally regarded as the criterion for diastolic pressure (Clancy, 1978), the disappearance of Korotokoff sounds in Phase V has also been used as the diastolic pressure criterion (Geddes *et al.*, 1966). Kirkendall *et al.* (American Heart Association, 1967) suggest the recording of the appearance of both Phase IV and Phase V. In terms of accuracy, the ascultatory method is at best an *estimate* of true (direct) arterial pressures. Assuming optimal measuring technique, the obtained systolic level and the obtained diastolic pressure will be 8 to 10 mm Hg higher than true systolic and diastolic levels (Geddes, 1970; Roberts, Smiley, & Manning, 1953; Steele, 1941). These errors are compounded by another factor: the lability and variability of blood pressure within and across patient populations. Tursky, Shapiro, and Schwartz (1972) demonstrated a 10–34 mm Hg range in systolic and diastolic pressure levels over a span of 50 consecutive heart beats. This beat-to-beat variability indicates the need for repeated measurement in attempting to arrive at meaningful determination of arterial blood pressure. Any measure of blood pressure derived from a single beat interval can result in a false assessment of a subject's average pressure (Tursky, 1974). Armitage, Fox, Rose, and Tiniter (1966) found that on the basis of a single sphygmomanometric reading, 33% of 722 men were falsely determined as hypertensive and 5% were falsely determined normotensive when compared to a mean value obtained based on four readings. Thus, whether assigning subjects to experimental conditions, such as hypertensive or normotensive; or assessing the effects of a particular manipulation, as in the voluntary control of blood pressure (Benson, Shapiro, Tursky, & Schwartz, 1971; Shapiro, Schwartz, & Tursky, 1972; Shapiro, Tursky, Gershon, & Stern, 1969); or assessing the effects of stressors (Obrist *et al.*, 1979; Obrist & Light, 1980), variability is a factor that the investigator must consider in the measurement of blood pressure.

*Early Automatic Indirect Techniques*

Automatic methods for the measurement and recording of systolic and diastolic pressures were developed in part to reduce the variability of obtained measurements between operators using the manual method

(London & London, 1966). For a detailed description of the earlier automatic methods, see Lywood (1967). Briefly, the first automatic systems included a program for the inflation and deflation of the occluding cuff, a means of recording cuff pressure, and a microphone system for Korotokoff sound detection. Typically, the cuff was rapidly inflated and cuff pressure was allowed to fall over a specified period of time, ranging from 25 sec (Gilson, Goldberg, & Slocum, 1941) to over 3 min (Rose, Gilford, Broida, Soler, Partenope, & Freis, 1953). The Korotokoff sounds, as detected by a crystal microphone, were amplified and superimposed on the continuously monitored cuff-pressure recording (Geddes, Spencer, & Hoff, 1959; see Figure 2-9).

These early systems all required the subsequent interpretation of the obtained recordings to determine systolic and diastolic pressures, with the first recorded sound indicating the systolic level and the last sound indicating the diastolic level. Systems employing a pulse detector (i.e., piezoelectric crystal) distal to the occluding cuff have also been employed to determine systolic pressure (Flanagan & Hull, 1968; Smyth, 1954).

Although some of these early systems made improvements in the detection of the Korotokoff sounds and in the procedures used to store and display the obtained measurements, the issue of beat-to-beat variability was still unresolved. The need for a blood pressure measure capable of beat-to-beat determinations intensified as psychophysiologists grew interested in demonstrating the voluntary control of blood pressure. The result was the development of several types of instruments capable of monitoring systolic and diastolic pressures on a semicontinuous basis: the servocontrolled tracking systems (Brener & Kleinman, 1970; Green, 1955; Miller, DiCara, Solomon, Weiss, & Dworkin, 1970), the constant-cuff-pressure system (Tursky et al., 1972; Tursky, 1974), a hybrid system incorporating features from both (Elder et al., 1977), and a recently reported computer-controlled tracking-cuff beat-to-beat system (Shapiro et al., in press).

*Servocontrolled Tracking and Constant-Cuff-Pressure Systems*

Both tracking and constant-cuff-pressure systems utilize the Korotokoff sound to regulate cuff pressure so that it approximates either systolic or diastolic levels. In the servocontrolled tracking system (Lee, Caldwell, & Lee, 1977; Miller et al., 1970), pressure in a standard cuff is adjusted across cardiac cycles to keep the intensity of Korotokoff sounds constant.

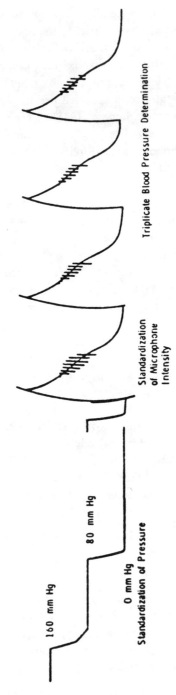

FIG. 2-9. Automated sphygmomanometer blood pressure recording. Korotokoff sounds are superimposed on calibrated recording of the deflation of blood pressure cuff.

This procedure is based on the fact that the relationship between Korotokoff sounds and systolic and diastolic pressures is a continuous, monotonic function (Tursky et al., 1972). In these systems a criterion Korotokoff sound level identifies the first systolic sound, and cuff pressure is then modulated to maintain that criterion sound intensity level constant. If sound intensity is too low, as determined by electronic level detectors, then cuff pressure is decreased; and if it is too high, cuff pressure is increased. By recording the modulated cuff pressure, a beat-to-beat approximation of systolic and diastolic levels can be achieved. The blood pressure tracking method has been successfully employed in the area of learned control of blood pressure (Goldman & Lee, 1978; Lee et al., 1977; Miller et al., 1970; Shannon, Goldman, & Lee, 1978).

Although this system is capable of continuous tracking of relative blood pressure, it can only be used for short periods of time (i.e., 2–3 min). Prolonged exposure to arterial occlusion leads to venous pooling, edema, and high levels of subject discomfort due to the elimination of venous return. Brener and Kleinman (1970) have described a tracking technique in which systolic blood pressure was continuously monitored from the finger instead of the upper arm. An occluding cuff which measured slightly less than the circumference of the finger was employed, with approximately ¼ inch of the dorsal side of the finger remaining unoccluded to permit venous return. Cuff pressure was modulated in 5-mm-Hg steps based on the detection of a pulse distal to the cuff. Thus cuff pressure oscillated about the subject's systolic pressure, with readings taken every two to three heartbeats. Drawbacks of this system included the fact that systolic levels are considerably higher in the finger than they are at the heart, diastolic pressures could not be determined, and alterations in pressure may be confounded with changes in the local vasculature (i.e., vasoconstriction).

In the constant-cuff-pressure technique (Shapiro, Tursky, Gershon, & Stern, 1969; Tursky et al., 1972), a standard cuff is inflated until the pressure approximates the systolic pressure level (or diastolic level); at this point Korotokoff sounds are recorded while cuff pressure is held constant for a period of 50 heartbeats. Using solid-state programming equipment and a highly regulated pressure source (see Figure 2-10), pressure is adjusted to a level at which Korotokoff sounds are detected on approximately 50% of the cardiac cycles. This cuff pressure corresponds to the median systolic (or diastolic) pressure. The number of R-K coincidences in a trial determines the cuff pressure for the next trial. For

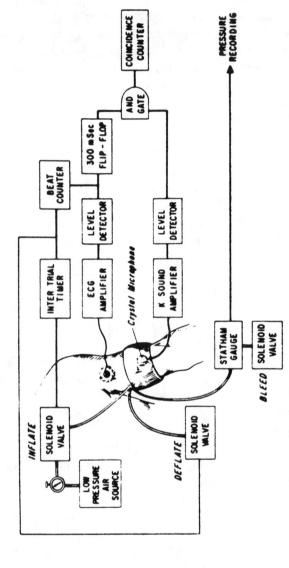

FIG. 2-10. Block diagram of constant-cuff blood pressure recording system (Tursky *et al.*, 1972). Percent presence or absence of Korotokoff sounds for a fixed number of heart cycles determines median systolic or diastolic pressure.

example, in determining systolic pressure, if the percentage of coincidence is between 25% and 75%, cuff pressure is assumed to be at median systolic pressure ±2 mm Hg. Cuff pressure is raised 2 mm Hg for coincidence levels above 75%, or lowered 2 mm Hg for levels less than 25%. Diastolic pressure is similarly determined. This system automatically adjusts cuff pressure on a trial-to-trial basis until R-K coincidences occur 50% of the time, thus providing a measure of median pressures to an accuracy of ±2 mm Hg. Pressure obtained in this manner compares favorably with median pressure values obtained from direct catheterization records (Tursky *et al.*, 1972). More importantly, the presence or absence of the Korotokoff sound at each heart cycle identifies whether arterial pressure for that heart cycle is above or below the median diastolic or systolic pressure, and makes it possible to reinforce an increase or decrease in pressure at each heart cycle.

The constant-cuff-pressure method has been successfully employed in the study of learned control of systolic (Benson *et al.*, 1971; Shapiro *et al.*, 1969) and diastolic (Shapiro *et al.*, 1972) pressures.

Elder *et al.*, (1977) proposed a hybrid apparatus combining the tracking system's cuff adjustment operations with the R-K coincidence detection system of the constant-cuff-pressure method. Cuff pressure is continually readjusted in response to detected Korotokoff sounds. This system employs two inflatable cuffs for both right and left arms that allow for the continuous tracking of either or both systolic and diastolic pressures.

Recently, Shapiro *et al.* (in press) utilized a computer-programmed constant-cuff system to automatically track arterial blood pressure by differentially altering cuff pressure at each heart cycle on the basis of the amplitude of the Korotokoff sounds.

*Ultrasonic Sphygmomanometry*

Stegall, Kardon, and Kemmerer (1968) described a method of indirect blood pressure measurement that makes use of ultrasonics to detect arterial vessel movements beneath a cuff. In this system, two piezoelectric crystals are attached to the bottom of a standard cuff (see Figure 2-11). One crystal is connected to a frequency generator and serves as an 8-MHz signal emitter. The second crystal detects the reflected signal. As the cuff pressure is lowered, the pulsatile movements of the brachial artery result in a reflected signal that is Doppler shifted in frequency, with the frequency shift proportional to the instantaneous wall velocity. When cuff

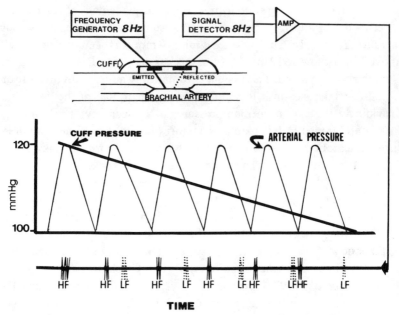

FIG. 2-11. Diagram of automated ultrasonic sphygmomanometric blood pressure measurement systems. Systolic/diastolic blood pressure levels are measureed as a function of detected Doppler shift in frequency proportional to turbulence in the artery. Systolic pressure is indicated by merger of high and low frequencies.

pressure is reduced to below systolic level, the opening of the artery results in wall movements which generate relatively high-frequency signals (200–500 Hz), whereas arterial wall movements associated with the closing of the artery produce low-frequency signals (20–100 Hz) (Cobbald, 1974). As can be seen in Figure 2-11, systolic pressure is signaled by the occurrence of a high-frequency audio signal. As cuff pressure is further reduced, the time separation between high and low signals initially increases and then decreases. The point at which the two signals merge is considered to be the diastolic pressure and is accompanied by a distinct change in the audible characteristics of the signal. All signals disappear when the artery remains open throughout the rest of the cardiac cycle.

The ultrasound method, because it uses ultrahigh frequencies, is able to identify systolic and diastolic pressures in noisy environments as well as in infants and hypotensives (Geddes, 1970).

*Oscillometric Techniques*

The oscillometric method was among the first attempts at indirectly determining human blood pressure. In this procedure, a counterpressure in the form of an occluding cuff (Geddes & Newberg, 1977; Papillo *et al.*, 1981), a fluid-filled chamber (Posey, Geddes, Williams, & Moore, 1969), or a pressure capsule (Krausman, 1975; Uzmann & Wood, 1950) is applied to an artery. As the counterpressure is reduced from above systolic to below diastolic, an orderly sequence of pressure oscillations can be observed in the mercury manometer. As cuff pressure is reduced, the point at which oscillations appear is noted as the systolic pressure. With further reductions in cuff pressure, the amplitude of the oscillations first increases, then decreases in strength. For many years there was a controversy as to whether maximum pressure oscillations represented diastolic pressure (Geddes, 1970). More recent investigations (Posey *et al.*, 1969) have demonstrated that mean arterial, not diastolic, pressure is closely associated with maximum pressure oscillations, and that oscillation amplitude is reduced as cuff pressure approaches the diastolic level.

The use of oscillometry in obtaining systolic or diastolic measures of a subject's blood pressure is rare in psychophysiology. However, the continuous measurement of pressure oscillation from a partially inflated cuff as a measure of relative blood pressure has been used extensively in the detection of deception. "Relative blood pressure" tracings, also referred to as "cardio" tracings by polygraphers, are not absolute measures of blood pressure, but rather refer to changes in the amplitude of pressure oscillations at a cuff pressure midway between systolic and diastolic pressures (Orne, Thackray, & Paskewitz, 1972). Geddes and Newberg (1977) demonstrated that when cuff pressure is below the point of maximum oscillation, increases in blood pressure result in a decrease in oscillation amplitude; while when cuff pressure is above the point of maximum oscillation, an increase in blood pressure produces an increase in oscillation amplitude. In a study with many practical implications for psychophysiology, Papillo, Tursky, and Friedman (1981) demonstrated that subjects are capable of discriminating the relative strengths of the pulsatile sensations produced by applying an occluding cuff to the upper arm. Subjects perceived maximum intensity pulsations approximately at the calculated mean arterial pressure (MAP), with the perceived intensity of the sensations symmetrically and monotonically decreasing as cuff pressure was either increased or decreased from MAP (see Figure 2-12). In support of earlier findings (Geddes & Newberg, 1977; Posey *et al.*, 1969) Papillo *et al.* found that when cuff pressure was held constant above the point of maximum oscillation, there was a direct relationship between an increase or decrease in arterial pressure and a corresponding increase or decrease in the perceived intensity of the pulsatile sensations. Their results suggest that these pulsatile sensations may provide a beat-to-beat measure of relative changes in arterial pressure.

*Pulse-Wave Velocity/Pulse Transit Time*

Pulse-wave velocity (PWV) as expressed in meters per second represents the speed at which a pressure pulse is propagated within the vascular system. Variables influencing PWV include elasticity and distensibility of

FIG. 2-12. Relationship between applied cuff pressure levels ranging from 10 mm Hg below diastolic to 10 mm Hg above systolic and the judgments of perception of arterial pulsations. Maximum pulsations are perceived at mean arterial pressure (MAP) (Papillo *et al.*, 1981).

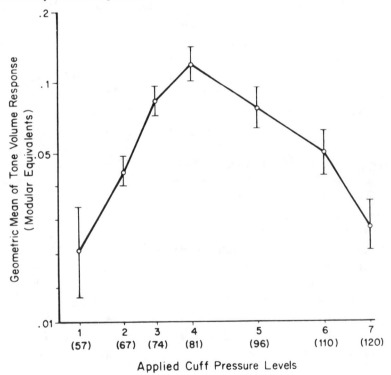

the vessel walls, phases of isovolumetric contraction, and intraarterial pressure. Pulse transit time (PTT) is a measure of the time interval of the movement of the pressure pulse between two fixed points in the arterial system.

PTT has been extensively employed in clinical evaluation of cardiac functioning (Tavel, 1976; Weissler & Garrard, 1971). PTT has been employed as a psychophysiological measure of cardiovascular activity by a number of investigators. Changes in PTT (in milliseconds) have been used in the study of psychophysiological responses to electric shock (Obrist et al., 1979), cold pressor (Obrist et al., 1979), reaction time tasks (Obrist et al., 1979; Steptoe, 1977, 1978), mental arithmetic (Steptoe, Smulyan, & Gribbin, 1976; Williams & Williams, 1965) visual stimuli (Obrist et al., 1979), and pharmacological agents (Obrist et al., 1979; Steptoe et al., 1976; Williams & Williams, 1965); and as a discriminative stimulus (Martin, Epstein, & Cinciripini, 1980). PTT has also been manipulated through the use of biofeedback (Martin et al., 1980; Newlin & Levenson, 1980; Steptoe, 1977, 1978).

Changes in PTT are also reported to be related to changes in blood pressure, with increases in blood pressure associated with decreases in PTT. Early investigators believed that PTT was an index of diastolic pressure (Williams & Williams, 1965). Steptoe and his associates believed PTT to be related to mean arterial pressure, but recent work seems to indicate that changes in PTT reflect changes in systolic pressure (Dale, Shapiro, & Greenstadt, 1980; Obrist et al., 1979). PTT is a distinct measure of cardiovascular activity and may be used as a measure of relative changes in, rather than absolute values of, blood pressure.

PTT values have been obtained using a number of techniques, all of which share the same underlying principles. The transit time interval spans from an initiation point—such as the appearance of a pulse detected by an inflatable cuff (Gribbin et al., 1976) or the peak of the R-wave component of the ECG (Newlin & Levenson, 1980; Obrist et al., 1979; Steptoe, 1978)—to the appearance of the pulse wave associated with the same cardiac cycle at some peripheral vascular site. Several investigators have measured PTT by measuring the interval between the peak of the R wave (acting as a trigger) and the foot of the systolic upstroke of the pulse detected at the radial artery (Steptoe, 1976, 1978; Vander-Hoeven, deMonchy, & Beneken, 1973), while others have suggested that the peak of the peripheral pulse should serve as the "marker" to reduce movement artifacts (Obrist et al., 1979).

Pulse detection techniques include the use of piezoelectric strain gauges strapped to a peripheral site (Obrist *et al.*, 1979; Steptoe, 1976, 1978), impedance plethysmographs (Williams & Williams, 1965), photoelectric plethysmographs which can be applied to the body surface with adhesive tape (Martin *et al.*, 1980; Williams & Williams, 1965), ear densitometers which are spring clipped to the pinna of the ear (Haffty *et al.*, 1977; Newlin & Levenson, 1979), and the use of low-frequency microphones (Tavel, 1976). Several peripheral vascular sites have been chosen for pulse detection, including R wave to radial artery (Obrist *et al.*, 1979; Rhodes & Schwartz, 1980; Steptoe, 1976, 1977, 1978; VanderHoeven *et al.*, 1973), R wave to brachial artery (Williams & Williams, 1965), R wave to ear lobe (Haffty *et al.*, 1977; Newlin & Levenson, 1979, 1980), and R wave to carotid artery (Tavel, 1972). The choice of pulse recording sites must be carefully considered. Williams and Williams (1965) suggested that the pulse wave should be measured from the earliest detectable point (e.g., brachial or carotid arteries) because of the artifact due to increased distortion of the waveform as it is propagated throughout the systemic system. Other investigators have not found this to be a problem (Lance & Spodick, 1977; Newlin & Levenson, 1979). Rhodes and Schwartz (1980), in comparing PTT as measured from brachial to radial pulse sites (PPTT) and R wave to brachial pulse site (RPTT), found that RPTT was more related to cardiac activity than was PPTT, but PPTT seemed to represent more of an index of peripheral blood flow.

Pressure pulse waves have a frequency spectrum ranging from .1 to 100 Hz (Peura, 1978). Thus the recording device used must be capable of delivering a linear output at these frequencies. Low-frequency piezoelectric crystal transducers are commonly used in PTT recording (Tavel, 1976), though strain gauges and plethysmographs have also been employed. Unlike the piezoelectric crystal, which generates its own output signal, these instruments require an external excitation power source.

In all instances the transducer must be in firm contact with the body surface. This may be accomplished with elastic straps, suction devices, or adhesive tape. Pulse transit time intervals can be determined by either using a computer algorithm (see Newlin & Levenson, 1979), or manually from a high-speed (100–150 mm/sec) chart recorder, or photographically from an electronic oscilloscope display (Steptoe *et al.*, 1976; Tavel, 1976; Yang, Bentivoglio, Maranhão, & Goldberg, 1972).

PTT promises to be a useful measure for the psychophysiologist. Although at present the relationship between PTT and blood pressure is uncertain, Steptoe (1976) attempted to calibrate PTT against catheter-obtained recordings of blood pressure and found that a 10-mm-Hg change in MAP was equivalent to approximately a 10-msec alteration in PTT. While it may be possible to calibrate the PTT of a given subject by measuring his/her own particular relationship between PTT and absolute levels of arterial pressure, between-group comparisons should be avoided, and PTT should be regarded as an intraindividual measure of cardiac activity. Research into the contributing components of PTT is currently under way, and with it, the possibility of its use as a continuous, relatively unobtrusive index of blood pressure.

## Physiological and Methodological Considerations for the Indirect Recording of Human Blood Pressure

Current cardiovascular psychophysiology still relies to a great extent upon pressurized occluding devices to provide an indirect determination of arterial blood pressure. Such procedures provide a sampling of arterial pressure instead of a continuous monitoring of beat-by-beat systolic and diastolic pressures. The psychophysiologist must therefore consider a number of factors which have a systematic influence upon this measurement. The first centers around the inflatable cuff itself; that is, there is an important relationship between the width of the occluding cuff and the circumference of the limb to which it is applied (Geddes, 1970). The use of a cuff that is too large or too small will produce inaccurate measurements (Ragan & Bordley, 1941). This is especially important when the subjects are obese (King, 1967) or very young (Robinow, Hamilton, Woodbury, & Volpitto, 1939). The recommended cuff width is 20% wider than the arm diameter. This corresponds to about 12 cm wide for the average adult arm, smaller cuff widths for a child's arm, and larger widths for the obese arm (American Heart Association, 1967).

A second consideration, especially in electronic detection, is the frequency range of the Korotokoff sounds. Geddes (1970) has suggested that 25–80 Hz is the frequency range that should be most useful, although the total frequency range of the Korotokoff sounds extends to 200 Hz. In addition, the amplitude of these signals is low, and thus recording must occur in the absence of extraneous environmental noise (Peura, 1978).

With the advent of automated sphygmomanometers (see previous section), intraoperator measurement differences were reduced, but measurements were still liable to errors due to individual differences in pressure lability. The tracking and constant-cuff procedures, while not as prone to this problem, still provide a sampling of pressures. The techniques which may provide continuous monitoring, such as oscillometry and PTTs, provide information only about the relative changes in pressure.

Finally, the question must be raised, What is actually being measured by recording blood pressure? Factors contributing to blood pressure include heart rate, stroke volume, distensibility and elasticity of the systemic system, and isovolumetric phases. The psychophysiologist must consider whether the information he/she requires may best be obtained from these contributing factors rather than from the complex measure of blood pressure. If this is true, then such measures as blood flow and pulse volume or systolic time interval may be the measures of choice. The answers to these questions can best be found by empirical research.

BLOOD FLOW AND VOLUME: OVERVIEW

The primary function of the cardiovascular system is metabolic: to maintain a minimum capillary pressure (i.e., 20–30 mm Hg) so that the diffusion of oxygen and metabolites to the various cell bodies and the removal of carbon dioxide and other metabolic byproducts can occur. The cardiovascular system also plays an important role in heat exchange. In addition, the cardiovascular system must pattern its flow distribution to different parts of the body in response to local demands, all of which vary with changes in metabolism associated with an increase in muscle and organ activity.

Blood flow reflects the primary measurement of oxygen concentration in the cells; that is, blood flow represents an index of metabolic activity (Webster, 1978). The direct measurement of blood flow is difficult to obtain and usually requires a surgical procedure to place a transducer either within the artery (Geddes, 1970) or snugly around it (e.g., flow probes; Cobbald, 1974). These traumatic preparations are not plausible in the research psychophysiological laboratory, and for this reason they are discussed in this chapter. The interested reader can find an extensive treatment of this topic in Geddes (1970), Cobbald (1974), and Webster (1978). Fortunately, there are several methods that can indirectly and relatively unobtrusively estimate blood flow to a particular segment of the body. These techniques are venous-occlusion plethysmography, impedance plethysmography, and photoplethysmography. These methodologies have been extensively employed in a number of psychophysiological investigations, which include the study of anxiety (Bloom, Houston, & Burish, 1976; Kelly, 1967; Knight & Borden, 1979; Mathews & Lader, 1971) sexual arousal (Geer, 1975; Hoon et al., 1976), response to simple auditory and tactile stimulation (Davis, Buchwald, & Frankmann, 1955), emotional stress (Brod, Fencl, Hejl, & Jirka, 1959), cold pressor (Lovallo & Zeiner, 1974), the voluntary control of peripheral circulatory activities (Kluger, Jamner, & Tursky, 1981; Quintanar, Cacioppo, Crowell, Sklar, & Snyder, 1981; Surwit & Fenton, 1980), classical conditioning (Lidberg, Schalling, & Levander, 1972; Shean, 1968), pain (Tursky & Greenblatt, 1967), and the orienting and defensive reflexes (Royer, 1966; Sokolov, 1963).

Plethysmographic techniques typically measure the tonic and phasic changes in volume of a particular segment of the body, with the change in volume taken as an indirect estimate of the amount of blood contained in that segment. The rate of change of volume provides the psychophysiologist with an index of blood flow.

Evolution of Plethysmography

The term "plethysmography" comes from Greek, meaning the measurement of enlargement. One of the earliest attempts to measure blood flow was conducted in the 1730s by curate Stephen Hales (Olmsted, 1967). Utilizing the bucket method, Hales opened an artery and measured the amount of blood collected in a graduated bucket for a given period of time. However, the forerunner of the modern plethysmograph was developed by Glisson and Swammerdam in the 17th century. These investigators employed a rigid, nondistensible container which encompassed a body segment or organ whose volume was to be measured. This container was water filled, and any swelling of the body organ or segment resulted in water displacement from the container into a volume-measuring system (Hyman & Winsor, 1961). The value of plethysmography was greatly enhanced when Brodie and Russell (1905) demonstrated that when venous occlusion (inflated cuff proximal to the plethysmograph) was employed with the plethysmographic technique, estimates of blood flow were possible. These findings were the predecessors of what is known today as "hydroplethysmography" (see Lewis & Grant, 1925). Pneumoplethysmography, in which the volume of displaced air is recorded, has also been employed with considerable success (Winsor, 1953). In an attempt to reduce artifacts due to limb movement within the enclosure, Lewis and Grant (1925) introduced an enclosure which encased only a portion of a body segment, such as the forearm or calf, so that limb movement would move the entire enclosure instead of introducing movement artifacts within the enclosure. This later became known as "chamber plethysmography," and measurements of blood flow to the forearm and calf became possible. However, it soon became evident that these measurements not only included blood flow to the segment but also blood draining into the segment from more distal portions of the extremities. An answer to this problem was offered by Grant and Pearson (1938), who suggested the use of an arterial occlusion cuff just distal to the plethysmograph, thus ensuring that blood flow was restricted to areas of interest.

The advent of electronics resulted in a profusion of volume detectors. These technological advances also led to alternate methods of measuring blood volume and flow. These included the use of impedance plethysmography which monitors changes in the electrical impedance of a region between two electrodes (Nyboer, 1950; Stewart, 1897); resistive transducers (strain gauges), which measure changes in electrical resistance resulting from changes in capacitance as a function of blood volume changes, and photoelectric transducers, which deliver varying output voltages proportional to volume changes in the body segment (Hertzman, 1938; Hertzman, Randall, & Jochim, 1946). The sophistication and refinement of these early methodologies grew with the development of more advanced detection and recording equipment. The methods most commonly employed in current psychophysiological investigations—such as photoplethysmography, impedance plethysmography, girth (strain gauge) plethysmography, and displacement plethysmography—are examined next.

## Plethysmographic Recording and Techniques

There are two components in the photoplethysmographic response. The first is a phasic measure referred to as blood volume pulse or pulse amplitude, which depicts the pulse wave produced by the pulsatile pumping action of the heart (see Figure 2-13). The rising front of the pulse wave reflects the systole inflow to the body segment under investigation, with the wave peak representing the peak volume. Pulse amplitude (PA) is measured from the trough of the preceding wave to the crest of the succeeding one. Inflow exceeds outflow prior to the systolic peak, they are

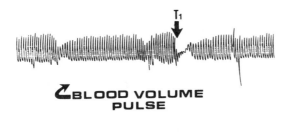

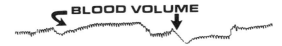

FIG. 2-13. Dynograph recording of photoplethysmographic record of blood volume (BV) and blood pulse volume (BPV).

equal at the peak, and decay after the peak represents the rate of outflow without inflow until the diastolic trough has been reached (Brown, 1967). Pulse volume can be AC recorded (.1 sec TC), but quantification of pulses requires the use of stable high-gain amplifiers (Lader, 1967).

The second component is a tonic signal, which is referred to as blood volume (BV) (see Figure 2-13). This measure represents the overall engorgement of the body segment. As can be seen in Figure 2-13, vasoconstriction, shown at $T_1$, is indicated by a diminution of the PA and a downward deflection of the BV tracing; the reverse process is true for vasodilation. In contrast to PA, BV measures can be DC recorded at lower levels of amplification.

*Volume-Displacement Plethysmography*

In volume-displacement plethysmography, the finger, hand, arm, or leg is placed within a rigid, inflexible chamber which is sealed tightly by snug-fitting rubber sleeves (Kelly, 1967) and a sealing compound (Winsor, 1953). In hydraulic plethysmography, the chamber is filled with an incompressible low-viscosity liquid (such as water). Tubing from the plethysmograph chamber, filled with the same liquid, connects to a transducer that converts volume change into an electrical output. Care must be taken that the temperature of the liquid is maintained at body temperature (34°C); otherwise a vasomotor response to the fluid stimulus may occur (Lader, 1967). Other inherent difficulties associated with this method include the hydrostatic effects of the liquid upon the limb, dampening of brief transient changes in volume, and fluid leakage. An alternative measure based on similar principles in pneumatic plethysmography, employing air as its medium, in which volume changes of the body segment are transmitted pneumatically to a distensible transducer. Rheoplethysmography is a variation of the pneumatic technique in which an airtight cup surrounds a finger tip, and alterations in digital volume are transmitted by the surrounding liquid (Brown, 1967) or air (Winsor, 1953) to the recording transducer.

When venous occlusion is used in conjunction with volume-displacement plethysmography, accurate measurements of blood flow are possible. "Venous-occlusion plethysmography," as it is referred to, entails the use of occluding cuffs proximal and distal to the plethysmograph, as in the case of forearm plethysmography. When the body segment is encased by the plethysmographic chamber, only one occluding cuff is placed proximal to the device, as is true in digital plethysmography.

In venous-occlusion plethysmography, the transducer is first calibrated by sealing off the chamber and injecting a known quantity of air with a syringe. The voltage changes, as given by microvolt of output per cubic millimeter of volume change, are then recorded. Following calibration, the venous-occluding cuff (proximal) is applied as close to the plethysmograph as is feasible and then inflated to a pressure of 50–60 mm Hg (Lader, 1967). This prevents venous blood from leaving the chamber but allows for the easy inflow of arterial blood. Thus, the increase in volume of blood within the body segment per unit time is equal to arterial inflow. If the plethysmograph encloses only a segment of the body, then an arterial-occlusion cuff is applied (distal) and inflated to a pressure of 180–200 mm Hg (Webster, 1978) so that volume changes in the chamber reflect only arterial inflow to that segment. By timing the volumetric changes, we can derive blood flow by constructing a Cartesian plot of volume change, and flow is equal to the rate of change of volume, or $F = dV/dt$ (see Figure 2-14).

A number of factors must be considered to ensure high-fidelity measures; one such factor is the position of the limb. In order to maintain the normal relationship between PA and BV, it is necessary for the limb under measurement to be at the same level as the heart. Raising the limb above the heart increases PA and decreases BV, while lowering the limb below heart level has the opposite effect (Cook, 1974). Another factor is the effect of environmental temperature and humidity. PA is increased

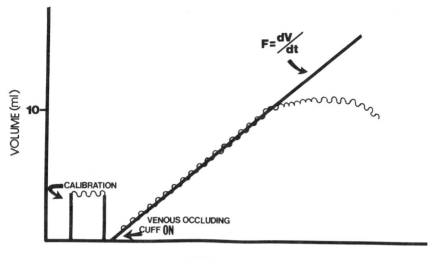

TIME min

FIG. 2-14. Diagram of volume-displacement plethysmograph record demonstrating an example of volume change recorded against time after venous-occluding cuff is applied. Calibration pulse and measure of rate of change (dV/dt) are depicted.

when environmental temperature rises above a "comfortable" level, and PA and BV both decrease when temperatures are below the "comfort zone" (Cook, 1974). Lader (1967) suggests a temperature between 24°C and 27°C ± 1°C and a humidity of approximately 50-60%. The location of the transducer is also important; recording from different sites may produce different physiological information. For example, sympathetically innervated skin blood flow is recorded when a plethysmographic record is obtained from the fingers; thus the effect of stimulation is vasomotor constriction. In contrast, forearm plethysmography primarily reflects blood flow to the muscle, and the effect of strong stimulation is vasodilation (Brod et al., 1959; Fencl, Hejl, Jirka, Madlafovsek, & Brod, 1959).

Plethysmographic records are systematically influenced by respiration. A number of investigators have reported that respiratory activity results in peripheral (digital) vasoconstriction (Engel & Chism, 1967). Stern and Anschel (1968) varied the depth and rate of respiration, and reported that deep and slow breathing produced maximum digital vasoconstriction. Shean and Strange (1971) reported the same finding and also reported that maximum digital vasoconstriction occurs within 4-8 sec following a deep breath. Thus it is advisable that the investigator consider concurrent respiratory measurement to distinguish respiratory artifact from experimental manipulations. For a review of nonpsychological influences upon the plethysmographic response, see Cook (1974) and Lader (1967).

## Impedance Plethysmography

Electrical-impedance plethysmogrpahy is based upon the principle that when electrodes are placed a certain distance apart on living tissue such as a limb, the current distribution between them is a function of the capacitive reactance and resistivity of the various intervening tissues and fluid. A particular body segment will exhibit a characteristic impedance to a high-frequency AC signal. This impedance is due to the summation of the segment's tissues (i.e., muscle and bone) and the volume of blood contained in the segment. Given the assumption that the amount of tissue present is relatively constant, changes in impedance ($\Delta Z$) are said to reflect alterations in the amount of blood contained within. As the volume of the body segment changes due to the pulsations of blood that pass through it, the impedance of that segment also changes, and the concomitant impedance pulse contours obtained are similar to pulse waves obtained by other plethysmographic techniques (Geddes & Baker, 1968). A major drawback of this method is that it provides only relative measures of blood volume changes. It is difficult to calibrate the obtained impedance pulse into absolute blood flow units, although attempts have been made by some investigators (Geddes & Hoff, 1964). Although only providing a relative measure of blood flow, impedance plethysmography remains an attractive measure to the psychophysiologist. Specialized electrodes are not required; the electrodes consist of flat metal plates of aluminum, stainless steel, or brass (Brown, 1967), or conductive tape applied to the area of interest (Abel & McCutcheon, 1979; Miller & Horvath, 1978). Unlike volume-displacement plethysmography, the impedance method allows for electrode placement anywhere on the body. This provides access to noninvasive relative blood flow measurements of the body trunk.

Typically, a tetrapolar electrode configuration is used in impedance plethysmography (see Figure 2-15). A high-frequency AC current (i.e., 100–200 kHz) is applied to the two outer electrodes ($Z_1$ and $Z_4$), which produces a uniform current density between the two interior electrodes

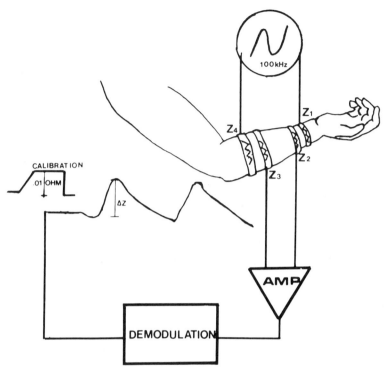

FIG. 2-15. Diagram of typical impedance plethysmograph circuit. Outer electrodes $Z_1$ and $Z_4$ are connected to 100-kHz oscillator; inner electrodes $Z_2$ and $Z_3$ record changes in impedance due to changes in blood volume.

($Z_2$ and $Z_3$). The use of a 100- to 200-kHz signal minimizes changes in the body segment's reactance component so that obtained impedance alterations reflect only the resistive component (Brown, Giddon, & Dean, 1965). Webster (1978) has suggested that the current employed be greater than 1 mA so that an adequate signal-to-noise ratio will be achieved.

Figure 2-15 shows a typical tetrapolar impedance plethysmograph circuit with its output. As mentioned previously, electrodes $Z_2$ and $Z_3$ are voltage-sensing and should be coupled to a high-input impedance voltage amplifier so that there is no current flow between $Z_2$ and $Z_3$. A medium-gain amplifier is sufficient, since when a 100-kHz, 1-mA signal is employed to excite $Z_1$ and $Z_4$, the voltage detected by $Z_2$ and $Z_3$ is approximately .16 V (Webster, 1978). The output from the amplifier is amplitude modulated by the current source I and impedance change $\Delta Z$. This signal is then demodulated, which produces an output of $Z + \Delta Z$, in which Z is the tissue's impedance to flow. $\Delta Z$ can then be extracted using a high-pass filter. The relationship between the change in volume and impedance alterations as a result of increased blood volume can be expressed by

$$\Delta V = \frac{-P_b L^2 \Delta Z}{Z^2}$$

where $\Delta V$ is the change in volume, $P_b$ is the resistivity of blood (= 150 $\Omega$-cm; Geddes & Baker, 1968), L is the length between the sensing electrodes, Z is the limb impedance, and $\Delta Z$ is the impedance change (Webster, 1978).

Although impedance plethysmography has not been employed to a large extent as a psychophysiological measure, the relative ease with which measurements can be obtained makes it a measure worthy of consideration in situations that require only the monitoring of relative changes in blood volume in response to various stimuli.

*Photoplethysmography*

The photoplethysmographic technique of measuring peripheral circulatory events is based on the fact that tissue and blood have very different light absorption coefficients. Body tissues are relatively transparent to wavelengths in the red and infrared portions of the spectrum (8000–9000 $\mu$m), to which blood is relatively opaque (Weinman, 1967). Thus when a constant-intensity light source is directed into or through a portion of tissue, the amount of light reflected is a function of both the volume of the interposed tissue, which can be assumed to be constant, and a variable component reflecting transient changes in blood volume within the illuminated region. Given that a linear function exists between the intensity of light that falls upon the photodetector and its electrical output, a derivative of the Lambert–Beer equation can be used to express the previous statement (Brown, 1967):

$$I = I_0 e^{-Ax}$$

where $I_0$ is the intensity of the incident light, I is the intensity of the reflected or emerging light, A is the mean absorption coefficient of the interposed tissue–blood composite, and x is the depth in centimeters of the interposed tissue.

Since the term A is the average absorption coefficient for both tissue and blood, and the absorption coefficient of the quantity of tissue is a constant (given fixed placement of the transducer), then I is dynamically modulated by alterations in both the color and quantity of blood. The variation in the photocell's electrical output can be divided into two components: modulation as a function of changes induced by the pulse pressure wave (blood pulse volume) and a slower component reflecting the level of engorgement of blood in the area.

Photoplethysmographically obtained measurements of pulse volume and blood volume are relative, rather than absolute. Whereas in volume-displacement plethysmography results can be stated in cubic centimeters, the output of photoplethysmography only allows for comparative evaluation (i.e., percent change), although attempts to demonstrate a quantitative correlation between cutaneous blood flow and a photoplethysmographically obtained pulse have been made (see Hertzman *et al.*, 1946). Despite this disadvantage, photoplethysmography is a frequently used measurement technique as it allows for the continuous recording of peripheral vascular changes at any bodily site. This is in contrast to venous-occlusion plethysmography, which provides only an intermittent measure of pulse amplitude and blood volume, and is also quite restrictive in transducer placement.

There are three different types of photoplethysmographic transducer techniques: the transillumined method, in which a body segment is "sandwiched" between the light source and the photodetector (Hertzman, 1938); the reflectance transducer, in which the photocell and light source are placed side by side (Depater, Vandenberg, & Bueno, 1962); and the fiber optic transducer, which also employs the side-by-side configuration of source and detector, and in which optical fibers are employed to illuminate the tissue from a remote source and to return the reflected light from the tissue to the photocell (Brown, 1967).

Although all are based on similar principles, each of these transducers possesses its own unique advantages and disadvantages. Hertzman (1938) was among the first to introduce "photoelectric plethysmography." Hertzman's and other early photoelectric transducers utilized the transillumined method. The advantage of this type of transducer is that circulatory changes deep within the tissue are monitored. This is in contrast to the reflectance transducer, which represents circulatory changes restricted to the superficial cutaneous vascular bed. However, the transillumined method can only be applied to the small extremities such as the fingers, toes, or ears. In addition, the required light intensity results in the heating of the area of interest, which elicits the vasomotor response of dilation. This may or may not be considered desirable, as this produces an enhanced pulse (Webster, 1978).

This problem was eliminated by the use of optical fibers to transmit and receive light from a removed source (Giddon, Goldhaber, Kushnir, & Gustafson, 1963; Tursky & Greenblatt, 1967), a side-by-side photocell light source configuration which permits the use of low-intensity lamps so that heating is minimal (Depater et al., 1962; Weinman & Manoach, 1962), and the development of new semiconductor materials such as the light-emitting diode (LED) and phototransistor. Lee, Tahmoush, and Jennings (1975); and Tahmoush, Jennings, Lee, Camp, and Weber (1976) have described a LED–transistor plethysmograph which eliminated many of the problems which plagued the frequently employed tungsten lamp–CdS photocell. These included the conventional CdS photocell's sensitivity to temperature, prior light history, and the difficulties of maintaining a constant intensity illumination. The photoplethysmograph they described is a reflective transducer in which the LED and the phototransistor are applied adjacent to one another. A gallium arsenide (GaAs) infrared LED, which produces a narrow radiation band with a peak spectral emission of .94 $\mu$m, is used in combination with a silicon phototransistor that is sensitive to radiation between .4 and 1.1 $\mu$m. This permits the LED to be operated at low power levels (.25 mW) so that heat output is minimal. The transducer can be AC coupled or DC coupled to record pulse volume and blood volume signals, respectively. Tahmoush et al., (1976) reported that the phototransistor provides a linear voltage output with respect to the intensity of light striking it, and that this linear relationship is relatively unaffected by temperature changes or the prior light history. In addition, the fact that the system employs the infrared portion of the spectrum negates the need for filters (which are otherwise required to prevent signal distortion due to varying blood oxygen concentrations) and prevents extraneous signals (i.e., fluorescent lamps) from being detected (Webster, 1978).

Photoplethysmography requires that the transducer be firmly affixed to the body surface. Extreme sensitivity to movement artifact may be the major deficiency of the technique (Brown, 1967; Webster, 1978; Weinman, 1967). The transducer may be attached to the body by the use of adhesive collars with the addition of adhesive tape. Depater et al. (1962) discussed the relationship between the pressure of transducer application and the resulting plethysmogram. They reported that as contact pressure is varied, the amplitude and shape of the plethysmogram are varied, possibly due to the altered volume and distensibility of the venous bed. They consider a contact pressure of between 10 and 40 mm Hg optimal.

Photoplethysmography has been extensively employed in both clinical and psychophysiological investigations. This may be due in part to the ease of applicability of the transducer to many body sites. This freedom has allowed reserachers to monitor previously inaccessible body sites, and it permits the investigator to begin to unravel the many interrelationships among cardiovascular variables. This may be illustrated in research pertaining to the voluntary control of peripheral circulation. A number of investigators have investigated voluntary vasoconstriction of the temporal artery (Elmore & Tursky, 1981; Quintanar *et al.*, 1981), digital vasoconstriction (Quintanar *et al.*, 1981), and digital vasomotor activity; and they reported that digital pulse volume dilatation achieved by finger temperature feedback was accompanied by a constriction in temporal pulse amplitude, while biofeedback of temporal pulse amplitude constriction was accompanied by digital pulse constriction.

Photoplethysmographs have also been used in the investigation of differential vascular responding to stimuli, as is demonstrated in the orienting and defensive reflexes. Sokolov (1963) demonstrated that the vascular system responded to mild stimuli with a characteristic pattern of cephalic vasodilation and digital vasoconstriction, which he called the "orienting reflex." If the stimulus intensity is increased or made noxious, a vascular response of vasoconstriction in both digital and cephalic vasculature occurs. This he termed the "defensive reflex."

*Strain-Gauge Plethysmography*

Strain-gauge plethysmography, like photoplethysmography, has proved to be a versatile, extensively employed instrument in the study of peripheral circulation. Strain-gauge plethysmography is based upon the principle that when a conductive element (such as a column of mercury contained within an elastic tube) is strained within its elastic limits, a lawful relationship exists between resistance changes and changes in the diameter, length, and resistivity of the element (Brown, 1967). Hallbook, Mansson, and Nilsen (1970) described this relationship as

$$\frac{\Delta V}{V} = 2(\Delta G / G) \tag{1}$$

in which $\Delta V$ is the percentage change of volume and $\Delta G$ is the percentage change in girth (circumference) of the limb.

Extension of the strain gauge results in an alteration in its length and cross-sectional area, with volume remaining constant. The relationship between resistance and length of the strain gauge can be given by

$$\frac{\Delta R}{R} = 2(\Delta L / L) \tag{2}$$

in which $\Delta R$ and $\Delta L$ are the percentage changes in the gauge's resistance and width. Given that the elastic gauge assumes the circumference of the limb, the percentage change of the circumference ($\Delta G$) is equal to the percentage change in the length of the gauge ($\Delta L$), giving

$$\frac{\Delta R}{R} = 2(\Delta G / G) \tag{3}$$

Combining Equations (1) and (3) gives

$$\frac{\Delta R}{R} = \frac{\Delta V}{V}$$

By this relationship, it is possible to derive volume changes by recording the corresponding alterations in resistance. The most commonly employed transducer is the mercury strain gauge introduced by Whitney (1949, 1953), although elastic strain gauges which employ other liquid conductors have been used (see Geddes & Baker, 1968).

Typically the mercury strain gauge consists of a silicon rubber tube ranging from 3 to 25 cm in length, with an inside diameter of .5 mm and a resistance of .02 to .20 $\Omega$/cm of length (Cobbald, 1974). Resistance changes are detected by including the strain gauge within a Wheatstone bridge circuit, which may be energized by a constant voltage (Brakkee & Vendrik, 1966) constant current (Cobbald, 1974; Hallbook et al., 1970). The typical output of a constant-voltage DC bridge is approximately a .24 mV signal per millimeter change in length per volt applied (Lawton & Collins, 1959), and an AC-energized bridge demonstrates a sensitivity of 1 mm of pen deflection per 2 $\mu$m of gauge extension. Typically in the mercury strain gauge, a 1% increase in gauge length results in a 2% change in resistance (Geddes & Baker, 1968). The major deficiencies of this method include the sensitivity of this transducer to thermal drift (Whitney, 1953), calibration difficulties (Brakkee & Vendrik, 1966; Hallbook et al., 1970), the corrosive effect of mercury on rubber tubing, and the fact that obtained measurements of circumference are invariably lower than those obtained by other methods such as ultrasonics (Cobbald, 1974).

Despite its deficiencies, mercury strain-gauge plethysmography can still be considered to be a good, relatively unobtrusive, continuous measure of blood volume. It has received particular attention in the psychophysiological investigation of male sexual arousal (Rosen & Keefe, 1978). For a theoretical review of strain-gauge plethysmography, the reader is referred to Sigdell (1969) and Brakkee and Vendrik (1966).

### Thermal Transcutaneous Flow Measurements

Local capillary flow can be detected by monitoring the rate at which heat is drawn from a heating element. When placed in contact with the skin, a heat source will lose heat both by means of thermal conductivity of the underlying tissue, which is a relatively constant factor, and by blood flow transport. The subcutaneous blood flow results in a thermal conductivity change whose magnitude is proportional to capillary flow (Cobbald, 1974).

Harding, Rushmer, and Baker (1967) have described a thermal transcutaneous flowmeter. Their transducer is ½ inch in diameter and contains two thermisters ¼ inch apart, one of which is enclosed in a tiny heating coil. A temperature difference of 1°C is maintained between the thermisters by a servocontrol which modulates the heating coil's power supply. Variations in the power required to maintain this difference were used as an index of conductive heat loss. Cook, Cohen, Gerkovich, Anderson, and Graham (1979) examined the utility of this device as a psychophysiological instrument and reported that the output of this device was related to blood flow and seemed to reflect a vascular process different from information obtained photoplethysmographically (pulse amplitude) or thermally (skin temperature).

In an interesting application of this method, Cohen and Shapiro (1971) mounted a transducer similar to the one described onto the ring of a vaginal diaphragm. With this system, they recorded vaginal blood flow changes in response to imagined sexual fantasies. Significant correlations were obtained between vaginal blood flow measures and reported subjective intensity of the fantasies.

Since the thermal transcutaneous flowmeter provides for the continuous monitoring of vascular functioning and is easily applied to any part of the body, its potential for use as a psychophysiological measurement device is great. Future research investigations into its calibration and quantification are needed.

## Summary and Theoretical Considerations

For the proper interpretation of obtained plethysmograms, the psychophysiologist should be aware of nonpsychological variables which systematically influence the vasculature. One simple but important factor is that when the transducer is placed over a major vein, no pulse amplitude recording will be obtained. Another relevant variable is the pressure with which the transducer is applied to the body surface, which systematically affects obtained results. In addition, the type of tissue over which the transducer is placed must be considered to account for tissue specificity of response. Because of these three variables, between-subject comparisons should be made with caution.

Another nonpsychological variable is the position of the limb being investigated. Blood flow is maximal when the limb is at heart level and decreases as the limb deviates from that position (Abel & McCutcheon, 1979; Guyton, 1976). In contrast, pulse amplitude increases above heart level and decreases below it, while blood volume does the opposite (Cook, 1974). This fact fails to support earlier claims that pulse amplitude represents an index of blood flow (Burton, 1972). Cook (1974) has suggested that pulse amplitude be considered a measure of blood flow only if the measurement site is maintained at heart level. Pulse amplitude and blood volume are also differentially affected by changes in environmental temperature.

This apparent lack of correlation between pulse amplitude and blood volume, and between pulse amplitude and blood flow should lead us to question what these measures represent. Weinman (1967) suggested that pulse amplitude represented a response to pulse pressure, which was modified by the distensibility of the vessel wall, when measured photoplethysmographically. Indeed, accumulating evidence appears to indicate that pulse amplitude is an index of arterial tone, whereas blood volume represents the capacitance of the local venous system (Cook, 1974).

From a measurement standpoint, psychophysiology remains in need of an adequate blood flow measure. While many advances have been made in the measurement of cardiodynamics, there is lack of development in the area of noninvasive flow measurement. Talbot and Gessner (1973) make an appropriate analogy that the study of hemodynamics without the aid of measurement of flow is comparable to the electrical engineer studying active networks but unable to monitor currents or impedances. Clearly, the need for a continuous measuring device is demonstrated.


## CONCLUDING REMARKS

An overview of the techniques and methodologies employed in the measurement of cardiovascular functioning has been presented. Although current methods will one day appear ancient and crude, the physical principles behind them will continue to serve as a guide for future developments. A brief history of the evolution of the various forms of measurement has been presented, illustrating the systematic advancement in the study of cardio- and hemodynamics from personal observations (e.g., curate Stephen Hales's observations of blood flow/pressure) through the employment of mechanical devices (e.g., Marey's determination of blood pressure), to the introduction of electricity and electronics (e.g., galvanometers) into the measurement process. With the advent of the miniaturization of electronic components and computers, psychophysiological instrumentation is at the beginning of a new phase.

As stated earlier, many technological advances in measurement equipment were the result of the psychophysiologist's special relationship with the bioinstrumentation engineer. Working together, unique transducers and instruments were developed to meet the needs of the researcher. This represented a time in which the byproduct of psychophysiological research was instrumentation. The past tense is used intentionally, as this process has seen a shift toward commercially available equipment determining the measurement technique. Tursky (1980) has suggested that the former symbiotic relationship between psychophysiologist and bioinstrumentation engineer should be reaffirmed. Technology today permits the construction of devices as small as the head of a pin that possess the capabilities of an instrument previously occupying hundreds of times as much space. This development greatly lessens the reactivity of the measurement processes; that is, because of their physical dimensions, previous methods affected the system that they were designed to measure. Now that instrument size constraints are virtually eliminated, issues in psycho-physiological measurement may be reexamined.

In the introduction to this chapter, the point was made that the investigator's ability to understand the functioning of the cardiovascular system bears a circular relationship to his/her capabilities of measuring the system's basic physical characteristics; as our understanding of cardio-dynamics and hemodynamics increases, new measurement instruments are developed which further our understanding of the cardiovascular system. Although some aspects of the cardiovascular system's performance and regulatory controls have been under investigation more intensively and for a longer period than other physiological systems, it still remains imperfectly understood. Talbot and Gessner (1973) made this point and called for a strong "give and take" relationship between the physiologist, medical scientist, and engineer.

The problem of elucidating the relationship among the many inter-dependent cardiovascular parameters is quite formidable. One possible solution is the adoption of a physiological systems approach to the cardiovascular system. As will be seen in the next chapter, a systems approach entails the study of a particular physiological system in terms of design of, and interaction among, its subsystems so that optimal task performance exists (Talbot & Gessner, 1973).

In order for the psychophysiologist to achieve the goal of specifying the relationships among behavior, emotion, and physiological parameters, he/she must first demonstrate the ability to faithfully measure them. In cardiovascular psychophysiology, progress has been made to accomplish this goal.

## ACKNOWLEDGMENTS

We wish to thank Ms. Abbe Herzig, whose contribution of time, effort, and skill made it possible to complete this chapter. We also wish to thank Dr. Richard Friedman for his editorial assistance.

This work was supported by National Institute of Mental Health Grant MH-22296-03 and National Science Foundation Grant 5-041125.

## REFERENCES

Abel, F. L., & McCutcheon, E. P. *Cardiovascular function: Principles and applications.* Boston: Little, Brown, 1979.

Alexander, A. A. Psychophysiological concepts of psychopathology. In N.S. Greenfield, & R. A. Sternbach (Eds.), *Handbook of psychophysiology*. New York: Holt, Rinehart, & Winston, 1972.

Allard, E. M. Sound and pressure signals obtained from a single intra-cardiac transducer. *IRE Transactions of Bio-Medical Electronics*, 1962, *BME-9*, 74–77.

American Heart Association (Kirkendall, W. M., Burton, A. C., Epstein, F. H., & Freis, E. D.). Recommendations for human blood pressure determinations by sphygmomanometers. *Circulation*, 1967, *36*, 503–509.

Armitage, P., Fox, W., Rose, G. A., & Tiniter, C. M. The variability of measurements of casual blood pressure: II. Survey experience. *Clinical Science*, 1966, *30*, 337–344.

Atzler, E. Neues Verfahren zur Funktionsbeurteilung des Herzens. *Deutsche Medizinische Wochenschrift*, 1933, *59*, 1347–1349.

Atzler, E. Dielektrographie: Handbuch der Biologie. *Arbeitsmethoden*, 1935, *5*, 1073–1084.

Ax, A. F., The physiological differentiation between fear and anger in humans. *Psychosomatic Medicine*, 1953, *15*, 433–449.

Bennett, C. A., & Franklin, N. L. *Statistical analysis in chemistry and the chemical industry*. New York: John Wiley & Sons, 1954.

Benson, H., Shapiro, D., Tursky, B., & Schwartz, G. E. Decreased systolic blood pressure through operant conditioning techniques in patients with essential hypertension. *Science*, 1971, *173*, 740–742.

Berger, L. Interrelationships between blood pressure responses to mecholyl and personality variables. *Psychophysiology*, 1964, *1*, 115–118.

Bloom, L. J., Houston, B. K., & Burish, T. G. An evaluation of finger pulse volume as a measure of anxiety. *Psychophysiology*, 1976, *13*, 40–42.

Bloom, L. J., & Trautt, G. M. Finger pulse volume as a measure of anxiety: Further evaluation. *Psychophysiology*, 1977, *14*, 541–544.

Brakkee, A. J. M., & Vendrik, A. J. H. Strain-gauge plethysmography: Theoretical and practical notes on a new design. *Journal of Applied Physiology*, 1966, *21*, 701–704.

Brener, J. Heart rate. In P. H. Venables & I. Martin (Eds.), *A manual of psychophysiological methods*. Amsterdam: North-Holland, 1967.

Brener, J., & Hothersall, D. Paced respiration and heart rate control. *Psychophysiology*, 1967, *4*, 1–6.

Brener, J., & Kleinman, R. Learned control of decreases in systolic blood pressure. *Nature*, 1970, *226*, 1063–1064.

Brod, J., Fencl, V., Hejl, Z., & Jirka, J. Circulatory changes underlying blood pressure evaluation during acute emotional stress (mental arithmetic) in normotensive and hypertensive subjects. *Clinical Science*, 1959, *18*, 269–279.

Brodie, T. G., & Russel, A. E. On the determination of the rate of blood flow through an organ. *Journal of Physiology*, 1905, *32*, 47–49.

Brown, C. C. The techniques of plethysmography. In C. C. Brown (Ed.), *Methods in psychophysiology*. Baltimore: Williams & Wilkins, 1967.

Brown, C. C. Instruments in psychophysiology. In N. S. Greenfield & R. A. Sternbach (Eds.), *Handbook of psychophysiology*. New York: Holt, Rinehart, & Winston, 1972.

Brown, C. C., Giddon, D. B., & Dean, E. D. Techniques of plethysmography. *Psychophysiology*, 1965, *1*, 253–266.

Burton, A. C. *Physiology and biophysics of the circulation* (2nd ed.). Chicago: Year Book Medical, 1972.

Cacioppo, J. T., Sandman, C. A., & Walker, B. B. The effects of operant heart rate conditioning on cognitive elaboration and attitude change. *Psychophysiology*, 1978, *15*, 330–338.

Clancy, F. Factors affecting correlation between direct and indirect arterial blood pressure measurements. *Journal of Clinical Engineering*, 1978, *3*, 49–51.

Clemens, W. J., & Shattock, R. J. Voluntary heart rate control during static muscular effort. *Psychophysiology*, 1979, *16*, 327–332.

Cobbald, R. S. C. *Transducers for biomedical measurements*. New York: John Wiley & Sons, 1974.

Cohen, H. D., & Shapiro, A. A method for measuring sexual arousal in the female. *Psychophysiology*, 1971, *8*, 251–252. (Abstract)

Cook, M. Peripheral vascular changes. In P. A. Obrist, A. H. Black, J. Brener, & L. V. DiCara (Eds.), *Cardiovascular psychophysiology*. Chicago: Aldine, 1974.

Cook, M. R., Cohen, H. D., Gerkovich, M. N., Anderson, F. H., & Graham, C. In vitro and in vivo tests of a continuous measure of cutaneous blood flow. *Psychophysiology*, 1979, *16*, 177.

Dale, A., Shapiro, D., & Greenstadt, L. *Systolic blood pressure biofeedback and the balloon stress test with pulse transit time correlates*. Paper presented at the meeting of the Society for Psychophysiological Research, Vancouver, B.C., October 1980.

Davis, R. C., Buchwald, M., & Frankmann, R. W. Autonomic and muscular responses and their relationship to simple stimuli. *Psychological Monographs: General and Applied*, 1955, *69*, 1–71.

Dawson, M. E., Schell, A. M., & Catania, J. J. Autonomic correlates of depression and clinical improvement following electroconvulsive shock therapy. *Psychophysiology*, 1977, *14*, 569–578.

Denniston, J. C., Maher, J. T., Reeves, J. T., Cruz, J. C., Cymerman, A., & Grover, R. F. Measurement of cardiac output by electrical impedance at rest and during exercise. *Journal of Applied Physiology*, 1976, *40*, 91–95.

Depater, L., Vandenberg, J., & Bueno, A. A. A very sensitive photoplethysmograph using scattered light and a photosensitive resistance. *Acta Physiologica Pharmacologica Neerlandica*, 1962, *10*, 378–390.

Dock, W., & Taubman, F. Some techniques for recording the ballistocardiograph directly from the body. *American Journal of Medicine*, 1949, *7*, 751–755.

Elder, S. T., Longacre, A., Welsh, D. M., & McAfee, R. D. Apparatus and procedure for training subjects to control their blood pressure. *Psychophysiology*, 1977, *14*, 68–72.

Elmore, A., & Tursky, B. A comparison of the psychophysiological and clinical response to biofeedback for temporal pulse amplitude reduction and biofeedback for increases in hand temperature in the treatment of migraine. *Headache*, 1981, *21*, 93–101.

Engel, B. T. Some physiological correlates of hunger and pain. *Journal of Experimental Psychology*, 1959, *57*, 389–396.

Engel, B. T. Operant conditioning of cardiac function: A status report. *Psychophysiology*, 1972, *9*, 161–177.

Engel, B. T., & Chism, R. A. Effect of increases and decreases in breathing rate on heart rate and finger pulse volume. *Psychophysiology*, 1967, *4*, 83–89.

Fencl, V., Hejl, Z., Jirka, J., Madlafovsek, J., & Brod, J. Changes of blood flow in forearm muscle and skin during an acute emotional stress (mental arithmetic). *Clinical Science*, 1959, *18*, 491–498.

Ferris, C. D. *Introduction to bioinstrumentation*. Clifton, N.J.: Humana Press, 1978.

Fey, S. G., & Lindholm, E. Biofeedback and progressive relaxation: Effects on systolic and diastolic blood pressure and heart rate. *Psychophysiology*, 1978, *15*, 239–247.

Fitchenbaum, M. Counter inverts period to measure low frequency. *Electronics*, 1976, *49*, 100.

Flanagan, G. J., & Hull, C. J. A blood pressure recorder. *British Journal of Anaesthesiology*, 1968, *40*, 292–298.

Freis, E. D., & Sappington, R. F. Dynamic reactions produced by deflating a blood pressure cuff. *Circulation*, 1968, *38*, 1085–1096.

Furedy, J. J. Teaching self-regulation of cardiac function through imaginational Pavlovian and biofeedback conditioning: Remember the response. In N. Birbaumer & H. D. Kimmel (Eds.), *Biofeedback and self-regulation*. Hillsdale, N.J.: Erlbaum, 1979.

Geddes, L. A. *The direct and indirect measurement of blood pressure.* Chicago: Year Book Medical, 1970.

Geddes, L. A. & Baker, L. E. *Principles of applied biomedical instrumentation.* New York: John Wiley & Sons, 1968.

Geddes, L. A., & Hoff, H. E. The measurement of physiological events by impedance change. *American Journal of Medical Electronics*, 1964, *3*, 16–27.

Geddes, L. A., Hoff, H. E., & Badger, A. S. Introduction of the ascultatory method of measuring blood pressure—Including a translation of Korotokoff's original paper. *Cardiovascular Research Center Bulletin*, 1966, *5*, 57–74.

Geddes, L. A., & Newberg, D. C. Cuff pressure oscillations in the measurement of relative blood pressure. *Psychophysiology*, 1977, *14*, 198–202.

Geddes, L. A., Spencer, W. A., & Hoff, H. E. Graphic recording of Korotokoff sounds. *American Heart Journal*, 1959, *57*, 1178–1180.

Geer, J. H. Direct measurement of genital responding. *American Psychologist*, 1975, *30*, 415–419.

Giddon, D. B., Goldhaber, P., Kushnir, H., & Gustafson, L. A. *Photoelectric monitoring of gingival vascular reactions.* Paper presented at the 41st meeting of the International Association of Dental Research, March 1963. (Abstract)

Gilson, W. E., Goldberg, H., & Slocum, H. C. An automatic device for periodically determining both systolic and diastolic pressure in man. *Science*, 1941, *94*, 194.

Goldman, M. S., & Lee, R. M. Operant conditioning of blood pressure: Effects of mediators. *Psychophysiology*, 1978, *15*, 531–537.

Graham, F. K. Normality of distributions and homogeneity of heart rate and heart period samples. *Psychophysiology*, 1978, *15*, 487–491.(a)

Graham, F. K. Constraints on measuring heart rate and period sequentially through real and cardiac time. *Psychophysiology*, 1978, *15*, 492–495.(b)

Grant, R. T., & Pearson, R. S. Blood flow in the human limb: Observations on the differences between the proximal and distal parts and remarks on the regulation of body temperature. *Clinical Science*, 1938, *3*, 119–139.

Green, J. H. Blood pressure follower for continuous blood pressure recording in man. *Journal of Physiology*, 1955, *130*, 37P–38P.

Gribbin, B., Steptoe, A., & Sleight, P. Pulse wave velocity as a measure of blood pressure change. *Psychophysiology*, 1976, *13*, 86–90.

Grings, W. W., & Schandler, S. L. Interaction of learned relaxation and aversion. *Psychophysiology*, 1977, *14*, 275–280.

Guyton, A. C. *Textbook of medical physiology.* Philadelphia: W. B. Saunders, 1976.

Guyton, A. C., Jones, C. E., & Coleman, T. G. *Circulatory physiology: Cardiac output and its regulation* (2nd. ed.). Philadelphia: W. B. Saunders, 1973.

Haffty, B. G., Kotilainen, P. W., Kobayashi, K., Bishop, R. L., & Spodick, D. H. Development of an ambulatory systolic time interval monitoring system. *Journal of Clinical Engineering*, 1977, *2*, 199–210.

Hallbook, T., Mansson, B., & Nilsen, R. A strain gauge plethysmograph with electrical calibration. *Scandanavian Journal of Clinical and Laboratory Investigations*, 1970, *25*, 413–418.

Harding, D. C., Rushmer, R. F., & Baker, D. W. Thermal transcutaneous flowmeter. *Medical and Biological Engineering*, 1967, *5*, 623–626.

Hertzman, A. B. The blood supply of various skin areas as estimated by the photoelectric plethysmograph. *American Journal of Physiology*, 1938, *124*, 328–340.

Hertzman, A. B., Randall, W. C., & Jochim, K. E. The estimation of the cutaneous blood flow with the photoelectric plethysmograph. *American Journal of Physiology*, 1946, *145*, 716–726.

Heslegrave, R. J., & Furedy, J. J. Carotid dP/dt as a psychophysiological index of sympathetic myocardial effects: Some considerations. *Psychophysiology*, 1980, *17*, 482–494.

Heslegrave, R. J., Ogilvie, J. C., & Furedy, J. J. Measuring baseline-treatment differences in heart rate variability: Variance versus successive difference mean square and beats per minute versus interbeat intervals. *Psychophysiology*, 1979, *16*, 151–157.

Hodges, W. F., & Spielberger, C. D. The effects of threat of shock on heart rate for subjects who differ in manifest anxiety and fear of shock. *Psychophysiology*, 1966, *2*, 287–294.

Hokanson, J. E., & Burgess, M. Effects of physiological arousal level, frustration, and task complexity on performance. *Journal of Abnormal and Social Psychology*, 1964, *68*, 698–702.

Hoon, P., Wincze, J., & Hoon, E. Physiological assessment of sexual arousal in women. *Psychophysiology*, 1976, *13*, 196–204.

Hyman, C., & Winsor, T. History of plethysmography. *Journal of Cardiovascular Surgery*, 1961, *2*, 506–518.

Jennings, J. R., Stringfellow, J. C., & Graham, M. A comparison of the statistical distributions of beat-by-beat heart rate and heart period. *Psychophysiology*, 1974, *11*, 207–210.

Jennings, J. R., & Wood, C. C. Cardiac cycle time effects of performance, phasic cardiac responses, and their intercollection in choice reaction time. *Psychophysiology*, 1977, *14*, 297–307.

Kahneman, D., Tursky, B., Shapiro, D., & Crider, A. Pupillary, heart rate, and skin resistance changes during a mental task. *Journal of Experimental Psychology*, 1969, *79*, 164–167.

Kelly, D. H. The technique of forearm plethysmography for assessing anxiety. *Journal of Psychosomatic Research*, 1967, *10*, 373–382.

Khachaturian, Z. S., Kerr, J., Kruger, R., & Schacter, J. A methodological note: Comparison between period and rate data in studies of cardiac function. *Psychophysiology*, 1972, *9*, 539–545.

King, G. E. Errors in clinical measurement of blood pressure in obesity. *Clinical Science*, 1967, *32*, 223–237.

Kinnen, E., Kubicek, W. G., & Patterson, R. *Thoracic cage impedance measurements: Impedance plethysmographic determination of cardiac output (a comparative study)* (SAM-TDR-64-15). San Antonio: U.S.A.F. School of Aerospace Medicine, Brooks Air Force Base, 1964. (also N64-21597)

Kluger, M. A., Jamner, L., & Tursky, B. A comparison of peripheral circulation feedback modalities. *Psychophysiology*, 1981, *18*, 179.

Knight, M. L., & Borden, R. J. Autonomic and affective reactions of high and low socially-anxious individuals awaiting public performance. *Psychophysiology*, 1979, *16*, 209–213.

Korotokoff, N. S. On the subject of methods of measuring blood pressure. *Bulletin of the Imperial Medical Academy of St. Petersburg*, 1905, *11*, 365–367.

Krausman, D. T. Methods and procedures for monitoring and recording blood pressure. *American Psychologist*, 1975, *30*, 285–294.

Kubicek, W. G., From, A. H. L., Patterson, R. P., Witsoe, D. A., Castenda, A., Lilleki, R. G., & Ersek, R. Impedance cardiography as a non-invasive means to monitor cardiac function. *Journal of the Association for the Advancement of Medical Instrumentation*, 1970, *4*, 79–84.

Lacey, B. C., & Lacey, J. I. Studies of heart rate and other bodily processes in sensorimotor behavior. In P. A. Obrist, A. H. Black, J. Brener, & L. V. DiCara (Eds.), *Cardiovascular psychophysiology*. Chicago: Aldine, 1974.

Lader, M. H. Pneumatic plethysmography. In P. H. Venables & I. Martin (Eds.), *A manual of psychophysiological methods*. Amsterdam: North-Holland, 1967.

Lambert, E. H., & Wood, E. H. The use of resistance wire strain gauge manometer to measure intra-arterial pressure. *Proceedings of the Society for Experimental Biology and Medicine*, 1947, *64*, 186–190.

Lance, V. Q., & Spodick, D. H. Systolic time intervals utilizing ear densitigraphy: Advantages and reliability for stress testing. *American Heart Journal*, 1977, *94*, 62–66.

Landis, C., & Wiley, L. E. Changes of blood pressure and respiration during deception. *Journal of Comparative Psychology*, 1926, *6*, 1–19.

Lang, P. J., Melamed, B. G., & Hart, J. H. A psychophysiological analysis of fear modification using an automated desensitization procedure. *Journal of Abnormal Psychology*, 1970, *76*, 220–234.

Lang, P. J., & Twentyman, C.T. Learning to control heart rate: Effects of varying incentive and criterion of success on task performance. *Psychophysiology*, 1976, *13*, 378–385.

Lawler, J. E., & Obrist, P. A. Indirect indices of contractile force. In P.A. Obrist, A. H. Black, J. Brener, & L. V. DiCara (Eds.), *Cardiovascular psychophysiology*. Chicago: Aldine, 1974.

Lawton, R. W., & Collins, C. C. Calibration of an aortic circumference gauge. *Applied Physiology*, 1959, *14*, 465–467.

Lee, A. L., Tahmoush, A. J., & Jennings, J. R. An L.E.D.–transistor photoplethysmograph. *IEEE Transactions on Biomedical Engineering*, 1975, *22*, 248–250.

Lee, R. M., Caldwell, J. R., & Lee, J. A. Blood pressure tracking systems and their application to biofeedback. *Biofeedback and Self-Regulation*, 1977, *2*, 435–447.

Lewis, T., & Grant, R. Observations upon active hyperemia in man. *Heart*, 1925, *12*, 73–76.

Lidberg, L., Schalling, D., & Levander, S. E. Some characteristics of digital vasomotor activity. *Psychophysiology*, 1972, *9*, 402–412.

Light, K. C., & Obrist, P. A. Cardiovascular response to stress: Effects of opportunity to avoid, shock experience, and performance feedback. *Psychophysiology*, 1980, *17*, 243–252

Lilly, J. C. The electrical capacitance diaphragm manometer. *Review of Scientific Instruments*, 1942, *13*, 34–39.

London, R. E., & London, S. B. Blood pressure survey of physicians. *Journal of the American Medical Association*, 1966, *198*, 981–984.

Lovallo, W., & Zeiner, A. R. Cutaneous vasomotor responses to cold pressor stimulation. *Psychophysiology*, 1974, *11*, 458–471.

Lykken, D. T. Range correction applied to heart rate and GSR data. *Psychophysiology*, 1972, *9*, 373–379.

Lywood, D. W. Blood pressure. In P. H. Venables & I. Martin (Eds.), *A manual for psychophysiological methods*. Amsterdam: North-Holland, 1967.

Mann, H. The capacigraph. *Transactions of the American College of Cardiology*, 1953, *3*, 162–175.

Manuck, S. B., & Garland, F. N. Coronary-prone behavior pattern, task incentive, and cardiovascular response. *Psychophysiology*, 1979, *16*, 136–142.

Manuck, S. B., Harvey, A. H., Lechleiter, S. C., & Neal, S. Effects of coping on blood pressure responses to threat of aversive stimulation. *Psychophysiology*, 1978, *15*, 544–549.

Martin, J. E., Epstein, L. H., & Cinciripini, P. M. Effects of feedback and stimulus control on pulse transit time discrimination. *Psychophysiology*, 1980, *17*, 431–436.

Mathews, A. M., & Lader, M. H. An evaluation of forearm blood flow as a psychophysiological measure. *Psychophysiology*, 1971, *8*, 509–524.

McKusick, V. A., Webb, G. N., Humphries, J. O., & Reid, J. A. On cardiovascular sound. *Circulation*, 1955, *11*, 849.

Miller, J. C., & Horvath, S. M. Impedance cardiography. *Psychophysiology*, 1978, *15*, 80–91.

Miller, N. E., DiCara, L. V., Solomon, H., Weiss, J. M., & Dworkin, B. Learned modifications of autonomic functions: A review and some new data. *Circulation Research*, 1970, *27* (Suppl. 1), 3–11.

Neuman, M. R., Biopotential amplifiers. In J. G. Webster (Ed.), *Medical instrumentation: Application and design*. Boston: Houghton Mifflin, 1978.

Newlin, D. B., & Levenson, R. W. Pre-ejection period: Measuring beta-adrenergic influences upon the heart. *Psychophysiology*, 1979, *16*, 546–553.

Newlin, D. B., & Levenson, R. W. Voluntary control of pulse transmission time to the ear. *Psychophysiology*, 1980, *17*, 581–585.

Nyboer, J. Electrical impedance plethysmography. *Circulation*, 1950, *2*, 811–818.

Obrist, P. A. Heart rate and somatic-motor coupling during classical aversive conditioning in humans. *Journal of Experimental Psychology*, 1968, *77*, 180–193.

Obrist, P. A., Gaebelein, C. J., & Langer, A. W. Cardiovascular psychophysiology: Some contemporary methods of measurement. *American Psychologist*, 1975, *30*, 277–284.

Obrist, P. A., Howard, J. L., Lawler, J. E., Sutterer, J. R., Smithson, K. W., & Martin, P. L. Alterations in cardiac contractility during classical aversive conditioning in dogs: Methodological and theoretical implications. *Psychophysiology*, 1972, *9*, 246–261.

Obrist, P. A., Lawler, J. E., Howard, J. L., Smithson, K. W., Martin, P. L., & Manning, J. Sympathetic influences on the heart in humans: Effects on contractility and heart rate of acute stress. *Psychophysiology*, 1974, *11*, 405–427.

Obrist, P. A., & Light, K. C. Comments on "Carotid dP/dt as a psychophysiological index of sympathetic myocardial effects: Some considerations." *Psychophysiology*, 1980, *17*, 495–497.

Obrist, P. A., Light, K. C., McCubbin, J. A., Hutcheson, J. S., & Hoffer, J. L. Pulse transit time: Relationship to blood pressure and myocardial performance. *Psychophysiology*, 1979, *16*, 292–301.

Obrist, P. A., Webb, R. A., & Sutterer, J. R. Heart rate and somatic changes during aversive conditioning and a simple reaction time task. *Psychophysiology*, 1969, *5*, 696–723.

Obrist, P. A., Webb, R. A., Sutterer, J. R., & Howard, J. L. The cardiac-somatic relationship: Some reformulations. *Psychophysiology*, 1970, *6*, 569–587.

O'Connell, D. N., & Tursky, B. Silver–silver chloride sponge electrodes for skin potential recording. *American Journal of Psychology*, 1960, *73*, 302–304.

Olmsted, F. Measurement of blood flow and blood pressure. In C. C. Brown (Ed.), *Methods in psychophysiology*. Baltimore: Williams & Wilkins, 1967.

Orne, M. T., Thackray, R. I., & Paskewitz, D. A. On the detection of deception: A model for the study of physiological effects of psychological stimuli. In N. S. Greenfield & R. A. Sternbach (Eds.), *Handbook of psychophysiology*. New York: Holt, Rinehart, & Winston, 1972.

Papillo, J. F., Tursky, B., & Friedman, R. Perceived changes in the intensity of arterial pulsations as a function of applied cuff pressure. *Psychophysiology*, 1981, *18*, 283–287.

Paul, G. Physiological effects of relaxation training and hypnotic suggestions. *Journal of Abnormal Psychology*, 1969, *74*, 425–437.

Peura, R. A. Blood pressure and sound. In J. G. Webster (Ed.), *Medical instrumentation: Application and design.* Boston: Houghton Mifflin, 1978.

Podlesny, J. A., & Raskin, D. C. Effectiveness of techniques and physiological measures in the detection of deception. *Psychophysiology*, 1978, *15*, 344–359.

Porges, S. W. Heart rate variability and deceleration as indexes of reaction time. *Journal of Experimental Psychology*, 1969, *81*, 497–503.

Posey, J. A., Geddes, L. A., Williams, H., & Moore, A. G. The meaning of the point of maximum oscillations in cuff pressure in the indirect measurement of blood pressure: Part I. *Cardiovascular Research Center Bulletin*, 1969, *8*, 15–25.

Quintanar, L. R., Cacioppo, J. T., Crowell, C. R., Sklar, J. A., & Snyder, C. W. Comparative effects of cranial vasoconstriction and digital vasodilation feedback on migraine. *Psychophysiology*, 1981, *18*, 159.

Ragan, C., & Bordley, J. The accuracy of clinical measurements of arterial blood pressure. *Bulletin of John Hopkins Hospital*, 1941, *69*, 504–528.

Reeves, J. L., Shapiro, D., & Cobb, L. F. Relative influences of heart rate biofeedback and instructional set in the perception of cold pressor pain. In N. Birbaumer & H. D. Kimmel (Eds.), *Biofeedback and self-regulation.* Hillsdale, N.J.: Erlbaum, 1979.

Rhodes, D. L., & Schwartz, G. E. *Pulse-to-pulse transit time is more related to peripheral blood flow than is R-wave to pulse transit time.* Paper presented at the meeting of the Society for Psychophysiological Research, Vancouver, B.C., October 1980.

Richards, J. The statistical analysis of heart rate: A review emphasizing infancy data. *Psychophysiology*, 1980, *17*, 153–166.

Roberts, L. N., Smiley, R. A., & Manning, G. W. A comparison of direct and indirect blood pressure determinations. *Circulation*, 1953, *8*, 232–242.

Robinow, M., Hamilton, W. F., Woodbury, R. A., & Volpitto, P. P. Accuracy of clinical determinations of blood pressure in children. *American Journal of Disabled Children*, 1939, *58*, 102–108.

Rose, R. C., Gilford, S. R., Broida, H. P., Soler, A., Partenope, E. A., & Freis, E. D. Clinical and investigative application of a new instrument for continuous recording of blood pressure and heart rate. *New England Journal of Medicine*, 1953, *249*, 615.

Rosen, R. C., & Keefe, F. J. The measurement of human penile tumescence. *Psychophysiology*, 1978, *15*, 366–376.

Roth, I. A self-retaining skin contact electrode for chest leads in electrocardiography. *American Heart Journal*, 1933–1934, *9*, 526–529.

Royer, F. I. The "respiratory vasomotor reflex" in the forehead and finger. *Psychophysiology*, 1966, *2*, 241–248.

Schacter, J. Pain, fear, and anger in hypertensives and normotensives. *Psychosomatic Medicine*, 1957, *19*, 17–29.

Schneiderman, N., Dauth, G. W., & VanDercar, D. H. Electrocardiogram: Techniques and analysis. In R. F. Thompson & M. M. Patterson (Eds.), *Bioelectric recording techniques.* New York: Academic Press, 1974.

Shannon, B. J., Goldman, M. S., & Lee, R. M. Biofeedback training of blood pressure: A comparison of three feedback techniques. *Psychophysiology*, 1978, *15*, 53–59.

Shapiro, D., Greenstadt, L., Lane, J. D., & Rubinstein, E. Tracing-cuff system for beat-to-beat recording of blood pressure, in press.

Shapiro, D., Schwartz, G. E., & Tursky, B. Control of diastolic blood pressure in man by feedback and reinforcement. *Psychophysiology*, 1972, *9*, 296–304.

Shapiro, D., Tursky, B., Gershon, E., & Stern, M. Effects on feedback and reinforcement in the control of systolic blood pressure. *Science*, 1969, *163*, 588–590.

Shean, G. D. Vasomotor conditioning and awareness. *Psychophysiology*, 1968, *5*, 22–30.

Shean, G. D., & Strange, P. W. The effects of varied respiration rate and volume upon finger pulse volume. *Psychophysiology*, 1971, *8*, 401–405.

Shimizu, H. Reliable and precise identification of R-waves in the EKG with a simple peak detector. *Psychophysiology*, 1978, *15*, 499–501.

Shipley, R. E., & Wilson, C. *Proceedings of the Society for Experimental Biology and Medicine*, 1951, *78*, 724.

Sigdell, J. A critical review of the theory of the mercury strain-gauge plethysmograph. *Medical and Biological Engineering*, 1969, *7*, 365–371.

Smyth, C. N. Electrical techniques in medicine. *Transactions of the Society of Instruments Technology*, 1954, *6*, 87–90.

Sokolov, E. N. *Perception and the conditioned reflex*. New York: Pergamon, 1963.

Sroufe, L. A. Learned stabilization of cardiac rate with respiration experimentally controlled. *Journal of Experimental Psychology*, 1969, *81*, 391–393.

Sroufe, L. A. Effects of depth and rate of breathing on heart rate and heart rate variability. *Psychophysiology*, 1971, *8*, 648–655.

Stallones, R. A. The rise and fall of ischemic heart disease. *Scientific American*, 1980, *243*, 53–59.

Starr, I. Progress towards a physiological cardiology: A second essay on the ballistocardiogram. *Annals of Internal Medicine*, 1965, *63*, 1079–1105.

Steele, J. M. Comparison of simultaneous indirect (ascultatory) and direct (intra-arterial) measurements of arterial blood pressure in man. *Journal of the Mount Sinai Hospital*, 1941, *8*, 1042–1050.

Stegall, H. F., Kardon, M. B., & Kemmerer, W. T. Indirect measurement of arterial blood pressure by ultrasonic sphygmomanometry. *Journal of Applied Physiology*, 1968, *25*, 793–798.

Steptoe, A. Blood pressure control: A comparison of feedback and instructions using pulse wave velocity measurements. *Psychophysiology*, 1976, *13*, 528–535.

Steptoe, A. Voluntary blood pressure reductions measured with pulse transit time: Training conditions and reactions to mental work. *Psychophysiology*, 1977, *14*, 492–498.

Steptoe, A. The regulation of blood pressure reactions to taxing conditions using pulse transit time feedback and relaxation. *Psychophysiology*, 1978, *15*, 429–438.

Steptoe, A., Smulyan, H., & Gribbin, B. Pulse wave velocity and blood pressure change: Calibration and applications. *Psychophysiology*, 1976, *13*, 488–493.

Stern, R. M., & Anschel, C. Deep inspiration as stimuli for responses of the autonomic nervous system. *Psychophysiology*, 1968, *5*, 132–141.

Sternbach, R. A. *Principles of psychophysiology*. New York: Academic Press, 1966.

Stewart, G. N. Researches on the circulation time and on the influences which affect it. *Journal of Physiology*, 1897, *22*, 158–183.

Surwitt, R. S., & Fenton, C. H. Feedback and instructions in the control of digital skin temperature. *Psychophysiology*, 1980, *17*, 129–132.

Tahmoush, A. J., Jennings, J. R., Lee, A. L., Camp, S., & Weber, F. Characteristics of a light emitting diode–transistor photoplethysmograph. *Psychophysiology*, 1976, *13*, 357–362.

Talbot, S. A., & Gessner, U. *Systems physiology*. New York: John Wiley & Sons, 1973.

Tavel, M. E. *Clinical phonocardiography and external pulse recording* (2nd ed.). Chicago: Year Book Medical, 1976.

Taylor, K., & Mandelberg, M. Precision digital instrument for calculation of heart rate and R-R interval. *IEEE Transactions of Biomedical Engineering*, 1975, *BME-22*, 255–257.

Thackray, R. I., & Orne, M. T. A comparison of physiological indices in detection of deception. *Psychophysiology*, 1968, *4*, 329–339.

Thauer, R. Circulatory adjustments to climatic requirements. In W. F. Hamilton & P. Dow (Eds.), *Handbook of physiology* (Vol. 3, Section 2: *Circulation*). Washington, D.C.: American Physiological Society, 1965.

Thorne, P. R., Engel, B. T., & Holmblad, J. B. An analysis of error inherent in estimating heart rate from cardiotachometer records. *Psychophysiology*, 1976, *13*, 269–272.

Tursky, B. The indirect recording of human blood pressure. In P. A. Obrist, A. H. Black, J. Brener, & L. V. DiCara (Eds.), *Cardiovascular psychophysiology*. Chicago: Aldine, 1974.

Tursky, B. An engineering approach to biofeedback. In L. White & B. Tursky (Eds.), *Clinical biofeedback: Efficacy and mechanisms*. New York: Guilford Press, in press.

Tursky, B., & Greenblatt, D. J. Local vascular and thermal changes that accompany electric shock. *Psychophysiology*, 1967, *3*, 371–379.

Tursky, B., Schwartz, G. E., & Crider, A. Differential patterns of heart rate and skin resistance during a digit-transformation task. *Journal of Experimental Psychology*, 1970, *83*, 451–457.

Tursky, B., Shapiro, D., & Schwartz, G. E. Automated constant cuff-pressure system to measure average systolic and diastolic blood pressure in man. *IEEE Transactions on Biomedical Engineering*, 1972, *BME-19*, 271–276.

Uzmann, J. W., & Wood, E. H. Oximeter earpiece for measurement of systemic blood content and arterial pressure in the human ear. *American Journal of Physiology*, 1950, *163*, 756–757.

Van Bergen, F. H., Weatherhead, D. S., Treolar, A. E., Dobkin, A. B., & Buckley, J. J. Comparison of indirect and direct methods of measuring arterial blood pressure. *Circulation*, 1954, *10*, 481–490.

VanderHoeven, G. M. A., deMonchy, C., & Beneken, J. E. W. Systolic time intervals and pulse wave transmission times in normal children. *British Heart Journal*, 1973, *35*, 669–678.

Walter, G. F., & Porges, S. W. Heart rate and respiratory responses as a function of task difficulty: The use of discriminant analysis in the selection of psychologically sensitive physiological responses. *Psychophysiology*, 1976, *13*, 563–571.

Webster, J. G. Measurement of flow and volume of blood. In J. G. Webster (Ed.), *Medical instrumentation: Application and design*. Boston: Houghton Mifflin, 1978.

Weinman, J. Photoplethysmography. In P. H. Venables & I. Martin (Eds.), *A manual of psychophysiological methods*. Amsterdam: North-Holland, 1967.

Weinman, J., & Manoach, M. A photoelectric approach to the study of peripheral circulation. *American Heart Journal*, 1962, *63*, 219–231.

Weiss, T., Delbo, A., Reichek, N., & Engelman, K. Pulse transit time in analysis of autonomic nervous system effects on the cardiovascular system. *Psychophysiology*, 1980, *17*, 202–207.

Weissler, A. M., & Garrard, C. L. Systolic time intervals in cardiac disease. *Modern Concepts of Cardiovascular Disease*, 1971, *40*, 1–7.

Welford, N. T. The SETAR and its uses for recording physiological and behavioral data. *IRE Transactions of Bio-Medical Electronics*, 1962, *9*, 185–189.

Whitney, R. J. The measurement of changes in human limb volume by means of a mercury-in rubber strain gauge. *Journal of Physiology*, 1949, *109*, 5P–6P.

Whitney, R. J. The measurement of volume changes in human limbs. *Journal of Physiology*, 1953, *121*, 1–27.

Williams, J. G. L., & Williams, B. Arterial pulse wave velocity as a psychophysiological measure. *Psychosomatic Medicine*, 1965, *27*, 408–414.

Williams, R. B., Kimball, C. P., & Willard, H. N. The influence of interpersonal interaction upon diastolic blood pressure. *Psychosomatic Medicine*, 1972, *33*, 465–473.

Williams, R. B., & McKegney, F. P. Psychological aspects of hypertension. *Yale Journal of Biology and Medicine*, 1965, *38*, 265–272.

Wilson, R. S. CARDIVAR: The statistical analysis of heart rate data. *Psychophysiology*, 1974, *11*, 76–85.

Winsor, T. Clinical plethysmography. *Angiology*, 1953, *4*, 134–164.

Yang, S. S., Bentivoglio, L. G., Maranhão, V., & Goldberg, H. *From cardiac catheterization data to hemodynamic parameters.* Philadelphia: F. A. Davis, 1972.

# 3

# Heart Rate as an Index of
# Anxiety: Failure of a Hypothesis

DON C. FOWLES

## INTRODUCTION

Heart rate (HR) has long been used in clinical research as an index of
anxiety (e.g., Borkovec, Weerts, & Bernstein, 1976; Martin & Sroufe,
1970; Mathews, 1971; Van Egeren, Feather, & Hein, 1971). It is the
purpose of the present chapter to call attention to certain difficulties
which are associated with this use of HR. At the same time, an alternative
conceptualization of the psychological significance of HR is proposed, by
elaborating points made in a recent theoretical paper by the author
(Fowles, 1980). This alternative conceptualization includes some elements
which are compatible with the view that HR is an index of anxiety, but it
is also incompatible with that view in several important respects. Thus the
present review has two goals which should not be confused: (1) to call
attention to difficulties with the simplistic notion that HR reflects anxiety
and (2) to propose a theoretical solution to the difficulties raised by those
results. Since the second goal involves a model offered for heuristic

Don C. Fowles. Department of Psychology, The University of Iowa, Iowa City, Iowa.

purposes which has not been tested, it must necessarily be viewed as highly speculative. Any possible weaknesses of this model should not, however, be allowed to obscure the importance of the data being cited as a challenge to a simplistic view of HR as an index of anxiety.

The model being proposed concerning the psychological influences on HR borrows constructs which have evolved from the literature on animal learning and motivation. In attempting to borrow constructs from this area to be applied to the analysis of HR, I rely almost exclusively on the work of J. A. Gray (e.g., 1973, 1975, 1976a, 1976b, 1977, 1978, 1979). Those aspects of Gray's work which are important to the present argument, however, overlap considerably with the theoretical analysis presented in the influential text by Mackintosh (1974).

GRAY'S MODEL

Gray postulates the existence of two motivational systems which mediate the effect of *conditioned* stimuli on behavior. The first of these is an appetitive, reward-seeking, or approach system which responds to positive incentives by activating behavior, and which can, therefore, be called a "behavioral activation system" (BAS). The second motivational system, which Gray calls the "behavioral inhibition system" (BIS), inhibits behavior in the presence of conditioned stimuli which indicate that aversive consequences would occur—for example, response-contingent punishment. In order to understand the functions of these two systems and their interaction, it is necessary to consider four basic paradigms.

The first paradigm is a simple reward-learning paradigm with 100% reinforcement, in which the animal learns to make a response in order to obtain a reward. In this situation, stimuli associated with reward (Rew-CSs) exert their control over behavior via the BAS. That is, the BAS activates reward-seeking behavior in response to Rew-CSs.

This simple reward-learning situation can be transformed into an approach–avoidance conflict by the introduction of response-contingent punishment, once the rewarded response has been established. This introduction of punishment (in addition to the reward) results in a reduction in the rate or probability of responding (passive avoidance). This passive avoidance in the approach–avoidance conflict situation is attributed to the inhibition of the approach response by the BIS in response to conditioned stimuli for punishment (Pun-CSs). Thus it can be seen that in this conflict situation, the BAS and the BIS act in opposition to each other: the BAS tending to activate approach behavior in response to Rew-CSs and the BIS tending to inhibit these responses in the face of Pun-CSs. Whether or not an approach response will occur depends on which of these mutually antagonistic systems is dominant, which, in turn, is influenced by the relative strength of the Rew-CS and Pun-CS inputs.

A similar mutual antagonism between the two systems is found in the case of extinction. In this analysis, it is assumed that the nonoccurrence of an expected reward produces frustration, the functional equivalent of punishment as far as the BIS is concerned. Stimuli in the extinction situation, then, become conditioned stimuli for frustrative nonreward ($\overline{\text{Rew}}$-CSs), which activates the BIS with a subsequent inhibition of the approach response. As the nonreward CSs increase in strength over extinction trials, BIS activity increases, eventually becoming strong enough to inhibit the approach response. This brief description shows that the approach–avoidance conflict and the extinction paradigms are similar in many respects, their major difference being in the source of the aversive unconditioned stimulus (UCS). In the conflict paradigm, the UCS is an externally applied punishment, whereas in the extinction paradigm it is the nonoccurrence of an expected reward.

The fourth paradigm is the one-way active-avoidance task, in which a conditioned stimulus is presented for several seconds prior to the onset of a shock. The animal will receive the shock if it does nothing, but if it makes a response during the CS which takes it out of the compartment, it can avoid the shock altogether. The avoidance response is maintained by the nonoccurrence of an expected punishment, the functional equivalent of a reward. Consequently, the avoidance response is activated by the BAS in response to conditioned stimuli for relieving nonpunishment ($\overline{\text{Pun}}$-CSs). This conclusion that the active-avoidance response is comparable to responses in a reward-learning situation is the most counterintuitive aspect of this analysis: A paradigm traditionally viewed as involving anxiety in response to the threat of shock is viewed, in this model, as primarily involving the activation of behavior under the control of positive incentive motivation. (See Mineka, 1979, for similar conclusions regarding the minimal role of fear in active avoidance.)

Several aspects of the analysis of the four paradigms in terms of the two motivational systems require comment. First, the crucial variable is what happens to behavior. If behavior is activated, the BAS is involved; if behavior is inhibited, the BIS is involved. Second, which system is involved depends on the appetitive or aversive nature of the UCS. Gray offers four terms to refer to the emotional or motivational state induced by each of these UCSs. The two aversive motivational states are called "frustration" (for extinction), and "fear" or "anxiety" (for punishment). The two appetitive motivational states are called "hope" (for rewards) and "relief" (for nonpunishment). These four different labels should not be taken to imply that there are four different systems involved. On the contrary, frustration and anxiety involve the same underlying motivational state, the difference between them being a matter of labeling based on the external stimulus conditions (Gray, 1973). Similarly, hope and relief involve a single motivational state, the differences again being attributable to the circumstances which induced that state. Third, in contrast to earlier S-R learning theories, this model incorporates an expectancy concept, which allows the theory to account for the effect of the nonoccurrence of rewards and punishments. This assumption is particularly important in the case of active avoidance, inasmuch as it is otherwise difficult to account for the maintenance of the response over many trials without extinction, and it plays an important role in the shift to viewing active avoidance as an appetitive response. Fourth, both systems are operating at all times. Even in the simple reward-learning situation the BIS is important in extinguishing irrelevant responses which do not lead to reward. In addition, the BIS is presumed to be involved in active avoidance with respect to signaling that the environment is dangerous in response to Pun-CSs (although this is a relatively weak role compared to the contribution of the BAS in this situation) (Gray, 1979). Consequently, it is the constant interaction between these two systems which regulates behavior from a motivational perspective.

It is of considerable relevance to the analysis of the effects of anxiety on heart rate that Gray views the BIS as the system which mediates anxiety. Two reasons for this have already been given: (1) Activation of the BIS is presumed to produce an aversive motivational state, and (2) it is the system which responds to aversive conditioned stimuli (Pub-CSs and $\overline{\text{Rew}}$-CSs). In addition to these reasons, Gray's (1977) review of research on the effect of antianxiety drugs has shown that these drugs appear to inhibit the activity of the BIS (Gray includes in the antianxiety drugs those pharmacological agents which appear clinically to reduce anxiety: alcohol, the barbiturates, and the minor tranquilizers). This conclusion is based on a theoretical analysis of the contribution of the BIS in various behavioral paradigms, combined with an examination of the effects of the drugs in these paradigms. For example, it is well established that in the approach–avoidance conflict situation, the antianxiety drugs have the effect of disinhibiting the passive avoidance response— that is, of reversing, or at least reducing, the effects of Pun-CSs (Beer & Migler, 1975; Bignami, 1978; Blackwell & Whitehead, 1975; Cook & Davidson, 1973, 1978; Houser, 1978; Sepinwall & Cook, 1978; Stein, Wise, & Belluzzi, 1977; Stein, Wise, & Berger, 1973). The antianxiety drugs have also been found to produce a resistance to extinction following continuous reinforcement. That is, the normal inhibition of behavior in response to $\overline{\text{Rew}}$-CSs is impaired by these drugs. Similar results have been obtained in three more complicated paradigms: fixed interval, fixed ratio, and differential reinforcement of low rate (DRL) schedules. All three have in common a predictable period of nonreward during which responding is partially inhibited under normal conditions, creating an approach–avoidance conflict between making a rewarded response and inhibiting that response in the presence of $\overline{\text{Rew}}$-CSs. Thus, the increase in response rate caused by the antianxiety drugs is attributable to an effect on the BIS. An extensive review of the literature on which these conclusions are based can be found in Gray (1977).

One implication of Gray's theory for the view that HR might serve as an index of anxiety is that, if this hypothesis were true, HR increases should be associated with BIS activity rather than BAS activity. Although it would be an oversimplification to require such a theory to always predict HR increases with behavioral inhibition, and decreases with behavioral activation, it should at least be possible to show a strong positive association between HR and BIS activity. As will be seen, this is not likely to be the case.

An important paradigm which has not yet been discussed is classical aversive conditioning. The noncontingent presentation of punishment would appear to be an excellent way to induce anxiety, and this has been the traditional interpretation of this paradigm. Although in the past Gray did not subscribe to the view that the BIS mediates the effect of classically conditioned Pun-CSs, his current position is not hostile to this assumption. This theoretical difficulty was discussed by Fowles (1980), who argued that it was reasonable to hypothesize that the BIS does respond to the anticipation of both response-contingent and response-noncontingent punishments. In any event, for the purposes of the present review, it will be assumed that Pun-CSs associated with aversive UCSs in a classical conditioning paradigm do constitute adequate stimuli for anxiety. Consequently, if HR is an index of anxiety it should *increase* in response to the stimuli.

## THE PSYCHOLOGICAL SIGNIFICANCE OF HEART RATE

### CARDIAC–SOMATIC COUPLING

In the late 1960s and early 1970s, rapidly accumulating evidence indicated that there was a substantial coupling between HR and somatic activity. The early influential paper by Obrist and his colleagues (Obrist, Webb, Sutterer, & Howard, 1970) summarized their own research, and more recent reviews have continued to underscore the strong association between HR and somatic activity (Brener, Eissenberg, & Middaugh, 1974; Elliott, 1974; Obrist, Howard, Lawler, Galosy, Meyers, & Gaebelein, 1974; Roberts, 1974). In general, these studies have shown that there is a strong parallelism between HR and somatic activity with respect to the direction, degree, and time course as a function of experimental manipulations (e.g., Obrist et al., 1970). This cardiac–somatic coupling has been demonstrated in a variety of situations—for example, classical aversive conditioning, classical appetitive conditioning, operant conditioning, and reaction time performance—and in a number of species, including rats, dogs, cats, and humans. Thus there can be no doubt as to the pervasiveness, reliability, and importance of cardiac–somatic coupling.

The theoretical interpretation of cardiac–somatic coupling is straightforward: Increased somatic activity requires increased blood flow to the working muscles (a variation in HR is one of the primary ways to alter cardiac output), thus creating a need for a "metabolically functional linkage between cardiac and somatic events" (Obrist et al., 1970, p. 572). This interpretation should not be taken to imply that HR is controlled directly by the metabolic needs of the muscles. To the contrary, it is assumed that HR and somatic activity both reflect the activity of some common control mechanism in the central nervous system (Brener et al., 1974; Obrist, 1976; Obrist et al., 1970, 1974).

Obrist's emphasis on cardiac–somatic coupling was not intended to exclude psychologically interesting processes, such as motivation and emotion. Rather, cardiac–somatic coupling served as a reference for emotional and motivational effects on HR in two respects (Obrist *et al.*, 1970). First, Obrist argued that such effects—whether normal or pathological—could be seen as exaggerated, exercise-like cardiovascular responses. That is, even emotional and motivational effects on the cardiovascular system appear to derive from the basic cardiac–somatic coupling but are exaggerations of this effect. Second, Obrist speculated that some somatic component may be required to trigger the exaggerated motivational and emotional effects. Thus, the influence of cardiac–somatic coupling can be seen even in psychologically interesting HR responses.

Psychological influences on HR can be inferred in those instances where the HR increase is greater than could be justified on the basis of the metabolic needs of the somatic activity, or when HR and somatic activity are affected in opposite directions. Such inferences are easy to make in the latter case, where there is a divergence of HR and somatic activity, but it is difficult to quantify total somatic activity and to estimate the HR change which is metabolically appropriate. As a result, when somatic activity and HR change in the same direction, it is only when there are large HR increases associated with small amounts of somatic activity (e.g., releasing a key in a reaction time experiment) that a clear inference can be drawn that motivational processes are involved.

Although an understanding of psychological effects on HR is important in evaluating the anxiety interpretation, cardiac–somatic coupling has implications in its own right. As already indicated, in the context of Gray's model, HR should show a strong positive association with the activity of the BIS. Cardiac–somatic coupling implies exactly the opposite. Insofar as HR tends to follow behavioral activation, it is positively associated with BAS activity and *negatively* associated with BIS activity. To the extent that Gray is correct in seeing the BIS as an anxiety system, therefore, cardiac–somatic coupling suggests that HR is negatively, rather than positively, associated with anxiety. Quite apart from Gray's model, the interpretation of cardiac–somatic coupling in terms of a response to metabolic needs suggests that HR is an index of the activity of the striate musculature, not of anxiety (Obrist *et al.*, 1974). Even if the inference of anxiety is to be limited to HR increases reflecting psychological factors, it is necessary to control for somatic activity in order to draw such inferences.

Unfortunately, it is not easy to control for somatic activity. Although HR and somatic activity are presumed to share a common control mechanism, the coupling between them is imperfect, even when this somatic control mechanism is responsible for HR changes. In particular, HR increases or decreases may precede the appearance of somatic activity, as in classical conditioning (Schneiderman, 1974). HR changes may even occur in the absence of the normally coupled somatic activity, as in the case when somatic activity is blocked with curare (Obrist et al., 1974). Thus, even in the absence of obvious somatic activity, it is possible that HR reflects covert somatic processes. This point will become somewhat clearer in the section on classical aversive conditioning, which follows.

CLASSICAL AVERSIVE CONDITIONING

As stated earlier, the classical aversive conditioning paradigm with shock (or an aversive auditory stimulus) as the UCS appears to be a prototype for an anxiety-producing situation. Not only is the subject faced with a threatening stimulus, but he/she is unable to do anything about it. Theories which stress that anxiety is increased when there is no coping response in the face of a threat (e.g., Mandler, 1972; Szpiler & Epstein, 1976) are particularly compatible with this view. A crucial test of the hypothesis that HR reflects anxiety, therefore, can be made in the classical aversive conditioning paradigm. According to this hypothesis, HR increases are to be expected in response to CSs paired with aversive UCSs.

The hypothesis has been disconfirmed in two important respects. First, HR acceleration often is not found in classical aversive conditioning. Second, explanations as to why HR decelerates in some cases, and accelerates in others, have centered around somatic influences rather than anxiety. The evidence for these conclusions comes from a variety of sources.

Both Obrist (1976) and Schneiderman (1974) have pointed to species differences in acceleration versus deceleration in classical conditioning. The expected HR acceleration has been found in dogs, monkeys, and pigeons; but paradoxical decelerations have been found in humans, cats, rabbits, and sometimes rats (Obrist, 1976). Obrist (1976) explained these differences in terms of the effect of inescapable aversive stimulation on behavior: those species which resort to immobility in such a situation show HR deceleration, whereas species who attempt to escape by struggling will show HR acceleration. Schneiderman (1974) proposed a somewhat similar explanation for the difference between monkeys and rabbits, though he was rather more guarded in the case of humans.

In addition to the between-species differences in HR response, variations can be seen within subjects in the response to CSs. Roberts and Young (1971) examined trial-by-trial HR responses using the conditioned emotional response (CER) paradigm, in which a CS previously paired with shock is superimposed on an operant schedule. Collapsing the data over all trials, they found that the CS elicted a decrease in both HR and overall movement. On the other hand, when the trials were subdivided in terms of whether the CS elicited an increase, decrease, or no change in overall movement, HR showed tight somatic coupling: HR increased if somatic activity increased, decreased if somatic activity decreased, and failed to change if somatic activity remained the same. In contrast, the CS elicited increases in skin conductance and skin potential regardless of somatic activity. These results make it clear that even within subjects there is not an invariant relationship between HR responses and CSs in an aversive conditioning paradigm.

Another examination of within-subjects variations in HR response during classical aversive conditioning was reported by Obrist, Howard, Lawler, Sutterer, Smithson, and Martin (1972). Commenting on that study, Obrist *et al.* (1974) reported that sympathetic effects were seen only on the first day of conditioning, when the dog appeared to be trying to escape, but that they disappeared as conditioning progressed and as the dogs appeared to become resigned to the inescapable nature of the situation (remaining immobile). It appears that these results included HR accelerations initially, followed by decelerations as conditioning progressed. Although the original paper did not explicitly report these results for HR, it did report them for cardiac contractility and stated that HR increases tended to be associated with increases in contractility (Obrist *et al.*, 1972). Elliott (1969) offered a similar interpretation of changes in the HR response in anticipation of shock in humans. He reported that subjects often show an increase of from 5 to 25 bpm in anticipation of shock, which he attributed to "the incipient organization of an avoidance, escape, or defensive response, one which would surely occur were it not for the constraints imposed by instructions" (p. 224). The HR acceleration is much diminished, on the other hand, once the subject has already experienced the shock and "is convinced that there is *no way to escape or avoid shock*" (p. 224, emphasis added). Thus, as Elliott argued, it is the instigation, anticipation, and initiation of responses which control HR acceleration, not the presence of anxiety per se.

Finally, in a study with humans employing fear-relevant and fear-irrelevant slide stimuli as CSs and electric shock as the UCS, Frederikson and Öhman (1979) found no conditioned HR responses, even though electrodermal activity showed reliable conditioning and differentiation between fear-relevant and fear-irrelevant stimuli. The authors attributed this failure to obtain HR conditioning to the use of too few trials. Whatever the reason for the failure to obtain HR conditioning, this study supports the Roberts and Young (1971) study in showing that HR is not a good index of classical aversive conditioning (whereas electrodermal activity is).

The conclusion from these studies is that HR acceleration is not a reliable response to classical aversive conditioning. Rather, HR changes tend to reflect the tendency to somatic activity. These somatic influences appear to be seen as in connection with actual changes in somatic activity during the CS interval, the anticipation of responses to the UCS, and even to motivational states involving a desire to make an avoidance response (even though that response is never actually made). This last possibility is suggested, of course, in Elliott's (1969) comment regarding the "incipient organization" of an avoidance response which is blocked by the constraints imposed by instructions. The possibility of a mobilization of the cardiovascular system for somatic activity without the actual execution of such activity is also discussed by Obrist et al. (1974). These authors suggest that such immobilization could result from: (1) the actual activation of unmeasured covert somatic activity, (2) simply the anticipation of somatic activity, or (3) a coupling with somatic activity in the past which has become uncoupled as a result of selective inhibition of somatic activity. Although these suggestions by Elliott and Obrist are necessarily somewhat speculative, they do point to the possibility that motivational states involving a disposition toward activity may affect HR in the absence of any observable response. Such cognitive or attitudinal effects on HR are important because they suggest that anxiety-like HR responses (i.e., HR acceleration in anticipation of shock) may be the result of covert cardiac-somatic coupling rather than anxiety per se.

ACTIVE AVOIDANCE

In the section just completed it was argued that HR increases in the face of a threatening stimulus are associated with avoidance responding, either actual or incipient. Indeed, a major point of the Elliott (1969) paper was that threatening or stressful situations affected HR only to the extent that they tended to instigate action. Although it was clear that Elliott was referring to motivational effects on HR associated with action instigation, the covariation between motivational and somatic influences admittedly made it difficult to unambiguously demonstrate that the effect on HR exceeded that required by the somatic activity per se. In fact, some years later, Elliott (1974) himself emphasized the difficulty of demonstrating motivational influences which could not be accounted for by the cardiac-somatic coupling hypothesis. It was, therefore, a major development when Obrist (1976), one of the foremost advocates of cardiac–somatic coupling, reported that what he called "active coping" had produced HR increases which exceeded any possible metabolic demand.

When subjects were placed in an unsignaled reaction time task in which shock avoidance and a monetary bonus were made contingent on their reaction time, large increases in HR relative to a resting baseline were obtained. When task difficulty was varied, there was an interaction with trials: HR remained more elevated over trials in a hard condition than in conditions involving either a very easy task or an impossible task. It was assumed that the hard task kept the subject more engaged, whereas they would give up on the impossible task and would find no challenge on the easy task.

In another experiment, subjects who were led to believe that they could avoid a shock by modifying some undesignated bodily activity showed greater HR increases than did subjects who believed there was nothing they could do. Neither group of subjects was, in fact, able to control the shock, the only difference between the groups being the perception that one group could actively control the situation. This study is interesting because it shows that the perception of, rather than the fact of, control affected HR.

Obrist (1976) commented that in one experiment on active coping, the average change in HR was 24 bpm, and that 25% of the subjects increased their HR in excess of 40 bpm. HR increases of this magnitude are not metabolically justified by the activity required in the typical experiment, such as performing a reaction time task. Obrist interprets this increase as a mobilization of the cardiovascular system for exercise—a fight or flight response—which somatically is either minimally executed or not executed at all.

Several differences between the active coping results and Obrist's previous work on cardiac–somatic coupling should be noted. First, there is a shift from looking at phasic HR changes to looking at tonic increases in level. Second, the earlier phasic effects were primarily attributable to vagal (parasympathetic) control of the heart, whereas the tonic active coping effects are primarily attributable to $\beta$-adrenergic (sympathetic) effects on the heart. Obrist (1976) suggested that these large tonic sympathetic effects are far more important in the etiology of pathological conditions, such as hypertension, than are the earlier phasic vagal effects, which he sees as biologically trivial. Third, the earlier classical aversive conditioning paradigm represents, in effect, the equivalent of the impossible condition in the shock-avoidance reaction time task. That is, when there is nothing a subject can do about an impending shock, he/she is effectively in a classical conditioning paradigm. Thus, the decrease in HR over trials in the impossible condition, compared to the hard condition, confirms the previous conclusion that helplessness in the face of a threatening stimulus does not produce HR increases. Finally, it should be stressed that these results, like the earlier cardiac–somatic results, appear to be quite reliable. The original results, published in more complete form by Obrist, Gaebelein, Teller, Langer, Grignolo, Light, and McCubbin (1978), have been replicated and extended (Light & Obrist, 1980; Obrist, Light, McCubbin, Hutcheson, & Hoffer, 1979).

The implications of this line of research for the formulation of HR as an index of anxiety are relatively straightforward: When anxiety is induced by the threat of punishment, the anxiety is reflected in HR only to the extent that the subject is motivated to make a response to avoid the punishment. If, on the other hand, no responses are seen as being potentially effective in avoiding the punishment, then HR will not reflect anxiety. At the other extreme, if avoidance of the punishment is extremely easy, HR will again not reflect the potential punishment. It is easy to see from this analysis why HR has often been viewed as an index of anxiety, but it is also clear that this is a very circumscribed phenomenon and one which is, at best, confounded with the subject's tendency to make an active-avoidance response.

From the perspective of Gray's model, it can be seen that the active coping paradigm used by Obrist overlaps considerably with a traditional active-avoidance paradigm, as described earlier. In the original study (Obrist, 1976; Obrist et al., 1978) using an unsignaled shock-avoidance reaction time procedure, subjects were rewarded for fast responses as well as punished for slow ones. In that study, then, reward incentives could also have been involved. Fortunatley, Light and Obrist (1980) have replicated that result using only shock avoidance. It is clear, therefore, that active coping effects are found in an active-avoidance paradigm. As indicated in the presentation of Gray's model, the BAS is the motivational system involved in the active-avoidance paradigm. Consequently, the literature on active coping, like that on cardiac–somatic coupling, strongly suggests that HR is positively correlated with the activity of the BAS rather than the BIS. There may also be a contribution of the BIS, however: in the hard task condition which elicits large HR increases there is a continuing threat of shock, which presumably is processed by the BIS. This point is discussed later, following a review of the literature on incentive effects on HR.

INCENTIVE EFFECTS

The hypothesis that HR responds to the incentive effects of rewards has been in the literature in some form for over two decades, and it was stated in its clearest form by Elliott in 1969. The well-known study by Bélanger and Feldman (1962), showing an effect of bar pressing for water on HR in water-deprived rats, was cited even prior to publication by Malmo (1958, 1959, 1962) and was discussed at considerable length by Malmo and Bélanger (1967). This study demonstrated that HR increases with the number of hours of water deprivation if it is measured when the animals are bar pressing for water, but not if heart rate is measured in the absence of Rew-CSs. This interaction between water deprivation and stimulating environmental cues led Malmo to develop his two-factor theory of arousal in the papers just cited and also to comment on the value of using physiological measures in experiments on appetitive functions (Malmo, 1958).

The Bélanger and Feldman paper stimulated a number of studies. The basic effect of water deprivation on HR has been replicated many times, particularly by Stern and his colleagues (Goldstein, Beideman, & Stern, 1970; Goldstein, Stern, & Rothenberg, 1966; Goldstein, Stern, & Sturmfels, 1969; Hahn, Stern, & Fehr, 1964; Hahn, Stern, & McDonald, 1962). Malmo and Bélanger (1967) cited a study from Bélanger's laboratory showing a similar effect of food deprivation on HR. All of these studies agreed that the effect of deprivation on HR was seen only under the stimulating conditions of access to water or food. Three of the studies from Stern's lab clearly demonstrated that HR increases could be seen in response to conditioned stimuli even in the absence of instrumental responding (Goldstein et al., 1966, 1969, 1970). In an important study Hahn, Stern, and Fehr (1964) showed that the force required for bar pressing did not affect HR, indicating that it is unlikely that somatic activity accounts for this phenomenon. A similar result was reported by Doerr and Hokanson (1968). Using less controlled observations, Goldstein et al. (1966, 1970) also argued that somatic activity was unlikely to account for this effect.[1]

These studies demonstrate that, at least in the case of water deprivation in rats, conditioned stimuli for rewards have a potent effect on HR which is not likely to be attributable entirely to somatic activity. This suggests strongly that HR responds to reward incentives, but it is desirable to demonstrate the generality of the phenomenon with regard to other species and other paradigms. Fortunately, other demonstrations of incentive effects on HR have been forthcoming.

Perhaps the closest demonstration at the human level to the incentive effects on animals just described is the impressive series of studies by Lipsitt and his colleagues on the neonatal HR response to sucrose solutions. These studies have shown that when a sucrose solution is presented to a neonate (within 2 hours prior to the morning feeding) it produces a HR increase. In the first study (Lipsitt, Reilly, Butcher, & Greenwood, 1976) HR increased when sucking produced a 15%-sucrose solution, as

---

1. One study (Doerr & Hokanson, 1968) was able to demonstrate the correlation between HR and deprivation levels only during the last 5 min of a 30-min response period. Several factors may account for the discrepancy between this and other studies. First, only one response in 13 was reinforced (fixed-ratio 13), whereas most experiments have used continuous reinforcement. Since fixed-ratio schedules tend to activate the behavioral inhibition system (Gray, 1977) according to the interpretation offered here, such a schedule may somewhat obscure simple appetitive effects on HR. Second, it appears that only one 30-min session was used at each deprivation level. Goldstein et al. (1966, 1969) showed that these conditioned HR effects required several trials to develop. Similarly, Bélanger and Feldman (1962) reported that previous exposure to different deprivation intensities is important. This suggests that the time required for the appearance of the effect in the Doerr and Hokanson study may have reflected the time required for conditioning to occur (a suggestion made by the authors themselves). Finally, the six deprivation levels were presented in counterbalanced order. The clearest results have been obtained when an ascending series is used (Bélanger & Feldman, 1962; Hahn et al., 1964). Thus, this exception to the otherwise reliable phenomenon does not seem to constitute a major challenge.

compared to sucking which produced no fluid at all. The sucrose solution also slowed the sucking rate within a burst while increasing burst duration. Thus, HR increased in response to sucrose, even though the rate of responding decreased. Although there were more total responses associated with the sucrose condition than the no-fluid condition, the authors commented that the HR increase occurred by the eighth or ninth suck in a series and thus could not be attributed to the longer bursts (see also Lipsitt, 1979). Consequently, they attributed the HR increase to a hedonic effect associated with the incentive value of the sucrose.

Crook and Lipsitt (1976) replicated the previous study with additional controls. Heart rate was measured only during bursts of sucking and was limited to the period after the eighth suck in order to avoid the initial lag between the onset of sucking and the fully developed HR response. In this experiment they compared a 5%- and a 15%-sucrose solution, and they found a higher HR with 15% sucrose. As before, the response rate during sucking bursts was lower for the 15% sucrose condition. This time there was no significant difference in the total number of sucking responses in the two conditions, eliminating this aspect of somatic activity as a potential explanation for the HR differences.

Crook (1976) compared the effect of delivering different amounts (.01 vs. .03 ml/suck) of 5% sucrose. Amount of liquid interacted with sequence, a significant increase for the larger amount being found in the sequence small–large, whereas there was no effect when the large dose was administered first. No differences were found in the total number of responses, though the distribution of responses was affected. In another analysis of the same data, HR was examined as a function of amount of sucrose delivered during the onset of a sucking burst—that is, for a short time at the beginning of a burst. As expected, the larger amount of sucrose produced a higher HR. This higher HR could be seen, however, during the second prior to the onset of sucking, suggesting that it reflected either an anticipation of the larger amount of sucrose or a tonic effect on level as a function of amount of sucrose delivered during that period. This analysis was important in showing that the HR effects were not due to longer bursts of sucking associated with higher-incentive conditions. More recently, Ashmead, Reilly, and Lipsitt (1980) attempted to eliminate additional somatic factors in a comparison of 15% sucrose with water. As before, there was a sequence effect, in which HR increased to sucrose in the water-first condition but failed to decline to water in the sucrose-first condition. In a thorough analysis of their data, they were able to show that the HR effects were not secondary to swallowing or to either "suction" (negative pressure) or "expression" (positive pressure exerted on the nipple) associated with sucking.

Throughout these papers, the authors have emphasized that the HR increases reflect a hedonic process, the pleasure associated with sweetness (Ashmead *et al.*, 1980), which offers a means to study basic incentive motivational processes in the newborn (Crook & Lipsitt, 1976). Given their many demonstrations that somatic variables did not account for this effect, their interpretation seems credible, particularly in view of the convergent evidence from animal studies already reviewed.

A study cited by Elliott (1969) also showed an effect of expectation of food-reward on HR in humans. In this study (Buckhout & Grace, 1966), resting HR was recorded in two groups of college students before and after 24-hour fasting. One group expected to eat food, which was visible to them, at the end of the second session; whereas the other group expected to fast for another 12 hours and had no food cues available. There was a greater increase in HR between the two sessions for the group which expected food (11.6 bpm) than for the control group (4.8 bpm).

Elliott's (1969) paper was one of the most explicit statements of the hypothesis that HR responds to incentives, and it was based largely on experiments with humans, many of which did not use biological reinforcers. Incentive and the tendency toward the instigation, anticipation, and initiation of responses were the two variables which affected HR. Elliott's concept of incentive was a broad one. Although never formally defined, incentive had to do with the importance of the situation for the subject. Incentive was referred to as "the major importance variable"; task involvement was mentioned as "a related importance variable" which referred to "the common incentive of performing to achieve certain standards, usually in the absence of external rewards" (p. 222).

Although no criticism is intended of Elliott's concept of incentive, for the purposes of the present review it is too broad. In order to distinguish between reward incentives versus anxiety associated with frustration or punishment, it is best to limit demonstrations of incentive effects to situations in which there is a minimum of threat of failure or punishment— for example, tasks in which subjects are rewarded on almost 100% of the trials and in which there is no threat of social disapproval or other punishment for failure. Under these circumstances, anxiety can be assumed to make a minimal contribution, allowing HR increases to be attributed to the incentive effects of rewards. From this perspective, two of the studies with human subjects cited by Elliott (Malmo, 1965; Schnore, 1959) are potentially contaminated by anxiety effects, since there was a strong emphasis on good performance in the high-incentive condition.

Two of the studies cited (Elliott, 1964, 1966b) did demonstrate small effects of *monetary incentives* on HR during a reaction time task for adults and children. However, only a transient effect was found in another study with adults (Elliott, 1966a), and this was not replicated in a follow-up (Elliott, 1966c), possibly because of a procedural change. On the other hand, Elliott (1969) reported an original study with a clear incentive effect. He compared HR as a function of monetary incentive during a reaction time experiment with college students. In the high-incentive condition, subjects received 5¢ for every successful response and were rewarded on approximately two-thirds of the trials for a total of $3-3.50 for the session. Low-incentive subjects did not receive money contingent on performance (they did receive money for participation). The average increase in HR as a function of incentive varied from 2.9 to 6.0 bpm, depending on sequence and the predictability of the reaction time preparatory interval.

From these results, it appears that incentive effects in humans are possible with monetary rewards, but they have been relatively small and are not always reliably found. They are important, nevertheless, because they suggest that incentive effects on HR are not limited to biological rewards. It should also be noted that these monetary incentive effects have not controlled for the contributions of somatic activity.

The results of these various studies involving reward incentive effects in humans are encouraging. It appears that in situations which approximate pure reward conditions, such as those utilized by Lipsitt, reliable effects on HR are obtained. The greatest unreliability appears to have been obtained with the use of monetary rewards. Two possibilities may account for this. First, the incentives were not very high, compared to the 48- or 72-hour deprivation conditions used in many animal studies. Second, the use of a reaction time paradigm requires that subjects inhibit responding in preparation for the imperative stimulus. This requirement for behavioral inhibition in order to obtain good performance quite likely involves the activation of the BIS (to inhibit unrewarded responses). Better results might be obtained in situations in which subjects can respond for rewards without having to inhibit responses.

## AN ALTERNATIVE HYPOTHESIS:
## THE BEHAVIORAL ACTIVATION SYSTEM

### Failure of the Anxiety Hypothesis

The preceding review has established that there are three factors which are known to influence HR. First, increases and decreases in somatic activity tend to be accompanied by corresponding changes in HR—the cardiac–somatic coupling phenomenon. Second, subjects placed in an active-avoidance paradigm, in which successful responding avoids punishment, show elevated heart rates. Third, subjects making approach responses for rewards show elevated heart rates. The common thread in these three situations is the activation of behavior, or at least a preparation for the activation of behavior. However, the notion that all of these HR increases are no more than a response to metabolic needs has been rejected. Interesting motivational or emotional effects have been demonstrated in both the active-avoidance and the simple reward paradigm. In spite of the strong tie to somatic activity, then, HR conveys information about the subject's motivational state which may not be obvious from overt behavior.

In contrast to the clear evidence in favor of the three factors just mentioned, attempts to show cardiac acceleration during a classical aversive conditioning procedure have yielded mixed results. When cardiac accelerations have been found, moreover, these have been attributed to somatic activity rather than to a direct effect of anxiety on HR. Consequently, the literature on classical aversive conditioning of HR is the most direct evidence against the hypothesis that HR is an index of anxiety. Along the same line, the evidence that HR increases in response to reward incentives argues against an exclusive anxiety hypothesis. This response to reward incentives, of course, need not imply that HR does not respond to anxiety. It only shows that HR responds to other variables. The results with an active-avoidance paradigm both support and contradict the anxiety hypothesis. Inasmuch as active avoidance takes place in the context of a threat of punishment, cardiac acceleration under these conditions does have something to do with anxiety. On the other hand, it has been argued that this HR increase is tied strongly to active responding rather than to anxiety per se, again contradicting the anxiety hypothesis. In view of these difficulties, the anxiety hypothesis appears to be a clearly inadequate formulation of the psychological significance of HR.

## HEART RATE AND THE BEHAVIORAL ACTIVATION SYSTEM

An alternative formulation of the psychological significance of HR was proposed by Fowles (1980). The crucial assumptions in this formulation are that responding in the active-avoidance paradigm is under the control of conditioned stimuli for relieving nonpunishment (Pun-CSs), and that the effect of these stimuli is mediated by the same system which activates reward-seeking behavior. With this assumption, it is possible to hypothesize that the psychological effects on HR reflect the activity of the BAS. Since both active-avoidance and reward-seeking behavior are manifestations of this system, this hypothesis readily explains the HR increases seen in these two paradigms. Similarly, this would explain why HR increases are seen in classical aversive conditioning only if there is a tendency toward behavioral activation: BAS activity increases in the face of threats of punishment only if active avoidance is possible. If the subject perceives that no avoidance is possible (extinction), the BIS is dominant. Thus, this simple hypothesis appears to account for most of the major findings on the psychological significance of HR.

It is difficult to estimate the degree to which the BAS influences on HR account for cardiac–somatic coupling. Given the assumption that the BAS influences both, it is certainly reasonable to argue that this is the central control mechanism which accounts for the coupling (with one exception to be discussed later). The question is whether the cardiac–somatic coupling seen over a range of behaviors (e.g., Elliott, 1975) reflects some independent metabolic demand, or whether it reflects a motivational (BAS) influence which covaries with the strenuousness of the somatic activity. With respect to the latter possibility, it is useful to quote Elliott (1969): "It is difficult, even paradoxical, to imagine situations in which a subject would make a response that is wholly unimportant" (p. 222). This suggests that more strenuous activity would require a greater motivation, thus producing a motivationally mediated cardiac–somatic coupling. On the other hand, there are homeostatic mechanisms under the control of metabolic feedback which affect HR, at least for extended activity. It seems most reasonable to propose, therefore, that motivational factors do account for some of the covariation between HR and somatic activity, but that metabolic needs are also involved.

One finding which may appear to contradict the BAS hypothesis is Obrist's (1976) finding that, in an active-avoidance paradigm, cardiac acceleration is greater for a difficult task than for an easy task (see discussion on p. 103). Since completely successful avoidance responding (easy task) should reflect BAS activity, HR increases should be found under these conditions. The explanation offered by Fowles (1980) for the higher HR with a moderately difficult task drew on a comparison with the Bélanger and Feldman (1962) results. High HRs were found only under conditions of high drive, produced by water deprivation of up to 72-hour duration. In an active-avoidance paradigm, the drive is induced by the threat of punishment. When the task is very easy, the threat is not very great. Consequently, the induced drive is lower than if there is a significant probability of punishment, as with a difficult task. This analysis suggests that Obrist's inverted U curve for HR as a function of task difficulty reflects the operation of two variables: Anxiety-induced drive decreases with probability of successful avoidance, whereas positive incentive effects increase with probability of successful avoidance. At one extreme (classical conditioning) there are no reward incentive effects, while at the other extreme (easy task) anxiety-induced drive is minimal. At intermediate points both variables operate to produce higher HRs. In support of this interpretation, it should be noted that the reward incentive effects on HR have been obtained with 100%-reinforcement schedules, suggesting that in the appetitive situation easy tasks do not eliminate HR increases.

If the analysis just offered is correct, it suggests that the association between HR and anxiety is not a fundamental one. Rather, it is a consequence of the fact that the motivation or drive must be induced in the case of punishment. According to Gray's model (e.g., Gray, 1975; Gray & Smith, 1969), the high states of arousal or drive induced by Pun-CSs are mediated by activity of the BIS, not the BAS. From this perspective, anxiety-inducing stimuli exert their effect through a system which does not directly control HR. It should be stressed, however, that what is intended here is a theoretical point about the system which exerts primary control on HR. It is not intended to imply that HR cannot reveal interesting information about anxiety, providing that the situation is carefully specified. Under the conditions of partially successful active avoidance, it is suggested that HR increases do reflect the degree of anxiety-induced drive. Unfortunately, it is essential to control the degree of active responding. For example, when subjects are simply presented with a threatening stimulus, as in many studies, HR increases will be a joint function of the degree of anxiety and the subject's tendency to actively avoid the situation. Thus it is necessary to find some means of holding constant the tendency toward active avoidance in order to draw inferences about anxiety. It remains to be seen whether such a paradigm can be developed. In the meantime, investigators should be aware that HR is a "noisy" index of anxiety, even when limited to experimental paradigms involving threatening stimuli.

## VAGAL VERSUS SYMPATHETIC INFLUENCES: MODIFICATION OF THE HYPOTHESIS

It was stated earlier that the common element in the activation of HR is somatic activity, and two of the paradigms (active avoidance and approach for rewards) strongly suggest that the BAS mediates this effect. This would make sense inasmuch as the BAS would be the logical system for HR increases which anticipate somatic activation. There is, however, evidence to suggest that some well-established HR phenomena cannot be subsumed under this simple hypothesis. In particular, Obrist (Obrist, 1976; Obrist, Langer, Grignolo, Sutterer, Light, & McCubbin, 1979) has shown that the phasic decelerations which constituted his original evidence for cardiac–somatic coupling are attributable to increased parasympathetic activity via the vagus. In contrast, his active coping effects are produced by $\beta$-adrenergic influences via the sympathetic branch innervating the heart. It is reasonable to hypothesize the $\beta$-adrenergic influences during active coping are manifestations of the BAS's activity, but it would be hard to maintain that the cardiac decelerations attributable to vagal influences were due simply to lessened activity of the BAS. Thus, it appears to be necessary to explain the cardiac decelerations in some other manner.

This explanation derives from the consideration that the conditions which produce these cardiac decelerations are the same conditions which would be expected to produce an increase in the activity of the BIS. The function of this system is to inhibit responses which will be punished or unrewarded, and it is the activity of this system which is associated with anxiety. The situations which Obrist found to induce cardiac decelerations seem to share these features. These situations are a signaled reaction time task, classical aversive conditioning, and vagal death.

In discussing the reaction time task, Obrist viewed both the cardiac deceleration and the decrease in somatic activity as "peripheral manifestations of a central mechanism concerned with the inhibition of ongoing, task irrelevant, activities" (Obrist et al., 1970, p. 574), an interpretation which has continued unchanged in his more recent publications (Obrist, 1976; Obrist *et al.*, 1974). This type of active inhibition of unrewarded (irrelevant) behavior is exactly the function attributed to the BIS.

A similar argument can be made in the case of classical aversive conditioning. Obrist's description of deceleration as occurring when the animals "appear resigned to the inescapable nature of the situation" (Obrist *et al.*, 1974, p. 158) and are "the helpless recipient of aversive events" (Obrist, 1976, p. 103) suggests the dominance of an extinction process. In addition, a case has already been made earlier in this discussion for the activation of the BIS in the classical aversive conditioning situation.

The most extreme case of vagal inhibitory influences on HR, and the one most explicitly involving extreme stress and anxiety, is the vagal death phenomenon, which Obrist (Obrist, Langer, Grignolo, Sutterer, Light, & McCubbin, 1979) sees as related to the vagal effects which he found in the other two paradigms. Vagal death was observed by Richter (1957) in wild rats who were forced to swim in a tank of water. The rats died either just before or immediately after being placed in the water. Unlike laboratory rats, the wild rats would not attempt to swim. Richter attributed this death to the animal's "giving up" and Obrist, Langer, Grignolo, Sutterer, Light, and McCubbin (1979) suggested that it occurs when the organism resorts to helplessness. Earlier, Obrist *et al.* (1970) quoted Engel in discussing a similar phenomenon in man, which Engel attributed to "a reaction which may result during experiencing of fear when action is inhibited or impossible" (Engel, 1950, p. 11). This vagal effect associated with immobilization is "exaggerated relative to any metabolic need" (Obrist, Langer, Grignolo, Sutterer, Light, & McCubbin, 1979, p. 72). In this respect, vagal death resembles the excessive HR changes in the opposite direction that have been the main focus on this review. As in the previous examples, this vagal effect on HR associated with immobility, helplessness, and anxiety seems to reflect activation of the BIS. It may even be the case that the exaggeration of vagal inhibition is a reflection of the extreme anxiety, just as it was argued that the large HR increases reflected appetitive motivational states in the active-avoidance and approach situations. In any event, these situations in which Obrist has found a vagally produced cardiac deceleration are such that they seem to implicate an activation of the BIS, leading to a tentative hypothesis that these vagal decelerations reflect an increase in the activity of the BIS.

The interpretation just offered supports the suggestion that the cardiac orienting response (OR) reflects BIS activity (Fowles, 1980). It is usually assumed that the cardiac OR involves a deceleration (Graham, 1973; Graham & Clifton, 1966; Graham & Jackson, 1970). If the phasic decelerations discussed previously are to be attributed to BIS activity, it is plausible to extend this hypothesis to the cardiac-decelerative OR. There is also independent evidence that the behavioral OR to novel stimuli is mediated by the BIS (Gray, 1977), providing additional support for the hypothesis.[2]

Although this analysis of HR changes has been based on Obrist's work, it should be noted that Schneiderman (1977) has proposed a similar distinction between two broad categories of cardiovascular adjustment. One is associated with HR increases in conjunction with the availability of a coping response and increased motor activity. The second is a vagally mediated HR decrease seen in situations where there is no control over impending aversive stimulation, and it is associated with decreased motor activity or behavioral freezing. The second pattern is also seen in the orienting responses of some species and during reaction time experiments, and it is assumed to be involved in the vagal death phenomenon reported by Richter (1957). Thus Schneiderman's (1977) evaluation of the literature on psychological influences on HR appears to correspond very closely to distinctions already drawn on the basis of Obrist's work, suggesting a substantial convergence of opinion on this important point.

THE BIS AND ANXIETY

The assumption that the BIS mediates anxiety has played an important role in the arguments presented. Two aspects of this connection between the BIS and anxiety require discussion by way of making explicit some of the complications and issues. The first of these concerns the consequences

---

2. This proposal that the BIS mediates cardiac decelerations under certain conditions, combined with Gray's description of the behavioral effects of BIS activity as the "inhibition of ongoing behavior, increased arousal, and *increased attention to environmental stimuli*, especially novel ones" (Gray, 1979, p. 315, emphasis added), suggests some overlap with the Laceys' intake–rejection hypothesis in which cardiac deceleration is associated with sensory intake. It would be difficult, however, to integrate two totally different theoretical formulations, and such a task is beyond the scope of the present chapter.

for anxiety of the interaction of the BAS and BIS in the approach–avoidance conflict situation. The second concerns the degree to which BIS activity increases physiological arousal (e.g., anxiety) in conjunction with the inhibition of overt responding.

Gray's model assumes that anxiety is proportional to BIS activity, which, in turn, is proportional to the strength of Pun-CSs input. When these assumptions are applied to the customary representation of the approach–avoidance conflict, in which approach and avoidance gradients both rise with proximity to the goal box (UCS) with the avoidance gradient being steeper, somewhat surprising predictions follow.

The first of these is shown in Figure 3-1, which depicts the effect of two different levels of approach motivation on anxiety. The solid line represents the avoidance gradient; the two dashed lines, the two levels of approach motivation. The two vertical arrows indicate the resulting points of equilibrium for approach and avoidance, with the length of the arrow reflecting BIS (and BAS) activity. The effect of the stronger approach motivation is to produce a state of equilibrium closer to the goal box, with the resulting *increase* in Pun-CS (and Rew-CS) intensity, BIS activity, and thus anxiety. Thus, to the extent that strong approach motivation brings the organism closer to potential punishment, it will increase anxiety.

The same phenomenon is illustrated in Figure 3-2, which compares the effect of two levels of avoidance motivation on anxiety. It can be seen

FIG. 3-1. Effect of strength of approach on anxiety (BIS activity) in an approach–avoidance conflict situation. Solid line = avoidance gradient. Dashed lines = approach gradients. ("CS strength" is used instead of the more familiar "distance from goal" for the abscissa.)

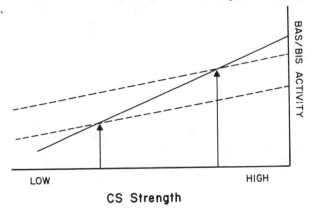

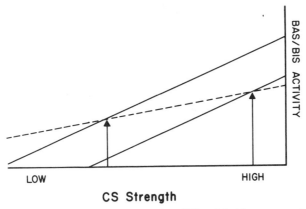

FIG. 3-2. Effect of strength of avoidance on anxiety (BIS activity) in an approach–avoidance conflict situation. Solid lines = avoidance gradients. Dashed lines = approach gradient. ("CS strength" is used instead of the more familiar "distance from goal" for the abscissa.)

that the stronger avoidance gradient will become dominant at a greater distance from the goal box, preventing the animal from encountering the strong Pun-CSs closer to the goal box. Consequently, the effect of a stronger avoidance motivation is to *reduce* Pun-CS input, BIS activity, and anxiety.

From these examples it can be seen that high anxiety may be associated with high levels of approach motivation and/or low levels of avoidance motivation, whereas low anxiety may be associated with low levels of approach motivation and/or high levels of avoidance motivation. This conclusion is true whether the levels of motivation derive from extrinsic rewards and punishments or from individual differences in the reactivity of the BAS and BIS. This analysis implies, therefore, that BIS-dominant situations (or individuals) may be associated with relatively *low* levels of anxiety, not with high anxiety as might be expected without considering the effects of proximity to the UCSs.

Another important example is the effects of antianxiety drugs, including alcohol. Gray (e.g., 1977) concluded that they reduce BIS activity, and thus they might be expected to reduce anxiety. However, Figure 3-2 shows that lowering the avoidance gradient (reducing BIS activity) can result in an actual *increase* in anxiety if the individual is facing an approach–avoidance conflict. It should be recalled that this tendency to approach the goal box more closely in a conflict situation is one of the most clearly demonstrated effects of the antianxiety drugs, suggesting that it is a likely consequence of reducing BIS activity. One could only expect these drugs to reduce anxiety if the circumstances were such that the strength of the Pun-CS input remained constant. This analysis may partially explain why there is such ambiguity as to whether alcohol reduces anxiety: it may, or may not, depending on circumstances.

These two examples do not exhaust the implications of the approach–avoidance conflict interactions of the BIS and BAS, but they do serve to illustrate that there can be a considerable uncoupling between the level of anxiety actually produced and the degree of dominance of BIS activity. No predictions can be made without a consideration of the strength of the Pun-CSs to be encountered in a given situation.

With the foregoing conclusion in mind, it is possible to discuss some of the ambiguities concerning the quietening or arousal consequences of the BIS. Throughout this review, the BIS has been said to inhibit behavior, and this might be taken to mean that the BIS inevitably produces an overall state of low physiological arousal along with a reduction in somatic activity. Although that might be true in some cases, it clearly is not true in general. The BIS as a system has one input and three outputs which are relevant to this question. The input consists of information concerning the presence and magnitude of Pun-CSs and $\overline{\text{Rew}}$-CSs. The outputs go to somatic activity (inhibitory), the BAS (inhibitory), and a nonspecific arousal system (excitatory) which Gray suggests is the reticular activating system. It has just been suggested that in some cases the BIS is so effective in preventing approach responses that Pun-CS (or Rew-CS) input is relatively weak. In that case, the output to the arousal system would presumably also be weak. If, on the other hand, strong Pun-CS cues are encountered, Gray's model predicts that the BIS will produce increased nonspecific arousal. Presumably the degree of nonspecific arousal contributes to the intensity of anxiety experienced with activation of the BIS, although Gray does not suggest this himself.

In Gray's use of the concept, the only explicit effect of nonspecific arousal is to increase behavioral vigor, such as increased running speed or a higher rate of bar pressing. For example, the partial reinforcement acquisition effect (Gray & Smith, 1969) refers to the fact that rats will run down an alley faster when they receive 50% reinforcement at the end than when they receive 100% reinforcement. The faster running cannot be attributed to greater activation of the BAS, since incentive is less on 50%

than on 100% reinforcement. Instead, it is attributed to the arousing effect of the Rew-CSs associated with partial reinforcement.

It is not possible to extrapolate from Gray's use of arousal to the measures of interest to psychophysiologists, but it does seem safe to conclude that BIS activity does not inevitably produce complete quiescence. Of particular interest is the question of what happens when there is no overt motor behavior. Gray (e.g., 1976a) comments that BIS-induced arousal increases behavioral vigor if the circumstances are such that responding occurs. He does not say what happens if the BIS succeeds in inhibiting responding. A step in the direction of extending Gray's model to the autonomic nervous system was offered by Fowles (1980), who proposed that electrodermal activity is associated with BIS activity (in addition to the HR-BAS hypothesis reviewed here), but no other measures have been considered. Somatic muscle tension is particularly of interest, since it would seem naturally to be tied to BAS activity, yet often is used to assess anxiety. Although it seems in keeping with the cardiac–somatic coupling literature to propose that muscle tension, like HR, would increase only if there is the incipient organization of a motor response (e.g., active avoidance), such a hypothesis could only be proposed after a review of the literature on muscle tension. It must suffice to alert readers to the gaps in our knowledge concerning the psychophysiological manifestations of activation of the BIS.

IMPLICATIONS FOR FUTURE RESEARCH

The HR response to aversive stimuli has been the focus of a great deal of research. The need to more sharply define this research in the direction of active coping or behavioral activation, rather than to focus only on the emotional state of anxiety, has already been discussed thoroughly. What has not been discussed is the potential fruitfulness of extending research on HR to paradigms involving appetitive stimuli. There are several possible areas of application for such research. Obrist (1976; Obrist, Langer, Grignolo, Sutterer, Light, & McCubbin, 1979) has pointed to large individual differences in the cardiovascular response in his active coping situation and has stressed the implications of an excessive response for the etiology of hypertension. Similarly, Schneiderman (1977) suggested that his active coping pattern might be seen in individuals showing the Type

A behavior pattern associated with coronary heart disease. It would be interesting to see if similar individual differences are found in appetitive situations. If so, it would suggest that the BAS was the primary contributor to the excessive reactivity in the active coping situation. Alternatively, the excessive responsiveness may be attributable to a higher level of drive (induced anxiety), in which case the excessive responsiveness should not generalize to appetitive situations.

Perhaps the most direct application to psychiatric problems is to those clinical formulations which emphasize a loss of appetitive motivation: "loss of interest or reinforcer effectiveness" in depression and "anhedonia" in schizophrenia. Loss of interest is a central symptom of depression—particularly autonomous or endogenous (Fowles & Gersh, 1979) or endogenomorphic (Klein, 1974) depression—and this has been attributed to loss of reinforcer effectiveness (e.g., Costello, 1972; Klein, 1974). On the other hand, the affective disorders are a heterogeneous group, presumably with multiple etiologies. An assessment of patients' cardiovascular responses to appetitive stimuli might provide a means for discriminating between those patients with a primary loss of interest and depressed patients with other etiologies, such as anxious depression (Gersh & Fowles, 1979) or reactive depression (Fowles & Gersh, 1979). Such research could be conducted in the context of the motivational theory used in the present review, which is quite similar to the formulation of depression offered by Eastman (1976) and overlaps with the biological substrates for reward and punishment discussed in the context of depression by Klein (1974) and Akiskal and McKinney (1975).

Anhedonia is a little-studied concept frequently used to describe some schizophrenics. Recently, however, Depue (1976) reported that anhedonia was characteristic of withdrawn schizophrenics but not of active schizophrenics. This suggests that the social withdrawal seen in some schizophrenics reflects, *in part*, a deficiency of the BAS. If so, it should be possible to show differences in the HR response to rewards in active versus withdrawn schizophrenics. Similarly, the recent development of an anhedonia scale for use with college students (Chapman, Chapman, & Raulin, 1976) makes it possible to investigate the relationship between HR and anhedonia in college populations.

It may be more complicated to investigate HR responses to appetitive stimuli at the other end of the continuum—that is, behavior which appears to be strongly reward seeking—because of the possibility that a lack of inhibitory control is extremely important, as suggested by Fowles

(1980) in the case of psychopathy. Nevertheless, a strong BAS would seem likely to be one contributor to phenotypic variance for behaviors described as stimulus seeking or impulsive.

CAVEATS

Numerous limitations of the formulation proposed here must be stressed in order to avoid appearing to claim more than is intended. In general, this review is concerned with motivational effects on HR under very circumscribed conditions. The hypothesis that HR reflects the activity of the behavioral activation system should not be taken to mean that it reflects only that. As Elliott (1974) noted, HR is affected by numerous variables other than motivation.

Even within the present theoretical system, the situation is quite complex. In Gray's model, the BAS and BIS have central mutual antagonism, which must be considered in addition to the peripheral sympathetic and parasympathetic effects discussed earlier. In addition, the model is quite complicated (e.g., see Gray & Smith, 1969), with many interconnections. Assuming individual differences at each stage in the model, correlations based on the model presented here may turn out to be relatively modest. For example, at an early stage for processing Rew-CSs the BAS might be quite responsive, but the output from the BAS to somatic activity might be weaker than normal. In such a case, there might be a HR response to rewards without a concomitant increase in reward-seeking behavior. Similarly, threatening stimuli might produce physiological responses associated with anxiety but fail to produce behavioral inhibition if the inhibitory output to somatic activity is deficient. Such cases may be of interest because the physiological activity tells us something which the behavior does not, but they do constitute exceptions to predictions based on the normal functioning of the two systems.

Another difficulty to be noted is that the present review suggests that cardiac decelerations in classical conditioning reflect activity of the BIS, whereas Fowles (1980) suggested that electrodermal activity reflect BIS activity. It is not intended to imply from this that there is an exact correspondence between electrodermal responses and cardiac decelerations. The study by Frederikson and Öhman (1979) showed that electrodermal activity conditioned more readily that did HR decreases, indicating differences between the two responses; and Roberts and Young (1971) showed a substantial uncoupling of HR and electrodermal activity. This could be due to any number of factors, but two are worth mentioning. First, the HR deceleration may be more difficult to develop because of antagonistic β-adrenergic effects on HR. Second, the two responses may reflect somewhat different aspects of the behavioral inhibition system. For example, it could be possible that electrodermal activity is more closely connected with the initial appraisal of threat and the immediate response to that, whereas the vagal effect on HR might be associated with the inhibitory output to somatic activity.

Finally, there is a need to develop paradigms for appetitive influences on HRs with humans. The clear evidence for appetitive effects has come largely from animal studies, and much work is needed in order to develop these paradigms for use with humans. Until that is done, the applications proposed in this discussion cannot proceed. Thus, our most urgent need is to begin to develop ways of assessing the HR response to rewards in human subjects.

# REFERENCES

Akiskal, H. S., & McKinney, W. T. Overview of recent research in depression: Integration of 10 conceptual models into a comprehensive clinical frame. *Archives of General Psychiatry*, 1975, *32*, 285–305.

Ashmead, D. H., Reilly, B. M., & Lipsitt, L. P. Neonates' heart rate, sucking rhythm, and sucking amplitude as a function of the sweet taste. *Journal of Experimental Child Psychology*, 1980, *29*, 264–281.

Beer, B., & Migler, B. Effects of diazepam on galvanic skin response and conflict in monkeys and humans. In A. Sudilovsky, S. Gershon, & B. Beer (Eds.), *Predictability in psychopharmacology: Preclinical and clinical correlations*. New York: Raven Press, 1975.

Bélanger, D., & Feldman, S. M. Effects of water deprivation upon heart rate and instrumental activity in the rat. *Journal of Comparative and Physiological Psychology*, 1962, *55*, 220–225.

Bignami, G. Effects of neuroleptics, ethanol, hypnotic–sedatives, tranquilizers, narcotics, and minor stimulants in aversive paradigms. In H. Anisman & G. Bignami (Eds.), *Psychopharmacology of aversively motivated behavior*. New York: Plenum Press, 1978.

Blackwell, B., & Whitehead, W. Behavioral evaluation of antianxiety drugs. In A. Sudilovsky, S. Gershon, & B. Beer (Eds.), *Predictability in psychopharmacology: Preclinical and clinical correlations*. New York: Raven Press, 1975.

Borkovec, T. D., Weerts, T. C., & Bernstein, D. A. Behavioral assessment of anxiety. In A. Ciminero, K. Calhoun, & H. E. Adams (Eds.), *Handbook of behavioral assessment*. New York: John Wiley & Sons, 1976.

Brener, J., Eissenberg, E., & Middaugh, S. Respiratory and somatal motor factors associated with operant conditioning of cardiovascular responses in curarized rats. In P.A. Obrist, A. H. Black, J. Brener, & L. V. DiCara (Eds.), *Cardiovascular psychophysiology: Current issues in response mechanisms, biofeedback, and methodology.* Chicago: Aldine, 1974.

Buckhout, R., & Grace, T. The effect of food deprivation and expectancy on heart rate. *Psychonomic Science*, 1966, *6*, 153–154.

Chapman, L. J., Chapman, J. P., & Raulin, M. L. Scales for physical and social anhedonia. *Journal of Abnormal Psychology*, 1976, *85*, 374–382.

Cook, L., & Davidson, A. B. Effects of behaviorally active drugs in a conflict-punishment procedure in rats. In S. Garattini, E. Mussini, & L. O. Randall (Eds.), *The benzodiazepines.* New York: Raven Press, 1973.

Cook, L., & Davidson, A. B. Behavioral pharmacology: Animal models involving aversive control of behavior. In M. A. Lipton, A. DiMascio, & K. F. Killam (Eds.), *Psychopharmacology: A generation of progress.* New York: Raven Press, 1978.

Costello, C. G. Depression: Loss of reinforcer or loss of reinforcer effectiveness. *Behavior Therapy*, 1972, *3*, 240–247.

Crook, C. K. Neonatal sucking: Effects of quantity of the response-contingent fluid upon sucking rhythm and heart rate. *Journal of Experimental Child Psychology*, 1976, *21*, 539–548.

Crook, C. K., & Lipsitt, L. P. Neonatal nutritive sucking: Effects of taste stimulation upon sucking rhythm and heart rate. *Child Development*, 1976, *47*, 518–522.

Depue, R. A. An activity-withdrawal distinction in schizophrenia: Behavioral, clinical, brain damage, and neurophysiological correlates. *Journal of Abnormal Psychology*, 1976, *85*, 174–185.

Doerr, H. O., & Hokanson, J. E. Food deprivation performance and heart rate in the rat. *Journal of Comparative and Physiological Psychology*, 1968, *65*, 227–231.

Eastman, C. Behavioral formulations of depression. *Psychological Review*, 1976, *83*, 277–291.

Elliott, R. Physiological activity and performance: A comparison of kindergarten children with young adults. *Psychological Monographs*, 1964, *78* (10, Whole No. 587).

Elliott, R. Effects of uncertainty about the nature and advent of a noxious stimulus (shock) upon distress. *Journal of Personality and Social Psychology*, 1966, *3*, 353–356. (a)

Elliott, R. Physiological activity and performance in children and adults: A two-year follow-up. *Journal of Experimental Child Psychology*, 1966, *4*, 58–80. (b)

Elliott, R. Reaction time and heart rate as functions of magnitude and incentive and probability of success: A replication and extension. *Journal of Experimental Research in Personality*, 1966, *1*, 174–178. (c)

Elliott, R. Tonic heart rate: Experiments on the effects of collative variables lead to a hypothesis about its motivational significance. *Journal of Personality and Social Psychology*, 1969, *12*, 211–228.

Elliott, R. The motivational significance of heart rate. In P. A. Obrist, A. H. Black, J. Brener, & L. V. DiCara (Eds.), *Cardiovascular psychophysiology: Current issues in response mechanisms, biofeedback, and methodology.* Chicago: Aldine, 1974.

Elliott, R. Heart rate, activity, and activation in rats. *Psychophysiology*, 1975, *12*, 298–305.

Engel, G. L. *Fainting: Physiological and psychological considerations.* Springfield, Ill.: Charles C Thomas, 1950.

Fowles, D. C. The three-arousal model: Implications of Gray's two-factor learning theory for heart rate, electrodermal activity, and psychopathy. *Psychophysiology*, 1980, *17*, 87–104.

Fowles, D. C., & Gersh, F. Neurotic depression: I. The endogenous-neurotic distinction. In R. A. Depue (Ed.), *The psychobiology of the depressive disorders: Implications for the effects of stress.* New York: Academic Press, 1979.

Frederikson, M., & Öhman, A. Cardiovascular and electrodermal responses conditioned to fear-relevant stimuli. *Psychophysiology,* 1979, *16,* 1–7.

Gersh, F., & Fowles, D. C. Neurotic depression: The concept of anxious depression. In R. A. Depue (Ed.), *The psychobiology of the depressive disorders: Implications for the effects of stress.* New York: Academic Press, 1979.

Goldstein, R., Beideman, L., & Stern, J. A. Effect of water deprivation and saline-induced thirst on the conditioned heart rate response of the rat. *Physiology and Behavior,* 1970, *5,* 583–587.

Goldstein, R., Stern, J. A., & Rothenberg, S. J. Effect of water deprivation and cues associated with water on the heart rate of the rat. *Physiology and Behavior,* 1966, *1,* 199–203.

Goldstein, R., Stern, J. A., & Sturmfels, L. Heart rate as a function of water deprivation and conditioning: Some additional controls. *Psychonomic Science,* 1969, *17,* 280–281.

Graham, F. K. Habituation and dishabituation of responses innervated by the autonomic nervous system. In H. V. S. Peeke & M. J. Herz (Eds.), *Habituation* (Vol. 1: *Behavioral studies*). New York: Academic Press, 1973.

Graham, F. K., & Clifton, R. K. Heart rate change as a component of the orienting response. *Psychological Bulletin,* 1966, *65,* 305–320.

Graham, F. K., & Jackson, J. C. Arousal systems and infant heart rate responses. In H. Reese & L. Lipsitt (Eds.), *Advances in child development and behavior* (Vol. 5). New York: Academic Press, 1970.

Gray, J. A. Causal theories of personality and how to test them. In J. R. Royce (Ed.), *Multivariate analysis and psychological theory.* New York: Academic Press, 1973.

Gray, J. A. *Elements of a two-process theory of learning.* New York: Academic Press, 1975.

Gray, J. A. The behavioural inhibition system: A possible substrate for anxiety. In M. P. Feldman & A. M. Broadhurst (Eds.), *Theoretical and experimental bases of behaviour modification.* New York: John Wiley & Sons, 1976. (a)

Gray, J. A. The neuropsychology of anxiety. In I. G. Sarason & C. D. Spielberger (Eds.), *Stress and anxiety* (Vol. 3). Washington, D.C.: Hemisphere, 1976. (b)

Gray, J. A. Drug effects on fear and frustration: Possible limbic site of action of minor tranquilizers. In L. L. Iversen, S. D. Iversen, & S. H. Snyder (Eds.), *Handbook of psychopharmacology* (Vol. 8: *Drugs, neurotransmitters, and behavior*). New York: Plenum Press, 1977.

Gray, J. A. The neuropsychology of anxiety. *British Journal of Psychology,* 1978, *69,* 417–434.

Gray, J. A. A neuropsychological theory of anxiety. In C. E. Izard (Ed.), *Emotions in personality and psychopathology.* New York: Plenum Press, 1979.

Gray, J. A., & Smith, P. T. An arousal-decision model for partial reinforcement and discrimination learning. In R. Gilbert & N. S. Sutherland (Eds.), *Animal discrimination learning.* New York: Academic Press, 1969. (Reprinted in Gray, 1975.)

Hahn, W. W., Stern, J. A., & Fehr, F. S. Generalizability of heart rate as a measure of drive state. *Journal of Comparative and Physiological Psychology,* 1964, *58,* 305–309.

Hahn, W. W., Stern, J. A., & McDonald, D. G. Effects of water deprivation and bar pressing activity on heart rate of the male albino rat. *Journal of Comparative and Physiological Psychology,* 1962, *55,* 786–790.

Houser, V. P. The effects of drugs on behavior controlled by aversive stimuli. In D. E.

Blackman & D. J. Sanger (Eds.), *Contemporary research in behavioral pharmacology*. New York: Plenum Press, 1978.

Klein, D. F. Endogenomorphic depression. *Archives of General Psychiatry*, 1974, *31*, 447–454.

Light, K. C., & Obrist, P. A. Cardiovascular response to stress: Effects of opportunity to avoid, shock experience, and performance feedback. *Psychophysiology*, 1980, *17*, 243–252.

Lipsitt, L. P. The newborn as informant. In R. B. Kearsley & I. E. Sigel (Eds.), *Infants at risk—Assessment of cognitive functioning*. Hillsdale, N.J.: Erlbaum, 1979.

Lipsitt, L. P., Reilly, B. M., Butcher, M. J., & Greenwood, M. M. The stability and interrelationships of newborn sucking and heart rate. *Developmental Psychobiology*, 1976, *9*, 305–310.

Mackintosh, N. J. *The psychology of animal learning*. New York: Academic Press, 1974.

Malmo, R. B. Measurement of drive: An unsolved problem in psychology. In M. R. Jones (Ed.), *Nebraska Symposium on Motivation*. Lincoln: University of Nebraska Press, 1958.

Malmo, R. B. Activation: A neuropsychological dimension. *Psychological Review*, 1959, *66*, 367–386.

Malmo, R. B. Activation. In A. J. Bachrach (Ed.), *Experimental foundations of clinical psychology*. New York: Basic Books, 1962.

Malmo, R. B. Finger-sweat prints in the differentiation of low and high incentive. *Psychophysiology*, 1965, *1*, 231–240.

Malmo, R. B., & Bélanger, D. Related physiological and behavioral changes: What are their determinants? *Research Publications of the Association for Research in Nervous and Mental Diseases*, 1967, *45*, 288–318.

Mandler, G. Helplessness: Theory and research in anxiety. In C. D. Spielberger (Ed.), *Anxiety: Current trends in theory and research* (Vol. 2). New York: Academic Press, 1972.

Martin, B., & Sroufe, L. A. Anxiety. In C. G. Costello (Ed.), *Symptoms of psychopathology: A handbook*. New York: John Wiley & Sons, 1970.

Mathews, A. Psychophysiological approaches to the investigation of desensitization and related procedures. *Psychological Bulletin*, 1971, *76*, 73–91.

Mineka, S. The role of fear in theories of avoidance learning, flooding, and extinction. *Psychological Bulletin*, 1979, *86*, 985–1010.

Obrist, P. A. The cardiovascular–behavioral interaction—As it appears today. *Psychophysiology*, 1976, *13*, 95–107.

Obrist, P. A., Gaebelein, C. J., Teller, E. S., Langer, A. W., Grignolo, A., Light, K. C., & McCubbin, J. A. The relationship among heart rate, carotid dP/dt, and blood pressure in humans as a function of the type of stress. *Psychophysiology*, 1978, *15*, 102–115.

Obrist, P. A., Howard, J. L., Lawler, J. E., Galosy, R. A., Meyers, K. A., & Gaebelein, C. J. The cardiac–somatic interaction. In P. A. Obrist, A. H. Black, J. Brener, & L. V. DiCara (Eds.), *Cardiovascular psychophysiology: Current issues in response mechanisms, biofeedback, and methodology*. Chicago: Aldine, 1974.

Obrist, P. A., Howard, J. L., Lawler, J. E., Sutterer, J. R., Smithson, K. W., & Martin, P. L. Alterations in cardiac contractility during classical aversive conditioning in dogs: Methodological and theoretical implications. *Psychophysiology*, 1972, *9*, 246–261.

Obrist, P. A., Langer, A. W., Grignolo, A., Sutterer, J. R., Light, K. C., & McCubbin, J. A. Blood pressure control mechanisms and stress: Implications for the etiology of hypertension. In G. Onesti & C. R. Klimt (Eds.), *Hypertension—Determinants, complications, and intervention.* New York: Grune & Stratton, 1979.

Obrist, P. A., Light, K. C., McCubbin, J. A., Hutcheson, J. S., & Hoffer, J. L. Pulse transit time: Relationship to blood pressure and myocardial performance. *Psychophysiology*, 1979, *16*, 292-301.

Obrist, P. A., Webb, R. A., Sutterer, J. R., & Howard, J. L. The cardiac-somatic relationship: Some reformulations. *Psychophysiology*, 1970, *6*, 569-587.

Richter, C. P. On the phenomena of sudden death in animals and man. *Psychosomatic Medicine*, 1957, *29*, 191-198.

Roberts, L. Comparative psychophysiology of the electrodermal and cardiac control systems. In P. A. Obrist, A. H. Black, J. Brener, & L. V. DiCara (Eds.), *Cardiovascular psychophysiology: Current issues in response mechanisms, biofeedback, and methodology.* Chicago: Aldine, 1974.

Roberts, L E., & Young, R. Electrodermal responses are independent of movement during aversive conditioning in rats, but heart rate is not. *Journal of Comparative and Physiological Psychology*, 1971, *77*, 495-512.

Schneiderman, N. The relationship between learned and unlearned cardiovascular responses. In P. A. Obrist, A. H. Black, J. Brener, & L. V. DiCara (Eds.). *Cardiovascular psychophysiology: Current issues in response mechanisms, biofeedback, and methodology.* Chicago: Aldine, 1974.

Schneiderman, N. Animal models relating behavioral stress and cardiovascular pathology: A position paper on mechanisms. In T. M. Dembroski (Ed.), *Proceedings of the forum on coronary-prone behavior.* Washington, D.C.: U.S. Government Printing Office, 1977.

Schnore, M. M. Individual patterns of physiological activity as a function of task differences and degree of arousal. *Journal of Experimental Psychology*, 1959, *58*, 117-128.

Sepinwall, J., & Cook, L. Behavioral pharmacolgy of antianxiety drugs. In L. L. Iversen, S. D. Iversen, & S. H. Snyder (Eds.), *Handbook of psychopharmacology* (Vol. 13: *Biology of mood and antianxiety drugs*). New York: Plenum Press, 1978.

Stein, L., Wise, C. D., & Belluzzi, J. D. Neuropharmacology of reward and punishment. In L. L. Iversen, S. D. Iversen, and S. H. Snyder (Eds.), *Handbook of psychopharmacology* (Vol. 8: *Drugs, neurotransmitters, and behavior*). New York: Plenum Press, 1977.

Stein, L., Wise, C. D., & Berger, B. D. Antianxiety action of benzodiazepines: Decrease in activity of serotonin neurons in the punishment system. In S. Garattini, E. Mussine, & L. Randall (Eds.), *The benzodiazepines.* New York: Raven Press, 1973.

Szpiler, J. A., & Epstein, S. Availability of an avoidance response as related to autonomic arousal. *Journal of Abnormal Psychology*, 1976, *85*, 73-82.

Van Egeren, L. F., Feather, B. W., & Hein, P. L. Desensitization of phobias: Some psychophysiological propositions. *Psychophysiology*, 1971, *8*, 213-228.

# 4

# Modification of Physiological and Subjective Responses to Stress through Heart Rate Biofeedback

DAVID SHAPIRO

JOHN L. REEVES II

Biofeedback research is now more than 15 years old, and considerable progress has been made in dealing with theoretical and empirical questions about the processes involved. The widespread emphasis on clinical applications, however, has tended to divert attention away from more systematic basic research on biofeedback (see Black, Cott, & Pavloski, 1977; Gatchel & Price, 1979; Shapiro, 1980). As a means of examining some of the mechanisms of biofeedback learning and of developing new ways of applying biofeedback clinically, the research discussed in this chapter poses different questions that have been asked in the past and utilizes a different experimental paradigm.

Typically in biofeedback, the individual's ability to modify physiological responses is evaluated under resting conditions. Feedback and reinforcement are given for spontaneously occurring responses, and no external stimuli are presented other than the tones, lights, or meters that make up the biofeedback displays. No demands are placed on the in-

David Shapiro. Department of Psychiatry and Biobehavioral Sciences, University of California, Los Angeles, California.

John L. Reeves II. Department of Anesthesiology, University of California, Los Angeles, California.

dividual other than those of the biofeedback task itself. The strategy employed in the present research is to present stimuli to the individual which elicit specific physiological responses, or changes in physiological arousal, and to determine whether such elicited physiological responses, or related anticipatory physiological responses, can be modified by means of biofeedback training procedures. Electric shock to the forearm and immersion of the hand in ice water were used as a means of arousing physiological and emotional responses.

A second aim of the research was to determine whether perceptions of the intensity of such stressful stimuli or other subjective reactions would also be modified as a consequence of the biofeedback training. This paradigm enables us to investigate the adapative or psychological significance of specific physiological component responses associated with emotional arousal and reactions to stress.

The use of biofeedback to alter a specific physiological response and thereby affect emotional arousal can be compared with the use of autonomic nervous system drugs for similar purposes. For example, a $\beta$-adrenergic blocking agent, propranolol, has been used in research on the modification of anxiety in chronically anxious patients (Tyrer, 1976). The aim was to determine if reductions in $\beta$-adrenergic functions, such as a reduction in heart rate, produced by the drug would be associated with reductions in anxiety. Tyrer found that propranolol led to reductions of anxiety, particularly in patients who report normally experiencing their anxiety in somatic or bodily terms. Biofeedback provides a behavioral means of studying similar processes. In the present research, the biofeedback procedure was oriented directly to the control of physiological responses which are part of the individual's total reaction to specific stressful stimuli, with the idea that such techniques may be useful to therapists in the management of anxieties, fears, and phobic reactions to such stimuli. Voluntary control of autonomic functions facilitated by biofeedback methods may be a useful strategy in the treatment of stress-related disorders. To the extent that physical symptoms are under the control of specific stress-related stimuli, then, it would be useful to adapt biofeedback training methods which involve the appropriate stimuli. For example, biofeedback training procedures could be adapted to help patients with Raynaud's disease reduce their abnormal vascular response to cold temperatures or to specific emotional or other triggering stimuli. Rather than having the biofeedback training occur in resting conditions, the task for the patient would be to increase skin temperature or blood flow while the stress-related stimuli are presented.

Two additional questions provided further impetus for the research described in this chapter.

1. We wanted to make a direct comparison of biofeedback effects under resting and stress conditions. Would it be more or less difficult for subjects to modify specific physiological responses associated with aversive stimuli or stress as compared with nonstress conditions?

2. Reductions in arousal-like activity (decrease in heart rate and blood pressure, increases in skin temperature) have been difficult to demonstrate in biofeedback studies. Would it be easier to obtain decreases in arousal when tonic levels are heightened under stressful conditions?

## CONTROL OF ELICITED ELECTRODERMAL RESPONSES

An empirical justification for the use of biofeedback as a means of altering elicited physiological responses to stressful stimuli derives in part from earlier studies in our laboratory on the control of electrodermal responses elicited by simple nonaversive stimuli. Shnidman (1970) examined the extent to which the skin-potential response elicited by presentation of a small red triangle for 5-sec periods could be instrumentally conditioned. One group of subjects was reinforced each time they showed a criterion skin-potential response to the stimulus. A second group was reinforced on the same trials as experimental subjects with whom they were matched for electrodermal responsivity, whether they responded or not. The reinforcers were slides of interesting landscapes and animals, equated with monetary bonuses. Significantly more skin-potential responses were shown in the experimental than in the control group. In related experiments, avoidance, punishment, and other conditioning procedures yielded further supporting evidence that electrodermal responses elicited by simple stimuli can be shaped instrumentally (Grings & Carlin, 1966; Kimmel & Baxter, 1964; Shnidman, 1969; Shnidman & Shapiro, 1971). Shnidman (1970) concluded: "The goal of desensitization is the modification of autonomic responses to specific stimuli and situations. Monitoring and conditioning autonomic responses to critical stimuli may effect desired changes in the autonomic activity and behavior" (p. 494). This anticipated the work to follow.

An unpublished pilot study from our laboratory attempted to follow this lead (Shapiro, Schwartz, Nelson, Shnidman, & Silverman, 1972). Volunteer subjects reporting moderate to intense fear of snakes were shown slides of snakes in order of increasing "fear" quality. Each slide was presented for 5 sec. Half the subjects were reinforced whenever the skin-resistance response elicited by a slide was larger than for the previous slide, and half the subjects were reinforced for smaller electrodermal responses. Both groups tended to show habituation in their elicited electrodermal responses, but the rate of habituation was greater in the decrease group. Before and after the conditioning trials, a snake- and spider-fear questionnaire was administered to subjects. Both groups showed a reduction in expressed fear, but the reduction was greater in the decrease group.

Mention should be made here of one of the first studies attempting to modify a physiological response as a means of modifying associated performance or behavior—in this case, problem solving and cognitive functioning (Kimmel, Pendergrass, & Kimmel, 1967). Children were reinforced with candy and approval when they showed decreases in skin resistance on the presentation of geometric stimuli used in the Seguin Form Board Task. It was found that the elicited electrodermal responses could be modified in this fashion. Moreover, although the results were quite complex, the conditioning appeared to transfer to the children's form board performance in a subsequent task (placing the forms in their proper places). Children reinforced for "orienting" did better on this "intelligence" test than those reinforced for not so responding.

For a further discussion of related biofeedback research on electrodermal, electromyographic, and electroencephalographic responses associated with emotional behavior, see McCroskery and Engel (1981). This chapter focuses on the control of heart rate responses and its consequences for behavior.


## CONTROL OF ANTICIPATORY HEART RATE RESPONSES

Heart rate was chosen for feedback training in the stress paradigm because of the ease with which subjects can learn voluntary control of this function (Brener & Hothersall, 1966; Engel & Hansen, 1966; Lang, 1974; Shapiro, Tursky, & Schwartz, 1970) and the oft-demonstrated empirical association between heart rate and fear or anxiety (Lang, Melamed, & Hart, 1970; Lang, Rice, & Sternbach, 1972).

Although psychophysiological research has closely linked together heart rate and emotional stimulation, it is not known whether heart rate merely reflects emotional responding or actually plays a more direct role in modulating the relative degree of such responding. DiCara and Weiss (1969) reported that curarized rats receiving operant training for heart rate increases demonstrated a deficit in subsequent skeletal shock avoidance and escape learning in the noncurarized state, when compared to rats given prior operant heart rate slowing training. Avoidance and escape performance were directly related to emotionality. Rats exhibited much more emotionality (as indexed by jumping, turning, and freezing behaviors) after operant training in heart rate speeding and less emotionality after operant heart rate slowing. A second experiment was reported in the DiCara and Weiss study on the degree to which the skeletal-avoidance learning was affected by shock intensity. It was hypothesized that the avoidance learning would become progressively disrupted at higher shock intensity levels. The results supported this hypothesis and suggested that "learning to speed up heart rate in a shock-avoidance situation had the effect of increasing fear or excitability" (1969, p. 372). The mechanism by which heart rate increase mediated fear (and poor avoidance learning) is uncertain. The authors proposed the fast heart rate learning produced strong fear, which led to unconditioned competing responses that interfered with avoidance learning. No data were presented concerning concurrent changes in other physiological responses or the degree to which the heart rate effects were specific or were associated with an overall physiological arousal pattern. In a related study in monkeys, classically conditioned changes in heart rate occurring in anticipation of electric shock could be significantly altered by operant reinforcement (Ainslie & Engel, 1974).

We examined the ability of human subjects to alter their heart rate in anticipation of receiving aversive stimuli. The first experiment (Sirota, Schwartz, & Shapiro, 1974) consisted of 72 15-sec trial periods, half followed by 2 sec of aversive electric shock stimulation to the forearm. Different colored lights remaining on for each 15-sec period signaled whether shock would follow or not. There were two groups of subjects ($n = 10$ per group). The first was instructed to increase heart rate and was given cardiotachometer feedback plus monetary bonuses for criterion heart rate increases. The second group was a heart rate decrease condition. Following each shock trial, subjects were asked to rate the intensity or painfulness of the stimulus on a 100-point scale. Significant differences both in tonic heart rate (heart rate per trial) and in phasic heart rate (change in heart rate during the 15-sec periods) were obtained between the two groups. The magnitude of the heart rate effects achieved was as large or larger than reported in typical biofeedback studies not involving specific eliciting stimuli. By and large, heart rate control was not interfered with when subjects were expecting to be shocked, compared with safe periods. In fact, rather than being disruptive of heart rate control, anticipation of shock seemed to result in larger bidirectional differences in phasic heart rate changes during the periods of anticipation.

Subjects in the increase group rated the shocks as more intense than subjects in the decrease group. The difference was present in the early trials and did not change appreciably over the course of training. A separate analysis of "cardiac-aware" versus "cardiac-unaware" subjects was undertaken, this variable defined by subjects' responses on an autonomic perception questionnaire adapted from Mandler, Mandler, and Uviller (1958) in which subjects were asked to indicate their awareness of physiological changes during fear situations in daily life. Two items dealing specifically with cardiac functioning—loud, pounding heart; increase in heart rate—defined the cardiac-awareness dimension. Cardiac-aware subjects rated these items as highly relevant to their fear. Reanalyzing the results in terms of this dimension, we found that cardiac-aware subjects in the increase group rated shocks as more and more intense over the course of training; cardiac-aware subjects in the decrease group tended to rate the shocks as less intense over trials. No differences between increase and decrease feedback conditions were obtained for the unaware subjects. These cardiac-aware–cardiac-unaware findings parallel Tyrer's (1976) results using pharmacological control of heart rate in somatically oriented anxious patients. Inasmuch as a no-feedback control group was not run in this study, there is no way to determine whether the biofeedback procedure served to facilitate a decrease in heart rate under the heightened conditions of arousal in this experimental situation. Nor were data available on associated physiological changes or respiration.

To replicate and extend these findings, Sirota, Schwartz, and Shapiro (1976) did an experiment which was divided into two parts, each consisting of a baseline period and 25 15-sec heart rate biofeedback trials. Four out of five trials ended with the presentation of an aversive electric shock. One group of subjects was instructed to increase heart rate during the first part of the experiment and decrease it during the second part. A second group of subjects was studied in the reverse order ($n = 10$ per group). Subjects were successful in increasing and decreasing their heart rate in anticipation of the aversive electric shock stimulation. In addition, the increases and decreases in heart rate were generally associated with parallel changes in subjective ratings of painfulness of the stimuli, especially in cardiac-aware subjects. In this experiment, heart rate was also measured during "blank trial" periods occurring between trials to assess whether bidirectional control was being achieved relative to nonspecific changes in heart rate over time. Generally, heart rate during increase trials was higher, and heart rate during decrease trials was lower, as compared with these control periods. The heightened arousal of this experimental situation may have helped demonstrate this bidirectional effect. No data were available on other physiological measures or respiration.

In this connection, DeGood and Adams (1976) compared the relative effectiveness of biofeedback for heart rate decreases, progressive relaxation, and a noncontingent music control group. Following an initial series of shock trials to determine pain levels, subjects received 25 min of training, and then were instructed to lower their heart rate during 10 tone–shock pairings. Reliable heart rate reductions were found during the tone–shock pairings for the biofeedback and progressive relaxation groups. Reliable reductions were also reported in pre-to-post-state anxiety and shock ratings, but no group differences emerged. Other techniques such as relaxation may be as effective as biofeedback in decreasing emotional arousal in this situation.

Taken together, the results support the notion that learned control of heart reactions to aversive stimulation may result in associated changes in subjective pain ratings. However, the actual role heart rate plays in affecting such perceptual changes remained unclear in light of evidence indicating that merely the belief that cardiovascular changes are occurring can result in changes in avoidance behavior and reports of pain (Borkovec, 1976; Holmes & Frost, 1976; Valins & Ray, 1967). It is conceivable that the belief that heart rate is increasing or decreasing may be sufficient in itself to alter subjective ratings of pain, particularly in cardiac-aware subjects. Moreover, the advantages of biofeedback over other methods of self-regulation remain an open question.

In an attempt to disentangle the relative effects of cognitive factors and heart rate on changes observed in subjective pain ratings, Sirota (1976) examined several unique combinations of heart rate feedback and instructions using a similar anticipatory shock paradigm. Four groups of cardiac-aware subjects were studied ($n = 10$ per group). Group 1 was given instructions to increase heart rate during Part 1 of the experiment and to decrease heart rate during Part 2, and was provided with veridical heart rate feedback during both parts. This group was intended to replicate their previous findings. Group 2 was given instructions to increase heart rate during Part 1 and then to decrease heart rate during Part 2, but were given feedback for heart rate stabilization in both parts. The purpose of this group was to make subjects believe that heart rate was changing while in fact it remained constant. Group 3 was given instructions to stabilize heart rate during Parts 1 and 2, but was given feedback for increasing heart rate during Part 1 and decreasing it during Part 2. This attempted to instill the belief that heart rate was not changing while in fact it was. Group 4 was given instructions to stabilize heart rate and provided with veridical feedback during both parts of the experiment. The results of this experiment were complicated since expected heart rate changes were not clearly obtained. Generally, subjects found it difficult to do one thing with their heart rate after being instructed to do another. A comparison of group heart rate changes suggested the prepotence of instructions over feedback in the control of heart rate with group shock ratings tending to parallel heart rate, particularly in Part 1. These results lent further support to the conclusion that a combination of physiological and cognitive factors is required for a learned heart rate response to transfer to a related perceptual change. The question of cognitive–physiological interactions is taken up again in a later section.

## CONTROL OF HEART RATE RESPONSE TO COLD-PRESSOR STRESS

The previous studies required subjects to control their heart rate in anticipation of an aversive stimulus. More recently, our research has focused on the ability of subjects to control their heart rate while actually experiencing aversive stimulation. Victor, Mainardi, and Shapiro (1978) investigated the effects of biofeedback training on heart rate and subjective reactions to the cold-pressor test—immersion of the hand in ice water for 30 sec. The cold-pressor test was chosen because it elicits reactions that are predictable, including tachycardia and pain in most human subjects. In addition, the test–retest reliability for heart rate changes and pain reports is high (Hilgard, 1975; Hilgard, Morgan, Lange, Lenox, Macdonald, Marshall, & Sachs, 1974; Lovallo, 1975). Following an initial 30-sec cold-pressor test, subjects were assigned to one of five experimental conditions ($n = 9$ per group): (1) meter biofeedback for heart rate increase, (2) meter biofeedback for heart rate decrease, (3) instructions to increase heart rate with no feedback, (4) instructions to decrease heart rate with no feedback, and (5) a habituation control group (no heart rate instructions or feedback). A second 30-sec cold-pressor test was given after 25 30-sec trials on training. Except for the habituation control condition, all groups were instructed to continue controlling their heart rate in the instructed direction during the second cold-pressor test. No feedback was given. A summary of the pain rating and heart rate effects is given in Table 4-1. Subjects in the feedback groups exhibited reliable heart rate increases and decreases as well as reporting parallel changes in subjective pain ratings. The no-feedback groups showed similar heart rate and pain-rating trends, but the differences failed to reach statistical significance. In this study, cardiac awareness was not significantly correlated with cold-pressor pain ratings (Shapiro, 1977).

Given a single session of biofeedback training, subjects were able to gain voluntary bidirectional control of heart rate while being subjected to the noxious stimulation of ice water. Inasmuch as the biofeedback training itself was carried out in ordinary resting-condition trials, the results indicate that the effects of such training can carry over to a stress situation. Moreover, it may be easier to demonstrate a decrease in arousal-like physiological activity with biofeedback training, in this case for heart rate, when it is assessed under stress conditions. In any case, the learned control was not interfered with.

Table 4-1 shows that the differences in pain rating generally paralleled the differences in heart rate observed during the second cold-pressor test; the higher the heart rate, the higher the report of painfulness. Of the five groups, only the decrease-feedback group showed a significant correlation between pain rating and heart rate and change in heart rate during the second cold-pressor test; the larger the reduction in heart rate, the lower the pain ratings in these subjects. Again, changes in other physiological measures or respiration were not available in this study.

In the next study, Reeves and Shapiro (in press) attempted to replicate the basic findings in the Victor *et al.* (1978) cold-pressor experiment while at the same time further exploring the interaction of instructional and physiological variables in affecting subjective ratings of pain. The study undertook to clarify further the relative contribution of changes in heart rate (by means of biofeedback training) and cognitive factors (instructionally induced belief that heart rate is changing in a specified

TABLE 4-1. Comparison of Mean Pain Ratings and Mean Heart Rate
Effects during the Second Cold-Pressor Test

| Group | Pain rating[b] | Heart rate indices (bpm)[a] | | |
|---|---|---|---|---|
| | | 1 | 2 | 3 |
| Increase—feedback | 6.7 | 88.6 | 11.5 | 11.6 |
| Increase—no feedback | 6.1 | 75.7 | 4.4 | 4.1 |
| Habituation—control | 6.3 | 74.3 | .2 | 4.1 |
| Decrease—no feedback | 5.4 | 73.5 | .1 | .5 |
| Decrease—feedback | 4.0 | 70.2 | −6.0 | −3.3 |

*Note.* From "Effect of Biofeedback and Voluntary Control Procedures on
Heart Rate and Perception of Pain during the Cold Pressor Test," by
R. Victor, J. A. Mainardi, and D. Shapiro, *Psychosomatic Medicine*, 1978,
*40*, 216–225. Reprinted by permission.

[a](1) Mean heart rate during 30 sec of Cold Pressor 2; (2) mean heart rate
during 30 sec of Cold Pressor 2 minus mean heart rate during 30 sec of
Cold Pressor 1; (3) mean heart rate in 30 sec of Cold Pressor 2 minus mean
heart rate in prior 5-sec base period, subtracting out parallel change in
Cold Pressor 1.

[b]1 = no pain; 10 = unbearably painful.

direction) in affecting subjective reports of pain during aversive ice water
stimulation. Four experimental conditions were studied ($n = 10$ per group).
Two conditions were essentially the same as the feedback conditions used
in Victor *et al.* (1978) and were an attempt to replicate their findings of
parallel changes in heart rate and pain during the cold-pressor test. Group
I-I was instructed to increase their heart rate and given veridical feedback;
Group D-D was instructed to decrease their heart rate and given veridical
feedback. In the other two conditions, subjects were also instructed either
to increase or decrease their heart rate, but the feedback display was
reversed: Group I-D was instructed to increase their heart rate but actually
given feedback for heart rate decrease; Group D-I was instructed to
decrease heart rate but given feedback for heart rate increase. Thus
Groups I-D and D-I were led to believe that their heart rate was changing
in the instructed direction, but an attempt was made to change it in the
opposite direction through reverse biofeedback.

Following a 10-min resting baseline, a 45-sec anticipation period
immediately preceded a 45-sec cold-pressor test. Subjects verbally reported
numerical pain values (0–10, open at the top) three times (each 15 sec)

during both anticipation and cold-pressor periods. Visual Analogue Scales (VASs) and psychophysically scaled descriptors were used to assess maximum pain, pain intensity, and reactivity. A second 3-min baseline was taken, and then 25 subject-initiated biofeedback training trials were given. Each trial consisted of a 15-sec no-feedback, no-control pretrial followed by 45 sec of visual feedback. Following feedback training, another 3-min baseline was recorded, and the final anticipation and cold-pressor test was administered. Subjects were instructed to control their heart rate in the same direction as instructed during training, while immersing their hand in the circulating ice water, but without the aid of feedback. Pain ratings were again taken.

Several methodological differences between this study and the Victor et al. (1978) study were introduced: (1) The cold-pressor stimulation was made more consistent and aversive by installing a circulating pump in the water in order to maintain a constant .5°C water temperature. The length of the cold-pressor test was also extended from 30 sec to 45 sec and was preceded by a 45-sec signaled anticipation period. (2) A computer graphics display (GT) was used to present heart period feedback. The visual feedback was presented in the form of a vertical feedback line, the height of which was linearly related to the time in milliseconds between successive R waves in the electrocardiogram. Each succeeding R-R interval generated a feedback line which appeared at equal intervals to the right of the preceding line on the display. The feedback lines remained on the GT display throughout each 45-sec training trial. The subject was therefore able to observe a history of his/her heart beat performance during each trial. Subjects were asked to try to make the vertical feedback lines as long or as short as possible, depending upon the condition. In order to control for individual heart rate variability, the display parameters and reward criteria were individualized for each subject. To equate for task difficulty, the display parameters for the increase and decrease feedback conditions were made equivalent in terms of the expected magnitude of heart rate effects. (3) A more precise attempt was made to accurately scale the subjects' pain ratings. In the previous studies, pain was verbally reported using a 0-10 numerical scale. In this study, subjects were required to report their pain using several different scales. Subjects verbally reported their pain levels when signaled by the computer three times (every 15 sec) during the cold pressor. The pain scale ranged from 0 (= no pain) to 10 (= intense pain). Numbers larger than 10 were permitted to be used for pain which increased beyond "intense." Thus, changes in pain during the cold pressor could be observed. This "open-ended" scale is similar to that previously used by Hilgard *et al.* (1974). In addition, an attempt was made to distinguish between the intensity (sensory) and affective components of the pain experience. Immediately following each cold-pressor test, two lists of 15 psychophysically scaled pain descriptors were presented, intended to assess: (a) intensity component—how much the pain hurts, and (b) affective component—how the pain feels. The subject chose the one word from each list of randomly ordered descriptors that best described his maximum experience during the cold-pressor tests (Gracely, McGrath, & Dubner, 1976). Since Gracely *et al.* calculated bias-free scale values for each descriptor using cross-modality scaling, numerical values could be recorded for the purposes of analysis. Table 4-2 shows the descriptors and corresponding psychophysically scaled values. A VAS was also given after each cold pressor. A VAS is a 10-cm, horizontal, straight line, the ends of which are anchored by the extreme limits of the sensation or response to the measure (Scott & Huskisson, 1976). The VAS was anchored by "no pain" on the left end and "pain as bad as it could be" on the right end of the line. Subjects were instructed to place a

TABLE 4-2. Intensity and Affective Pain Descriptors and Psychophysically Scaled Values

| Intensity scale | | Affective scale | |
| --- | --- | --- | --- |
| Extremely intense | 60.2 | Excruciating | 30.2 |
| Very intense | 47.0 | Intolerable | 23.5 |
| Very strong | 34.4 | Unbearable | 20.7 |
| Intense | 33.8 | Agonizing | 19.0 |
| Strong | 25.4 | Horrible | 16.0 |
| Slightly intense | 21.1 | Dreadful | 14.6 |
| Barely strong | 16.1 | Frightful | 13.1 |
| Moderate | 11.2 | Awful | 11.6 |
| Slightly moderate | 9.0 | Miserable | 10.9 |
| Very moderate | 8.9 | Oppressive | 10.7 |
| Mild | 5.1 | Distressing | 6.4 |
| Very mild | 3.3 | Uncomfortable | 4.0 |
| Weak | 2.6 | Unpleasant | 3.8 |
| Very weak | 1.3 | Distracting | 3.1 |
| Extremely weak | 0.7 | Bearable | 2.9 |

vertical "hash mark" somewhere on the line indicating their maximum experience during the cold-pressor test. The position of the hash mark was measured in centimeters to yield a pain score.

The main results of the study are summarized in Table 4-3. For ease of presentation, the data are discussed here in terms of heart rate rather than heart period. Biofeedback training resulted in heart rate increases for Group I-I and small heart rate decreases for Groups D-D, I-D, and D-I. These heart rate changes seemed to be parallelled by concomitant changes in frontal EMG, respiration period, and inspiration time, implicating possible somatic influences on heart rate changes during biofeedback training. The biofeedback data do not suppport the notion that instructions, and not biofeedback, are solely responsible for heart rate changes since Groups I-D and D-I failed to produce substantial heart rate changes in the instructed direction. The cold-pressor results showed that subjects can increase and decrease their heart rate during painful stimulation following heart rate biofeedback training. Group I-I, for whom instructions and feedback were veridical, showed substantial increases in heart rate during the second cold pressor, as compared with Group I-D, who were also instructed to increase heart rate but were given decrease biofeedback training. However, both groups instructed to decrease their heart rate showed comparable heart rate reductions, regardless of the

TABLE 4-3. Heart Period and Pain Rating Data

| Group | Heart period | | | Pain rating[d] | |
| | Feedback trials[a] | Feedback trials[b] | Cold pressor[c] | Verbal pain rating | Visual analogue scale |
|---|---|---|---|---|---|
| I-I | +67 | 808 | +48 | + .9 | +1.39 |
| D-D | −28 | 871 | −42 | −1.0 | −1.13 |
| I-D | −15 | 858 | −16 | − .1 | + .21 |
| D-I | −20 | 859 | −55 | − .3 | + .66 |

[a]Difference in mean heart period in milliseconds between 15-sec pretrial and 45-sec trial period (positive number means a decrease in interbeat interval or increase in heart rate).

[b]Mean heart period in milliseconds collapsed across trials.

[c]Difference in mean heart period in milliseconds between Cold Pressor 1 and Cold Pressor 2 (positive number means a decrease in interbeat interval or increase in heart rate).

[d]Difference in pain rating scales between Cold Pressor 1 and Cold Pressor 2 (positive sign means increase in pain).

direction of their prior biofeedback training. With the exception of Group D-I, who showed marked increases in respiration period and inspiration time, no other concomitant physiological changes were observed during the final cold pressor.

When feedback and instructions were veridical, reliable changes in verbal pain ratings and the VAS were found during the cold pressors. Group I-I increased and Group D-D decreased their pain ratings from the first to the second cold pressor. Groups I-D and D-I did not show changes in pain reports. No differences were found for the intensity and affective scales, although trends similar to the VAS and verbal scales were found. Perhaps more sensitive measures of the intensity and affective components of pain will help determine whether self-regulated heart rate changes during the cold pressor alter pain through arousal (affective) mechanisms or through actual sensory (intensity) threshold changes.

Correlational analysis indicated that changes in pain perception are associated with heart rate changes during the cold pressor in the veridical conditions, especially in Group I-I ($r = +.81$) and to a lesser extent Group D-D ($r = +.68$). Correlations also showed pain perception to relate to the magnitude of heart rate change during biofeedback training for Group I-I ($r = +.82$). Data from the groups given feedback opposite to instructions suggest that the pain perception effects are not a function of instructions per se (belief that heart rate is changing in the instructed direction). When instructions and feedback are opposite, pain ratings do not appear to depend on instructions or on heart rate changes observed during the cold-pressor test. Group D-I effectively reduced their heart rate response from the first to the second cold pressor by significantly slowing their respiration rate. However, Group D-I did not exhibit parallel changes in pain perception. A recent dissertation by J. D. Lane (1979) may provide an answer. Lane's dissertation showed that deliberately increasing or decreasing respiration rate during the cold pressor results in parallel increases and decreases in heart rate but does not affect pain perception. Thus, a subject may be able to voluntarily alter elicited heart rate responses in a variety of ways, but not all of these will necessarily result in associated behavioral or subjective changes.

The previous studies by Sirota et al. (1974, 1976) using a shock stimulus showed the importance of cardiac awareness in predicting changes in pain reports. This study, along with the Victor et al. (1978) study, used the cold-pressor test and failed to find a reliable relationship between cardiac awareness and pain. These results are perplexing but consistent, and possibly point to fundamental differences in the mechanisms underlying or mediating behavioral and subjective reactions to different laboratory stressors.

These data coupled with a previous pilot study reporting similar results (Reeves, Shapiro, & Cobb, 1979) suggest that a combination of veridical instructions and feedback is necessary for heart rate control during biofeedback and pain perception changes during cold-pressor stimulation. At least for the veridical conditions, heart rate changes during biofeedback may be related to changes in pain perception. Our previous research has not determined whether these heart rate and pain perception changes are a function of the subject's ability to actually control phasic heart rate during cold-pressor stress or whether the changes reflect a more tonic shift in heart rate reactivity following biofeedback training. The final study (Reeves & Shapiro, 1981) proposed to clarify this issue by giving veridical heart rate biofeedback for increasing (Group I) and decreasing (Group D) heart rate, and then testing heart rate reactivity and pain perception during cold-pressor stress. All procedures in this study were identical to the previous study (Reeves & Shapiro, in press) except subjects were specifically instructed not to alter their physiological reactions during the second cold-pressor stress—rather, they were to focus on accurately and honestly reporting their pain experiences. The results indicated that Group I increased their heart rate and Group D decreased their heart rate during biofeedback. Frontal EMG, but not skin conductance, showed a similar and reliable pattern. Both groups showed reliable reductions in heart rate, frontal EMG, and skin conductance from the first to the second anticipation and cold-pressor stress, with no reliable effects involving groups found. No group differences in pain ratings were found. Both groups showed a reliable increase in pain ratings on the second cold-pressor stress. These data suggested that single-session heart rate biofeedback training under resting conditions does not by itself alter subjects' heart rate reactivity to cold-pressor stress. The previously reported differential control of heart rate during cold-pressor stress probably reflects an acquired ability to alter phasic heart rate during cold-pressor stress and not simply an alteration in tonic reactivity related to an overall change in physiological arousal.

Finally, a recently completed study conducted by Greenberg (1981) provides further evidence regarding the functional significance of heart rate for perception of cold-pressor pain. This study employed the same experimental paradigm as Reeves and Shapiro (1981) except that feedback was given for systolic blood pressure rather than heart rate. A beat-to-beat tracking-cuff method of measuring blood pressure was used to provide feedback (Shapiro, Greenstadt, Lane, & Rubinstein, 1981). Two groups were run, an increase and a decrease blood pressure condition ($n = 10$ per group). The hypothesis that learned changes in blood pressure would be facilitated under stress conditions received partial support. Of interest to this discussion was the finding that heart rate varied along with blood pressure during the feedback trials, relatively increasing for the increase group and decreasing for the decrease group. In the final cold-pressor test, however, both groups showed a comparable decrease in heart rate as compared to their initial cold-pressor response. Thus, the specificity of blood pressure training effects, at least with respect to heart rate, did not become apparent until the subject was placed under the cold-pressor stress. Similar results were obtained in the Reeves and Shapiro (in press) study. That is, EMG and respiration tended to follow heart rate during bio-feedback trials, but during the final cold pressor only heart rate showed reliable changes in Groups I-I and D-D. As to pain perception, only one of six measures (reactivity) showed a significant effect (higher for the increase group). Assuming that the increase and decrease blood pressure instructions are comparable in their "emotional" implications to those used in the earlier heart rate research, these results lend support to the hypothesis that heart rate biofeedback (with appropriate instructions) may be critical to the repeatedly observed pain perception effects occurring after heart rate biofeedback training.

## DISCUSSION

This chapter has described a program of research on the use of biofeedback techniques to augment or reduce heart rate changes occurring in anticipation of aversive electrical stimulation or in response to the painful stimulation of the cold-pressor test. These laboratory stressors were chosen because they elicit relatively consistent increases in physiological and emotional arousal. The experiments were intended to provide a laboratory analogue of the behavioral control of pain, fear, and acute anxiety. Pain and fear are seen as complex patterns of physiological responses, overt actions, and various cognitive processes as indexed by verbal reports. The experiments attempted to demonstrate the utility of biofeedback methods as a means of selectively modifying physiological components of response to the two laboratory stressors and the effects of such modification on the individual's appraisal of the intensity or painfulness of the stimuli. The research was seen as a means of elucidating interactions between cognitive and physiological processes under conditions of stress and emotional arousal, and experiments were conducted in which the relative contributions of these two classes of events were evaluated.

The two sets of experiments described in this chapter involved control of heart rate in anticipation of electric shock and control of heart rate in response to the cold-pressor test. By and large, similar trends, and hypotheses for further study, emerged from the two kinds of experiments. The cold-pressor design appears to have certain advantages over the one used in the electric shock studies and is emphasized in this discussion. The design involved an initial assessment of the individual's physiological and subjective responses to the stressor prior to feedback training as well as a reassessment of the same responses after the intervening period of feedback training. During the training, instructions and feedback were manipulated independently. Moreover, with this design, feedback can be given for variables other than heart rate to examine the adaptive significance of one function over another in the control of perception of pain or in reports of fear or anxiety. This last strategy has not as yet been explored extensively in our research. The biofeedback training was carried out under nonstress conditions, and the aim was to determine whether the training could transfer effectively to the condition in which the stress was presented.

Now to summarize the major findings. There is no question that the heart rate acceleration normally associated with response to immersion of the hand in ice water can be potentiated by means of heart rate biofeedback training combined with appropriate instructions. For example, in Victor *et al.* (1978), the increase in heart rate after feedback training was almost three times greater than prior to training. Subjects not given such training and simply instructed to increase their heart rate during the ice water immersion also potentiated their heart rate response but to a much lesser degree. The same is true for similarly instructed subjects who were given prior heart rate decrease training (even though instructed to increase their heart rate) (Reeves & Shapiro, in press). Moreover, subjects given appropriate feedback training but instructed *not* to change their heart rate did not show an augmentation of their heart rate response (Reeves & Shapiro, 1981).

Evidence has also been presented that biofeedback training methods can be used to attenuate the heart rate response to ice water stress. It is not clear, however, that biofeedback offered any special advantage over simple instructions to reduce heart rate (Reeves & Shapiro, in press; Victor et al., 1978; see also Rupert & Holmes, 1978). Biofeedback is basically an active problem-solving procedure, involving information processing and presentations of stimuli and reinforcers which are arousing in and of themselves. In nondemanding conditions, heart rate may readily decelerate. Not trying actively to do anything or to achieve goals or rewards may be a good way to reduce physiological arousal. Subjects instructed to lower their heart rate during the cold-pressor test, even though they were given prior increase feedback training (without their explicit knowledge), seemed to be able to decelerate their heart rate (Reeves & Shapiro, in press). Subjects given either increase *or* decrease feedback training but instructed *not* to change their heart rate actually reduced their tonic heart rate, and to equivalent degrees, when given the cold water stimulation. Their phasic response to the stimulus was apparently not affected. Subjects given no special instructions (Victor et al., 1978), a no-treatment control, showed little or no change in their heart rate.

Thus, training with appropriate instructions and feedback can effectively transfer to a stress condition, providing the individual a means of augmenting or reducing his/her normal response to the stress. It requires an active attempt on the part of the individual to apply the skill learned from the prior training. It is clear that prior appropriate biofeedback training plus the use of the acquired skill can facilitate a potentiation of heart rate when the individual is put under stress. In the case of response attenuation, however, an active attempt to reduce heart rate may lead to the desired, result, regardless of the direction of prior feedback training. Such a reduction may be accomplished primarily through respiratory control, rather than being associated with a particular learned skill. Therefore, the experimental paradigm seems to offer an additional means of differentiating mediational processes involved in the voluntary control of physiological functions. This is supported by further evidence on the differential patterning of physiological changes that occurs during biofeedback training and during the stress-transfer trials.

Although biofeedback training appears to offer advantages over simply instructing subjects to alter their heart rate, various forms of relaxation, hypnosis, suggestion, meditation, and coping self-statements may also by effective in modifying physiological and emotional arousal

(Benson, 1975; Chaves & Barber, 1974; Davidson & Schwartz, 1976; Goleman & Schwartz, 1976; Grimm & Kanfer, 1976; Hilgard, 1977; Meichenbaum, 1977; Reeves, 1976). Biofeedback techniques are primarily oriented to selective control of specific individual responses, and it seems more likely that such specificity will evolve as a result of biofeedback training than from such other procedures. If we can determine which physiological systems in an individual are particularly relevant to physiological and emotional arousal under conditions of stress, then it may be possible to tailor the feedback procedure accordingly.

When we turn to the pain perception data, complex interrelationships of cognitions and physiological changes become evident. The strategy of altering a physiological component of the individual's reaction to a stressfull stimulus appears effective in altering reports of its painfulness. The perceptual effects depend on appropriate instructions as well as on the individual making a deliberate attempt to control his/her reactions on the basis of the instructions and prior feedback training. A reduction in tonic heart rate has no necessary consequence in and of itself for the individual's subjective response to stress, as is indicated by the results of Reeves and Shapiro (1981). The combination of appropriate instructions and veridical feedback is necessary for heart rate biofeedback training to exert a significant influence on pain perception.

One implication is that biofeedback or relaxation training for the purpose of reducing physiological arousal has no necessary effects on emotional reactions to stress or on anxiety (see Rupert & Holmes, 1978). Such decreased arousal has to be utilized by the individual as a deliberate and active coping skill, and the training has to be made directly relevant to the conditions eliciting the anxiety or emotionality.

Finally, comments are in order on the adaptive significance of heart rate for pain and stress reactivity. In general, we found some association between heart rate and subjective response to stress—increase associated with increased emotionality and decrease with decreased emotionality, especially when appropriate instructions and feedback were coupled. Additional research will have to be carried out comparing the effects of feedback training for other physiological variables. McCroskery and Engel (1981) reviewed related research concerning the effects of electromyographic and electroencephalographic biofeedback training as a means of coping with stress. The research to date has been inconclusive. The difficulties and complications that beset research in EMG and EEG biofeedback in relation to emotional behavior also concern the research we have described in this chapter. The significance of a biofeedback strategy for elucidating cognitive and emotional processes depends on knowledge of what physiological responses or patterns of responses are related to the particular psychological state and the reliability of such a relationship. Moreover, the target state or behavior has to be reliably assessed. The choice of heart rate in our work does not eliminate some of the complex issues of interpretation. Our research focused on heart rate increases associated with presentation of an aversive stimulus. But it is well known that heart rate also increases during mental effort, positive emotional behaviors, feeding, and exercise. The advantage of the strategy described in this chapter derives mainly from the choice of appropriate stimulus conditions that reliably elicit the target physiological change, the emphases on transferring training directly to the stress, and a suitable design for evaluating the physiological and subjective effects of the biofeedback training.

The demonstrated consequences of physiological change for emotional arousal are also consistent with peripheral conceptions of emotion derived from the James–Lange theory (Fehr & Stern, 1970; James, 1890). The finding that individual differences in cardiac awareness can be important in the obtained pain perception effects supports this interpretation. However, the degree to which individual differences in autonomic awareness plays a critical role in stress response requires further experimentation.

The importance of autonomic feedback is also reinforced by the common experience of an association between anxiety, fear, and other reactions to stress and an increase in heart rate or physiological arousal (see Harris & Katkin, 1975). The occurrence of such physiological arousal may serve as a cue for emotionality. In contrast, reduced heart rate or other autonomic deactivation may be less compatible with emotionality. Systematic desensitization is based on this relationship (Wolpe, 1958).

Biofeedback training for individually relevant physiological changes occurring in association with stressful stimuli has served as a behavioral strategy for changing anxiety and fear reactions. Several reports of clinical research have appeared which utilize these kinds of procedures (Blanchard & Abel, 1976; Gatchel & Proctor, 1976; Nunes & Marks, 1975; Prigatano & Johnson, 1972). More recent systematic research on the use of heart rate biofeedback in reducing anxiety suggests that expectancies and other nonspecific placebo effects probably have a major influence on the therapeutic benefits obtained with these methods (see Gatchel, 1979). The research described in this chapter has only touched upon the many complex issues that may be involved in clinical situations. Moreover, it is difficult to generalize from the reported laboratory research on physical stressors to situations involving psychological stressors or clinical pain. Nonetheless, this research provides some systematic experimental support for further research on and clinical applications of the use of biofeedback in the management of stress reactions. The research calls attention to the importance of appropriate instructions, the need to bring the critical environmental stimuli into the therapeutic situation, the significance of developing an active coping skill to facilitate transfer of training, and the potential role of individual differences in autonomic awareness in bringing about desired benefits. Hopefully, the methods and research findings described in this chapter will lead to further productive basic research on the psychophysiology of stress, pain, and anxiety, and to more effective clinical approaches to their management.

## ACKNOWLEDGMENTS

This research was supported by National Institute of Mental Health Research Grant MH26923; Office of Naval Research Contract N00014-75-C-0150, NR201-152; National Institute of Mental Health NRSA Institutional Grant MH14646; and Neuropsychiatric Institute Biomedical Research Support Grant RR5756. Computing assistance was provided by the Office of Academic Computing, UCLA.

## REFERENCES

Ainslie, G. W., & Engel, B. T. Alteration of classically conditioned heart rate by operant reinforcement in monkeys. *Journal of Comparative and Physiological Psychology*, 1974, *87*, 373–382.

Benson, H. *The relaxation response*. New York: William Morrow, 1975.

Black, A. H., Cott, A., & Pavloski, R. The operant learning theory approach to biofeedback training. In G. E. Schwartz & J. Beatty (Eds.), *Biofeedback: Theory and research*. New York: Academic Press, 1977.

Blanchard, E. B., & Abel, G. G. An experimental case study of the biofeedback treatment of a rape-induced psychophysiological disorder. *Behavior Therapy*, 1976, *7*, 113–119.

Borkovec, T. D. Physiological and cognitive processes in the regulation of anxiety. In G. E. Schwartz & D. Shapiro (Eds.), *Consciousness and self-regulation: Advances in research* (Vol. 1). New York: Plenum Press, 1976.

Brener, J., & Hothersall, D. Heart rate control under conditions of augmented sensory feedback. *Psychophysiology*, 1966, *3*, 23–28.

Chaves, J. F., & Barber, T. X. Cognitive strategies, experimenter modeling, and expectation in the attenuation of pain. *Journal of Abnormal Psychology*, 1974, *83*, 356–363.

Davidson, R. J., & Schwartz, G. E. The psychobiology of relaxation and related states: A multi-process theory. In D. I. Mostofsky (Ed.), *Behavior control and modification of physiological activity.* Englewood Cliffs, N.J.: Prentice-Hall, 1976.

DeGood, D. E., & Adams, A. S., Jr. Control of cardiac responses under aversive stimulation. *Biofeedback and Self-Regulation,* 1976, *1*, 373-385.

DiCara, L. V., & Weiss, J. M. Effect of heart-rate learning under curare on subsequent non-curarized avoidance learning. *Journal of Comparative and Physiological Psychology,* 1969, *69*, 368-374.

Engel, B. T., & Hansen, S. P. Operant conditioning of heart rate slowing. *Psychophysiology,* 1966, *3*, 176-187.

Fehr, F. S., & Stern, J. A. Peripheral physiological variables and emotion: The James-Lange theory revisited. *Psychological Bulletin,* 1970, *74*, 411-424.

Gatchel, R. J. Biofeedback and the treatment of fear and anxiety. In R. J. Gatchel & K. P. Price (Eds.), *Clinical applications in biofeedback.* New York: Pergamon Press, 1979.

Gatchel, R. J., & Price, K. P. (Eds.). *Clinical applications in biofeedback.* New York: Pergamon Press, 1979.

Gatchel, R. J., & Proctor, J. D. Effectiveness of voluntary heart rate control in reducing speech anxiety. *Journal of Consulting and Clinical Psychology,* 1976, *44*, 381-389.

Goleman, D. J., & Schwartz, G. E. Meditation as an intervention in stress reactivity. *Journal of Consulting and Clinical Psychology,* 1976, *44*, 456-466.

Gracely, R. H., McGrath, P., & Dubner, R. Ratio scales of sensory and affective verbal pain descriptors. *Pain,* 1976, *2*, 19-29.

Greenberg, W. Unpublished study, University of California-Los Angeles, 1981.

Grimm, L., & Kanfer, F. H. Tolerance of aversive stimulation. *Behavior Therapy,* 1976, *7*, 593-601.

Grings, W. W., & Carlin, S. Instrumental modification of autonomic behavior. *The Psychological Record,* 1966, *16*, 153-159.

Harris, V. A., & Katkin, E. S. Primary and secondary emotional behavior: An analysis of the role of autonomic feedback on affect, arousal, and attribution. *Psychological Bulletin,* 1975, *82*, 904-916.

Hilgard, E. R. The alleviation of pain by hypnosis. *Pain,* 1975, *1*, 213-231.

Hilgard, E. R. *Divided consciousness: Multiple controls in human thought and action.* New York: Wiley-Interscience, 1977.

Hilgard, E. R., Morgan, A. H., Lange, A. F., Lenox, J. R., Macdonald, H., Marshall, G. D., & Sachs, L. B. Heart rate changes in pain and hypnosis. *Psychophysiology,* 1974, *11*, 692-702.

Holmes, D. S., & Frost, R. O. Effects of false heart rate feedback on self-reported anxiety, pain perception and pulse rate. *Behavior Therapy,* 1976, *7*, 330-334.

James, W. *The principles of psychology.* New York: Holt, Rinehart, & Winston, 1890.

Kimmel, H. D., & Baxter, R. Avoidance conditioning of the GSR. *Journal of Experimental Psychology,* 1964, *68*, 482-485.

Kimmel, H. D., Pendergrass, V. E., & Kimmel, E. B. Modifying children's orienting reactions instrumentally. *Conditional Reflex,* 1967, *2*, 227-235.

Lane, J. D. *The effects of self-control of respiration upon experimental pain.* Unpublished doctoral dissertation, University of California-Los Angeles, 1979.

Lang, P. J. Learned control of human heart rate in a computer directed environment. In P. A. Obrist, A. H. Black, J. Brener, & L. V. DiCara (Eds.), *Cardiovascular psychophysiology.* Chicago: Aldine, 1974.

Lang, P. J., Melamed, B. G., & Hart, J. A psychophysiological analysis of fear modification using an automated desensitization procedure. *Journal of Abnormal Psychology*, 1970, *76*, 220-234.

Lang, P. J., Rice, D. G., & Sternbach, R. A. The psychophysiology of emotion. In N. S. Greenfield & R. A. Sternbach (Eds.), *Handbook of psychophysiology*. New York: Holt, Rinehart, & Winston, 1972.

Lovallo, W. The cold pressor test and autonomic function: A review and integration. *Psychophysiology*, 1975, *12*, 268-282.

Mandler, G., Mandler, J. M., & Uviller, E. T. Autonomic feedback: The perception of autonomic activity. *Journal of Abnormal and Social Psychology*, 1958, *56*, 367-373.

McCroskery, J. H., & Engel, B. T. Biofeedback and emotional behavior. In M. Christie & P. Mellett (Eds.), *Psychosomatic approaches in medicine* (Vol 1: *Behavioral approaches*). Chichester, England: John Wiley & Sons, 1981.

Meichenbaum, D. H. *Cognitive-behavior modification: An integrative approach*. New York: Plenum Press, 1977.

Nunes, J. S., & Marks, I. M. Feedback of true heart rate during exposure in vivo. *Archives of General Psychiatry*, 1975, *32*, 933-936.

Prigatano, G. P., & Johnson, H. J. Biofeedback control of heart rate variability to phobic stimuli: A new approach to treating spider phobia. In *Proceedings, 80th Annual Convention, APA, 1972*. Washington, D.C.: American Psychological Association, 1972.

Reeves, J. L. EMG-biofeedback reduction of tension headache: A cognitive skills training approach. *Biofeedback and Self-Regulation*, 1976, *1*, 216-225.

Reeves, J. L., & Shapiro, D. Heart rate reactivity to cold pressor stress following biofeedback training. *Psychophysiology*, 1981, *18*, 154. (Abstract)

Reeves, J. L., & Shapiro, D. Heart rate biofeedback and cold pressor pain. *Psychophysiology*, in press.

Reeves, J. L., Shapiro, D., & Cobb, L. F. Relative influences of heart rate biofeedback and instructional set in the perception of cold pressor pain. In N. Birbaumer & H. D. Kimmel (Eds.), *Biofeedback and self-regulation*. Hillsdale, N.J.: Erlbaum, 1979.

Rupert, P. A., & Holmes, D. S. Effects of multiple sessions of true and placebo heart rate biofeedback training on the heart rates and anxiety levels of anxious patients during and following treatment. *Psychophysiology*, 1978, *15*, 582-590.

Scott, J., & Huskisson, E. C. Graphic representation of pain. *Pain*, 1976, *2*, 175-184.

Shapiro, D. A monologue on biofeedback and psychophysiology. *Psychophysiology*, 1977, *14*, 213-227.

Shapiro, D. Theory of operant learning and biofeedback. In A. Agnoli, R. Anchisi, & A. Tamburello (Eds.), *Il biofeedback in neuropsichiatrica e medicina psicosomatica*. Rome: Centro Italiano Congressi, 1980. (In Italian)

Shapiro, D., Greenstadt, L., Lane, J. D., & Rubinstein, E. Tracking-cuff system for beat-to-beat recording of blood pressure. *Psychophysiology*, 1981, *18*, 129-136.

Shapiro, D., Schwartz, G. E., Nelson, S., Shnidman, S., & Silverman, S. Operant control of fear-related electrodermal responses in snake phobic subjects. *Psychophysiology*, 1972, *9*, 271. (Abstract)

Shapiro, D., Tursky, B., & Schwartz, G. E. Differentiation of heart rate and systolic blood pressure in man by operant conditioning. *Psychosomatic Medicine*, 1970, *32*, 417-423.

Shnidman, S. R. Avoidance conditioning of skin potential responses. *Psychophysiology*, 1969, *6*, 38-44.

Shnidman, S. R. Instrumental conditioning of orienting responses using positive reinforcement. *Journal of Experimental Psychology*, 1970, *83*, 491-494.

Shnidman, S., & Shapiro, D. Instrumental modification of elicited autonomic responses. *Psychophysiology*, 1971, *7*, 395–401.

Sirota, A. D. *Heart rate feedback and instructional effects on subjective reaction to aversive stimuli.* Unpublished doctoral dissertation, Pennsylvania State University, 1976.

Sirota, A. D., Schwartz, G. E., & Shapiro, D. Voluntary control of human heart rate: Effect on reaction to aversive stimulation. *Journal of Abnormal Psychology*, 1974, *83*, 261–267.

Sirota, A. D., Schwartz, G. E., & Shapiro, D. Voluntary control of human heart rate: Effect on reaction to aversive stimulation: A replication and extension. *Journal of Abnormal Psychology*, 1976, *85*, 473–477.

Tyrer, P. *The role of bodily feelings in anxiety.* London: Oxford University Press, 1976.

Valins, S., & Ray, A. A. Effects of cognitive desensitization on avoidance behavior. *Journal of Personality and Social Psychology*, 1967, *7*, 345–350.

Victor, R., Mainardi, J. A., & Shapiro, D. Effect of biofeedback and voluntary control procedures on heart rate and perception of pain during the cold pressor test. *Psychosomatic Medicine*, 1978, *40*, 216–225.

Wolpe, J. *Psychotherapy by reciprocal inhibition.* Stanford, Calif.: Stanford University Press, 1958.

# 5

# *A Biosocial Model of Attitude Change*

JOHN. T. CACIOPPO

RICHARD E. PETTY

## INTRODUCTION

The field of social psychology deals with the manner in which a person's feelings, verbalizations, and behaviors are influenced by the presence, characteristics, and behavior of other people. Social psychologists have become increasingly interested in psychophysiology because, though social psychology has traditionally focused on the influence of situational factors (e.g., Bem, 1972), a person's bodily responses have been found to be an important determinant of social behavior (cf. Cacioppo & Petty, in press; Schwartz & Shapiro, 1973; Shapiro & Crider, 1969; Shapiro & Schwartz, 1970). This interdisciplinary focus has already led to advances in the areas of aggression (e.g., Zillmann, Johnson, & Day, 1974), emotions (Schachter & Singer, 1962), cognitive dissonance (Kiesler & Pallak, 1976), social facilitation (Geen & Gange, 1977), attitude assessment (Cacioppo &

John T. Cacioppo. Department of Psychology, The University of Iowa, Iowa City, Iowa.

Richard E. Petty. Department of Psychology, The University of Missouri, Columbia, Missouri.

Petty, 1979a; Cacioppo & Sandman, 1981), sexual arousal (e.g., Cantor, Zillmann, & Bryant, 1975; Kelley & Byrne, in press), and competitive decision making (Blascovich, Nash, & Ginsburg, 1978).

A variety of physiological responses have been monitored in these studies, including the measurement of electrodermal (EDA) (cf. Schwartz & Shapiro, 1973), electromyographic (cf. Cacioppo & Petty, 1981a), pupillographic (e.g., Collins, Ellsworth, & Helmreich, 1967), and differential hemispheric alpha activity (Cacioppo, Petty, & Snyder, 1979). Nevertheless, the measurement of responses arising from the cardiovascular system has tended to be the focus of the initial and the preponderance of contemporary social psychophysiological investigations (e.g., heart rate [HR]— Buckhout, 1966; Cacioppo, Sandman, & Walker, 1978; blood pressure [BP]—Cantor et al., 1975; vasomotor activity [VA]—Acker & Edwards, 1964; Gerard, 1967; body temperature [BT]—Dabbs & Moorer, 1975). In addition, cardiovascular measures have been used (along with EDA) to gauge the extent of physiological arousal (e.g., Lazarus, 1966; Mewborn & Rogers, 1979; cf. J. I. Lacey, 1967); HR has commonly been "manipulated" bogusly to assess the role of cognitive factors per se in the modification of feelings (e.g., Valins, 1966); and HR has been manipulated exogenously and without the subject's awareness to examine the role of actual (but unperceived), momentary, and specific HR changes in intellective performance and attitude change (Cacioppo, 1979).

## BODILY RESPONSES AND ATTITUDE CHANGE

In this chapter we consider the contributions of cardiovascular psychophysiology to the study of attitudes in social psychology. Attitudes are people's general and enduring likes and dislikes of objects and issues. Gordon Allport (1935) stated in the first edition of the *Handbook of Social Psychology* that attitude is "the most distinctive and indispensable concept in contemporary social psychology" (p. 798). As we shall demonstrate in this chapter, principles and measurements from cardiovascular psychophysiology have contributed greatly to the present understanding of the influence of bodily responses on attitudes specifically and on social behavior generally.

There is a strong precedent for focusing on the cardiovascular system when studying people's likes and dislikes about objects and issues. A century ago Carl Lange contended:

We owe all the emotional side of our mental life, our joys and sorrows, our happy and unhappy hours, to our vasomotor system. If the impressions which fall upon our senses did not possess the power of stimulating it, we would wander through life unsympathetic and passionless, all impressions of the outer world would only enrich our experience, increase our knowledge, but would arouse neither joy nor anger, would give us neither care not fear. (in Dunlap, 1922, p. 73)

Similarly, William James (1890) stated:

If one should seek to name each particular emotion of which the human heart is the seat, it is plain that the limit to their number would lie in the introspective vocabulary of the seeker. (p. 485)

Although the specific hypothesis advanced by James and Lange that various emotions arise from the elicitation and perception of distinctive patterns of somatovisceral activity has been challenged seriously (e.g., Cannon, 1927; Schachter & Singer, 1962), it is interesting to note that the language people use daily to describe their feelings of liking and disliking hints that there at least are *accompanying* bodily responses. People sometimes describe their positive feelings toward someone or something as being "warm" or "hot," whereas they sometimes describe their negative feelings as being "cool" or "cold."[1]

In this chapter we refer more often to the concept of affect, or nonspecific *feelings* of liking/disliking typically accompanied by bodily responses, than to the concept of emotion, which covers a much wider

1. Pennebaker (1979) has reported evidence in four studies that distinctive constellations of perceived sensory changes are used to describe/identify specific emotional states. For instance, the sensations of pressure in the head, tightness in the jaw, and tense muscles were used to describe anger; whereas light headedness, the absence of a queasy stomach, no pressure in the head, no tension in the stomach, and no tightness in the jaw were the sensations used by subjects to describe joy. What is not clear from these data is whether these descriptions are characterized by actual constellations of physiological changes, whether they are the result of actually perceived sensory changes, or whether they are the consequence of social learning regarding what specific emotional states "should" feel like or be described as. Surprisingly little is known about the relationship between actual and perceived physiological changes (cf. Mackay, 1980; Mandler, Mandler, & Uviller, 1958; Shields & Stern, 1979). Generally, verbal and autonomic measures converge following rather dramatic environmental events, such as exposures to frightening films (Lang, 1971; Lazarus, Averill, & Opton, 1970; Mewborn & Rogers, 1979), but dissociate soon afterward, with perceptions of physiological arousal subsiding prior to the return to basal levels of physiological indices (e.g., HR, systolic blood pressure—cf. Cacioppo & Petty, in press; Zillmann, 1978).

spectrum of behavior and experience and which subsumes the dimension of affect.[2] The approach here is based on the fact that the concepts of attitude and affect have been equated by some (e.g., Fishbein & Ajzen, 1975; Thurstone, 1931) and are considered to be related closely by most social psychologists (e.g., Cacioppo, Harkins, & Petty, 1981; Oskamp, 1977; Triandis, 1971). A brief discussion should clarify the relationship between these concepts.

First, attitude development and change are thought to involve the arousal of new positive or negative *feelings* about the attitude object or issue. Hence, we might say that affect is involved during the development or change of an attitude (cf. Norman, 1976; Ostrom, 1969). But consider a person whose attitude toward some object was developed long ago and has not undergone change recently (e.g., an attitude toward an old, favorite movie). It is conceivable that should this person be asked to indicate his/her attitude toward the object, the person would recall his/her previous *evaluation* of the object. The person might even recall that he/she had felt a noticeable liking or disliking for the object long ago, but this memory could be accessed without the person experiencing the feelings at the moment (see Harris & Katkin, 1975, for a similar distinction between primary and secondary emotions). In instances such as this, the attitude is akin to a general belief of one's evaluation of the object. Furthermore, since (1) attitudes are typically defined as relatively enduring favorable or unfavorable reactions to a stimulus, (2) people hold many attitudes simultaneously (which they must in this complex world if attitudes endure), and (3) people cannot possibly maintain as many feelings (affects) simultaneously as they retain attitudes, it seems reasonable that attitudes are maintained in the form of general beliefs (or memories) of one's evaluations of and affective reactions to objects rather than in the form of affective reactions per se.

One interesting implication of this distinction is that psychophysiological assessments of an existing attitude that are designed to tap the

2. For instance, Willhelm Wundt (1905; see Mackay, 1980) proposed a three-dimensional theory of emotion based upon introspective reports. Wundt postulated that emotional states could be characterized along the dimensions of pleasantness–unpleasantness, aroused–subdued, and tense–relaxed. Harlow and Stagner (1933) proposed four dimensions (pleasure, unpleasantness, excitement, and depression), which Stagner (1948) subsequently collapsed to form two dimensions of emotional experience (pleasantness–unpleasantness and excitement–depression). The dimension of positive–negative feelings (i.e., pleasantness–unpleasantness) continues to play a major role in theories of emotion (cf. Grings & Dawson, 1978; Izard, 1976; Strongman, 1973).

affective "roots" of the attitude will generally be insensitive. The evidence to date seems to support this implication (cf. Cacioppo & Sandman, 1981). A second point is that attitude development and change (but less so, attitudes per se) should involve affective reactions. Hence, the present view concerns primarily studies of bodily responses and *attitude change.* We have categorized the studies on bodily responses and attitude change as follows: (1) physiological responses that are detected internally (symptoms), (2) physiological responses that are detected externally (signs), and (3) physiological responses that are undetected.

## SYMPTOMS, SIGNS, AND UNDETECTED RESPONSES

Before proceeding to a discussion of bodily responses and attitude change, we should comment briefly on the nature of this tripartite. The tripartite of symptoms, signs, and undetected bodily responses was developed to serve as a heuristic following our initial review of the literature on bodily responses and attitude change. Subsequently, we found that this tripartite has much in common with the gross distinctions made among bodily responses in applied pathologic physiology. In their textbook in this area, MacBryde and Blacklow (1970) note that:

> The word *symptom* is used to name any manifestation of disease. Strictly speaking, symptoms are subjective, apparent only to the affected person. *Signs* are detectable by another person and sometimes by the patient himself. . . . Some phenomena, like fever, are both signs and symptoms. (p. 1)

In our tripartite, signs and symptoms are partially overlapping categories of physiological responding, whereas these categories do not overlap with undetected physiological responses. Symptoms refer to the subjective component of a physiological reaction (whether that reaction be constituted by changes in a single system or multiple effector systems), but the physiological reaction need not refer to a manifestation of disease. Hence, our use of the term "symptom" is compatible with, but more general than, that characterizing the field of applied pathologic physiology. "Signs" in the present tripartite refer to the objective component of a physiological reaction that the affected person detects him/herself. Thus, signs are physiological reactions that are verifiable by others and about which the person learns through an objective procedure, perhaps with the aid of sophisticated instrumentation. Signs differ from symptoms in that the former are open to public verification or disconfirmation, whereas the latter are not. Signs differ from *undetected* physiological responses, not in each's potential for being quantified, but rather in the person's awareness that a change in physiological functioning has occurred. For instance, a slight speeding of the heart beat might be detected by an investigator using an electrocardiogram but go undetected by the individual whose heart rate is being monitored. This response would be termed an "undetected response." If the investigator provided feedback to the individual about his/her heart rate, however, then the physiological response would act as a sign to the individual even if the feedback were unveridical. Finally, if the individual felt a "speeding" of his/her heart beat, possibly because of its association with a concomitant increase in stroke volume, then the feeling of a speeding heart beat would serve as a symptom even if this perception were inaccurate. In the following sections we elaborate upon these distinctions and relate symptoms, signs, and undetected responses to processes underlying attitude change.

SYMPTOMS: PHYSIOLOGICAL RESPONSES
THAT ARE DETECTED INTERNALLY

People are aware of sensory changes in both their internal and the external environment. Included under the heading "symptoms: physiological responses that are detected internally" are experiments in which subjects report perceiving sensorial changes arising from within their own bodies, such as changes in pulse pressure or beat, or changes in feelings of overall arousal. As Mackay (1980) has noted, the physiological basis of these perceptions tends to militate against the accurate identification of their organic source. For instance, visceral perception derives from four different subtypes of receptors (mechanoreceptors, chemoreceptors, osmoreceptors, and thermoreceptors) that monitor the state of the *milieu intérieur*. Although the visceral afferent system is not grossly different from other afferent systems (Newman, 1974), the cortical projection areas tend to be small and nonspecific with respect to topography and function (Brener & Jones, 1974; Van Toller, 1979). Mackay (1980) further noted that proprioceptive receptors—which monitor the striate musculature, tendons, joints, and nonauditory parts of the inner ear—provide gross information about posture, balance, and movement, while providing somewhat more specific information about controlled (skilled) movements. Together, these factors act against accurate identifications of the source of visceral activity (see also Footnote 1).

SIGNS: PHYSIOLOGICAL RESPONSES
THAT ARE DETECTED EXTERNALLY

Included in this category are studies in which subjects obtain information (usually bogus) through exteroceptive channels regarding the status of their bodies' reactions to a stimulus. These "bodily reactions" generally come as a "discovery"—such as finding one's heart rate increased by viewing a feedback display when the name of an acquaintance was mentioned—rather than as a sensation that feels as if it derived from within the body.

PHYSIOLOGICAL RESPONSES THAT ARE UNDETECTED

Of course, a further distinction can be drawn between bodily responses that are detected (by whatever means and whether real or not) and those that influence phenomenological reactions but are themselves not detected. The few studies that deal with the effects of actual but undetected changes in heart rate on people's thoughts and feelings toward stimuli are discussed in the section headed "physiological responses that are undetected."

When the existing research on attitude development and change is examined in light of these categories, there emerges a fairly clear pattern of results that suggests the mechanism by which each type of bodily response (i.e., detected interoceptively, detected exteroceptively, undetected) influences attitude change. Furthermore, likely interrelationships among these mechanisms are revealed.

SYMPTOMS: PHYSIOLOGICAL RESPONSES
THAT ARE DETECTED INTERNALLY

Most of the research on bodily responses and attitude change falls under the first of the tripartite: bodily reactions that are "felt." This includes studies on emotional plasticity (e.g., Marshall & Zimbardo, 1979; Schachter, 1971), studies on cognitive dissonance, its phenomenology (Cooper, Fazio, & Rhodewalt, 1978; Cooper, Zanna, & Taves, 1978; Higgins, Rhodewalt, & Zanna, 1979; Rhodewalt & Comer, 1979) and its domain Fazio, & Rhodewalt, 1978; Cooper, Zanna, & Taves, 1978; Higgins, & Greenwald, 1979), and research on self-attention (e.g., Scheier & Carver, 1977; Scheier, Carver, & Matthews, in press).

## EMOTIONAL PLASTICITY

Schachter and Singer (1962) argued that regardless of the nature of the causal relationships between cognitive and physiological factors in naturally occurring emotional states, these links are not necessary for the initiation of emotional states. According to Schachter and Singer, the sensation of physiological arousal, if unaccounted for, creates an "evaluative need" and initiates an active search for cognitive sources that could plausibly be the cause of, and provide a verbal label for, the experienced bodily state. That is, what begins as ambiguous signals from the body can be transformed into strong feelings or, more specifically still, emotional experiences with the addition of an appropriate situational label (i.e., a cue that provides a plausible causal link between the bodily experience, which is presumably the consequence of actual physiological responses, and a specific emotional state).

Schachter and Singer (1962) tested their theory by injecting subjects with a small amount of epinephrine. Some subjects knew that the injection would make them aroused, whereas others did not. Each subject then was placed in a room with another person, who was a confederate of the experimenter, and both were asked to complete questionnaires. Just about the time that the drug began to take effect, the confederate began acting as if filling out the questionnaire had made him/her either very angry or very euphoric. Schachter and Singer expected that the subjects who knew their arousal was due to the injection would not be affected greatly by the situational cues (i.e., the confederate's behavior). Conversely, subjects who experienced unexplained arousal were expected to use the situational cues to determine a verbal label for what they were feeling. Consistent with this reasoning, subjects who were paired with the "angry" confederate believed themselves to be more angry when they did not know the injection would cause arousal than when they did know the injection had caused their felt arousal.

Contrary to Schachter and Singer's expectations, though, whether or not subjects knew in advance that the injection would cause them to feel aroused did not especially affect them if they were paired with the "euphoric" confederate. This latter result suggests that a sudden onset of unexplained arousal may not be experienced as neutral but rather as a distressful or apprehensive bodily state (cf. Maslach, 1979). This point has been the topic of debate (Marshall & Zimbardo, 1979; Maslach, 1979; Schachter & Singer, 1979), but Schachter and Singer's formulation has nevertheless been important in drawing attention to the influence of attributional processes on people's feelings and emotions.

COGNITIVE DISSONANCE

The research on cognitive dissonance builds upon this earlier research and specifies conditions under which people change their attitudes as a result of experiencing unpleasant bodily sensations.

According to Leon Festinger (1957), two elements of information (cognitions) are dissonant when knowing one suggests the opposite of the other to an individual (see also, Aronson, 1969). More recently, researchers have specified dissonance as being aroused when people accept personal responsibility for an action that leads to negative consequences that were either foreseeable or could have been foreseeable (i.e., retrospective foreseeability—see recent reviews by Cialdini, Petty, & Cacioppo, 1981; Wicklund & Brehm, 1976).

Festinger (1957, p. 3) described dissonance as a motivational tension that is unpleasant. This description points to three dimensions along which dissonance might be characterized: the physiological, phenomenological, and motivational. The physiological effects of dissonance are not very well understood yet. Gerard (1967) found that the dissonance created by deciding between two attractive alternatives leads to a constriction of the blood vessels in the hand, a response typically indicative of the activation of the sympathetic nervous system (SNS). Quanty and Becker (1974) monitored skin conductance while subjects anticipated painful electric shocks. In an induced-compliance paradigm, half of the subjects were given the perception that they freely chose to incur the painful electric shocks (high-dissonance-arousal condition), whereas half were given no choice whatsoever but to endure the electric shocks (low-dissonance-arousal condition). Quanty and Becker found that the subjects in the high-dissonance group exhibited greater skin conductance following their decision than the subjects in the low-dissonance group. On the basis of this sparse evidence, we tentatively suggest that cognitive dissonance is accompanied by increased SNS activity, though it is possible too that the specific pattern of physiological effects depends at least in part upon the individual and upon the procedures used to arouse cognitive dissonance (cf. J. I. Lacey, 1967; J. I. Lacey & Lacey, 1958).

Research on the motivational properties of cognitive dissonance indicates that dissonance arousal is associated with a drive-like behavioral state. In a review of the literature, Kiesler and Pallak (1976) pointed out that dissonance tends to enhance the performance of simple tasks (e.g., noncompetitive paired-associate learning), whereas it tends to damage the performance of complex tasks (e.g., competitive paired-associate learning). These observations, too, are consistent with the notion that cognitive dissonance enhances SNS activity since they are congruent with the known effects of SNS arousal on simple and complex task performance.

How does cognitive dissonance *feel* to a person? A number of procedures have been used to examine the phenomenology of dissonance. These procedures range from asking people to describe how they feel after dissonance induction (Shaffer, 1975) to assessing people's misattribution of dissonance to drug-induced states (Cooper, Zanna, & Taves, 1978). The most common procedure involves the subject ingesting a placebo that he/she believes has specific (experimenter-specified) side effects. This misattribution procedure is based upon the principle that people search for causes of an unexplained internal state, such as a sudden feeling of tension or arousal. In their search, people consider external as well as internal causes and sometimes misattribute the true cause of a felt bodily state (e.g., increased SNS activity caused by cognitive dissonance) to something that seems to be a reasonable cause at the time (e.g., a pill they recently ingested). Of course, only when a stimulus can have the same effects on a person as he/she is experiencing at the moment can misattribution occur. The nature of the internal state that the people are experiencing, therefore, can be inferred indirectly by determining the type of stimuli that elicits misattribution. Thus, in the misattribution paradigm, subjects are either exposed or not to treatments that are believed to arouse cognitive dissonance and are either exposed or not to a possible external cause for their felt internal sensations.

Zanna and Cooper (1974) were the first to employ the misattribution procedure to study how dissonance felt to people. Zanna and Cooper gave people a drug to ingest and told them that the experiment concerned the effects of the drug on learning. Some subjects were told that the drug had no side effects, others were told that it might cause them to feel tense, and still others were told that it might cause them to feel relaxed. Finally, subjects were told that any side effects would occur quickly, though the effects of the drug on learning would not occur for some time. Subjects were asked to assist the experimenter in another study to allow time for the drug to take full effect. The "other study" involved the subject writing a counterattitudinal message under either choice (high-dissonance) or no-choice (low-dissonance) conditions.

Zanna and Cooper had in fact given all of the subjects a placebo—a pill made of milk powder, which had absolutely no side effects. If dissonance caused the subjects to feel tense, then only the group of subjects who believed the pill might cause them to feel tense *and who chose* to write the counterattitudinal essay (i.e., in the high-dissonance group) would be in a position to misattribute the felt internal sensations induced by cognitive dissonance to the pill. Typically, subjects who engage in attitude-discrepant behavior under conditions of high choice are forced to realign their attitudes with their dissonant behavior to reduce the dissonance (e.g., Linder, Cooper, & Jones, 1967). But if subjects misattribute the dissonance-created feelings to the pill, then they should show no attitude change since they no longer have responsibility for doing anything about these feelings. These subjects, by their misattribution, have decided that the tension has been induced externally (i.e., by the pill) and is only temporary. Hence the subjects in the high-dissonance conditions who believe the pill may cause them to feel tense should show no attitude change. The results of Zanna and Cooper's study, which are presented in Figure 5-1, are consistent with this reasoning. They concluded that dissonance felt something like "tension."

Several subsequent studies using similar misattribution procedures were taken as evidence that cognitive dissonance felt "arousing" (e.g., Cooper, Fazio, & Rhodewalt, 1978; Cooper, Zanna, & Taves, 1978; cf. Zanna & Cooper, 1976), but the results of the studies could be explained as parsimoniously by the proposition that dissonance simply felt "unpleasant." Higgins *et al.* (1979) conducted a study to determine which, or if both, of these phenomenological reactions characterized a dissonant cognitive state. The study was similar to Zanna and Cooper's (1974), but this time subjects were told that the pill might cause them to feel "unpleasantly sedated" (unaroused–unpleasant), "relaxed" (unaroused–pleas-

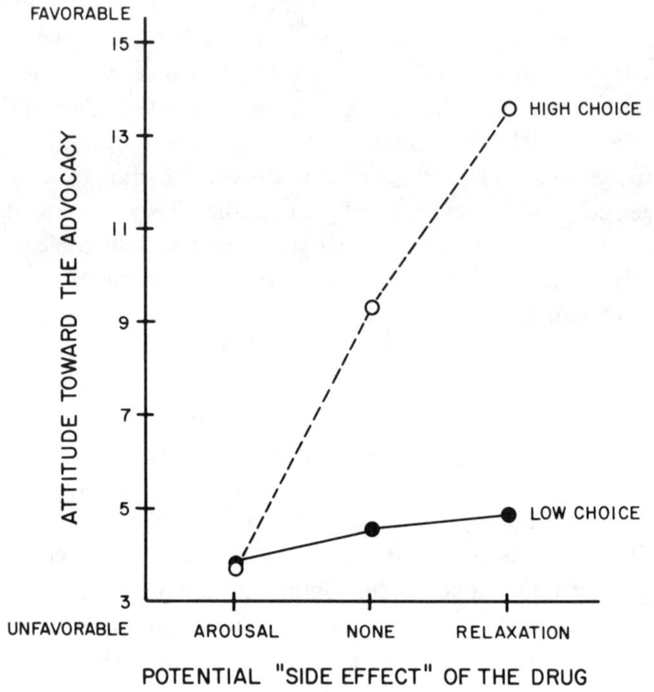

FIG. 5-1. Mean of subjects' attitudes toward banning speakers on campus as a function of decisional freedom and potential side effect of the drug. Adapted from "Dissonance and the Pill," by M. P. Zanna and J. Cooper, *Journal of Personality and Social Psychology,* 1974, *29,* 703–709. Used with permission.

ant), "tense" (aroused–unpleasant), "pleasantly excited" (aroused–pleasant), or nothing in particular (no-side-effects control group). These subjects voluntarily wrote a counterattitudinal message while supposedly waiting for the pill to take full effect.

The results are presented in Table 5-1. Higgins *et al.* (1979), like Zanna and Cooper (1974), found that a pill (a placebo) with the possible side effect of making the person feel "tense" lessened attitude change. More importantly, however, they found that a pill described as possibly causing a feeling of unpleasant sedation blocked attitude change even more completely. Overall, the characteristic of felt unpleasantness was more effective in eliciting the misattribution of dissonance to the pill than was the characteristic of felt arousal (see also Comer & Rhodewalt, 1979; Rhodewalt & Comer, 1979). Of course, there may be large discrepancies between the fact and the phenomenology of one's bodily reactions. Cognitive dissonance, for instance, may have sympathetic-like physiological effects but not *feel* "arousing."

There are important implications of these data for the role of bodily processes in the arousal of affect and the modification of attitudes. As we noted, Schachter and Singer (1962) suggested that emotional states result from a combination of neutral and unexplained physiological arousal, and a cognitive labeling process, which involves the person searching his/her situation for information that might help identify the cause and significance of the felt physiological reactions. Maslach (1979) and Marshall and Zimbardo (1979) recently have questioned Schachter and Singer's model and have suggested that an unexpected surge of autonomic activity, such as that induced by an injection of epinephrine, is perceived as being unpleasant rather than neutral. Hence, they suggested, there is a *negative biasing* in subjects' search for information and in their deductions regarding the meaning of their felt bodily reactions. The literature on cognitive dissonance supports the notions that bodily responses can feel unpleasant and thereby limit the inferences that are deemed as plausible causes (cf. Fries & Frey, 1980).

SELF-ATTENTION

It seems reasonable that physiological responses can feel pleasant as well as unpleasant, that they can vary in terms of the initial availability of verbal labels for them, and that positive rather than negative biasing of the labeling process can ensue when unexpected but pleasurable sensa-

TABLE 5-1. Mean Attitude Change at End of Session as a Function of "Drug Side Effects"

| High choice (dissonance conditions) | | | | | Low choice (no-dissonance control condition) |
|---|---|---|---|---|---|
| High arousal | | Low arousal | | | |
| Pleasant | Unpleasant | Pleasant | Unpleasant | No side effects | No side effects |
| 7.3 | 1.7 | 5.9 | .4 | 4.7 | −.6 |

*Note.* Adapted from "Dissonance Motivation: Its Nature, Persistence, and Reinstatement," by E. T. Higgins, F. Rhodewalt, and M. P. Zanna, *Journal of Experimental Social Psychology*, 1979, *15*, 16–34. Used with permission.

tions are felt to arise from one's body. Consistent with this reasoning, Carver, Scheier, and their colleagues have found in a number of studies that self-attention compared to environment-attention (either assessed dispositionally or varied experimentally by using mirrors or cameras to induce self-attention) leads to more polarized attitudes, feelings, and emotions, whether experienced as positive or negative initially. For instance, self-attention enhances (1) the accuracy of the reported arousing properties of female nudes and the acuity of taste (Scheier, Carver, & Gibbons, 1979), (2) the affective reactions to pleasant and unpleasant pictures and the induction of moods (Scheier & Carver, 1977), (3) the arousal of (the unpleasant state of) psychological reactance (Carver, 1977; Scheier et al., in press), and (4) the perceived symptom intensity (e.g., racing heart, headache, upset stomach) that results from exposures to noise (Matthews, Scheier, Brunson, & Carducci, 1980).

## THE MECHANISM OF ATTITUDE CHANGE

### Initial Reaction

From these data we can piece together a mechanism relating felt physiological responses, affect, and attitude change (see Figure 5-2). Beginning with physiological reactions that are felt, we first arrive at a branching in the flowchart that is controlled automatically by the valence of the initial phenomenological reaction accompanying the detection of the physiological response (cf. Zajonc, 1980).[3]

As we found earlier, perceived bodily reactions can be felt as distinctively pleasant or unpleasant even before the person attempts to determine the significance of the sensations. If the physiological reactions are felt to be unpleasant, then the subsequent search for a label should be biased negatively; if the physiological reactions are perceived as being pleasant, then the subsequent search should be biased positively; and if the physiological reactions are perceived as being neither pleasant nor unpleasant, then the labeling process should be unconstrained.

---

3. Zajonc has argued that external stimuli can elicit positive or negative affective responses that require neither autonomic input nor elaborate cognitive processes. Zajonc's argument is consistent with our reasoning that detected physiological responses may initiate preattentive processing in the same manner as do external stimuli and thereby be perceived as either distinctively pleasant or unpleasant prior to the onset of the labeling process and constrain the subsequent search for a suitable verbal label.

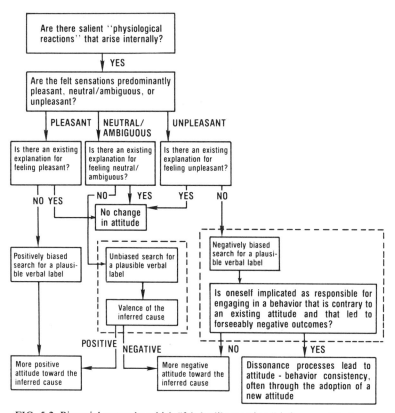

FIG. 5-2. Biosocial routes by which "felt bodily reactions" influence attitudes.

## Labeling Processes

The search for possible causes is inhibited if the person possesses a plausible explanation for the felt physiological responses prior to their detection (i.e., the search begins but is terminated immediately). If, however, the sensations are inexplicable at their onset, then the evaluative need is not immediately satisfied, thought about plausible causes ensues, and attitude change is potentiated. As we noted, this search can be biased (depending upon the initial affective reaction), which would limit the cognitive search to causes that are consonant in the effects with the affective reaction that initiated the search. The search terminates when an acceptable cognitive label has been obtained. Furthermore, we assume that explanations (labels) for felt physiological reactions that are parsimonious and impute favorable characteristics to the person are selected over equally available alternatives. That is, people generally seek explanations for their behaviors that provide a plausible account for an event while allowing them to maintain personal freedom and positive self-regard. In many instances, this means that people first seek explanations outside themselves for an event (or their responses), and when they cannot find a suitable external cause they look to internal causes (e.g., attitudes).

Attitudinal Consequences

As illustrated in Figure 5-2, the attitudinal consequence of this decision regarding the cause of the felt bodily reaction is that people will come to like people, objects, and stances that they inferred have caused them to feel pleasantly, and they will come to dislike people, objects, and positions that they inferred have caused them to feel unpleasantly.[4] In addition, the research on cognitive dissonance theory highlights an exception to this principle. Specifically, if in the course of a negatively biased search for a verbal label, an individual implicates him/herself as responsible for acting in a manner (1) that was contrary to a preexisting attitude and (2) that led to foreseeable (or retrospectively foreseeable) and undesirable outcomes, then a counterhedonic rather than hedonic effect on attitudes results in order for the person to maintain self-esteem (cf. Greenwald & Ronis, 1978).


## SIGNS: PHYSIOLOGICAL RESPONSES
## THAT ARE DETECTED EXTERNALLY

As we mentioned in a previous section, bodily reactions can be "discovered" through exteroceptive channels, such as by viewing a (bogus) feedback display for heart rate, as well as or in place of "feeling" changes that (presumably) travel visceral and proprioceptive afferents. The second

4. The research on self-attention suggests that there are individual differences in people's sensitivity to internal cues (e.g., proprioceptive feedback) and, in addition, that fairly common environmental stimuli (e.g., mirrors, cameras) can alter people's sensitivity to their internal sensations. The mechanism outlined in Figure 5-2, therefore, might be predictably more important to particular types of individuals and to all individuals in particular (self-focusing) situations.

general perspective on the role of bodily responses in the development and change of attitudes focuses on these "discovered" bodily responses. The work that falls under this heading was stimulated initially by Valins's (1966) contention that people need not feel physiological changes, but need only to *believe* that they occurred, for emotional experiences to be initiated.

THE VALINS EFFECT

The initial evidence for Valins's (1966) hypothesis was provided in a study in which men were asked to look at pictures of *Playboy* centerfolds while they listened to what they believed was their HR. The men's "heart rate" beat steadily as they viewed half of the pictures, whereas half the men heard their "heart rate" increase and the other half of the men heard it decrease as they viewed the remaining pictures. Afterward, the men rated the attractiveness of each picture. The results are presented in Table 5-2. Valins found that men rated as most attractive the pictures that were accompanied by bogus feedback indicating that their HR had changed (either increased or decreased). Valins (1967) replicated this finding and demonstrated further than the affective ratings by relatively emotional men were influenced more by the false physiological feedback regarding HR than were the ratings by nonemotional men. These data suggested that externally detected changes in physiological activity, whether real or bogus, enhance the positive regard for pleasant stimuli.

Subsequent research indicates that believing one's bodily responses are altered by attending to an unpleasant stimulus (e.g., pictures of accident victims) leads to more negative evaluations of the stimulus (e.g.,

TABLE 5-2. Mean Attractiveness Ratings of Photographs

|  | No change in sound accompanied slide onset | Change in sound accompanied slide onset |
|---|---|---|
| Sound indicated HR increase | 54.11 | 72.42 |
| Sound indicated HR decrease | 62.57 | 69.26 |
| Sound indicated extraneous noise (increase + decrease) | 63.76 | 60.86 |

*Note.* Adapted from "Cognitive Effects of False Heart-Rate Feedback," by S. Valins, *Journal of Personality and Social Psychology*, 1966, *4*, 400–408. Used with permission.

Hirschman, 1975; Stern, Botto, & Herrick, 1972). The impact of the bogus feedback on attitudes in this research is again more apparent in relatively emotional than nonemotional people (Hirschman & Hawk, 1978).

## THE MECHANISMS OF ATTITUDE CHANGE

In each of these studies, the "physiological reactions" (or lack thereof) signaled by the bogus feedback were sufficiently unexpected that they piqued the subjects' interest (cf. Liebhart, 1979). Subjects searched their environment for an explanation and particularly focused on the stimulus whose presentation was contiguous to their discovered bodily reaction. Thus, subjects may have attended to and thought more about a stimulus that was introduced contiguous to information that their bodies' responses had changed in an unexpected manner. Increased thought about stimuli makes initially likable ones (e.g., photographs of attractive women) more liked, and dislikable stimuli (e.g., photographs of atrocity victims) more disliked (cf. Tesser, 1978). Hence externally detected physiological reactions may serve as a cue that (1) piques the subjects' curiosity regarding the cause and import of the discovered physiological reactions, (2) leads subjects to search and think about aspects of their situation that covaried with the unexpected changes in bodily functioning, and (3) consequently leads to a change in attitudes in accord with the inferences that are drawn. This mechanism is depicted in the right portion of Figure 5-3.

### Externally Detected Changes That Are Also Felt

Of course, individuals might detect bodily reactions proprioceptively *and* exteroceptively. For example, people might both feel and see their face flush. Several experiments have recently been conducted in which actual physiological activities (e.g., HR, EDA) were measured while subjects received bogus physiological feedback (e.g., Hirschman & Hawk, 1978; Kerber & Coles, 1978; Stern *et al.*, 1972; cf. Harris & Katkin, 1975). The results indicate that bogus information about bodily processes often alters actual physiological activity, which *may be felt* by individuals. Although the actual changes do not appear to be necessary for obtaining the reported effects of bogus physiological feedback on attitudes (cf. Liebhart, 1979), there nevertheless may be a consonant biasing of the labeling

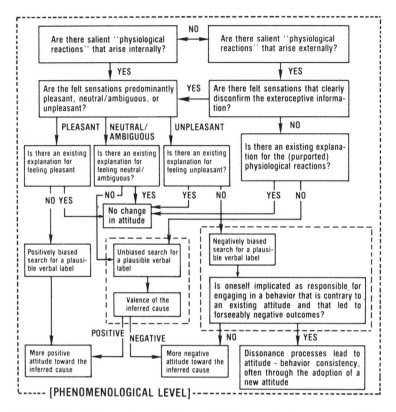

FIG. 5-3. Biosocial routes by which "detected bodily reactions" influence attitudes.

process and attitude change if the bodily reactions are felt to be distinctively pleasant or unpleasant. Unfortunately, it has seldom been specified in these studies whether bogus feedback led to actual bodily reactions, and whether these actual changes altered what bodily cues subjects detected internally as a result of what they detected externally through bogus feedback in the experimental setting (see Figure 5-3).

### Situational Cues Biasing the Labeling Process

In addition, if situational cues place some directive significance on an externally detected physiological response (and assuming there are no contradictory felt physiological responses), then the cognitive search for a verbal label and attitude change could be consonantly biased. Consider a

study by Pittman, Cooper, and Smith (1977). Subjects manually maneu-
vered the distance between two metal rods to move a metal ball up an
inclined plane. Each subject was given ten trials at the task to accumulate
as many points as possible. Electrodes were attached to each subject,
presumably so that the experimenters could measure "arousal." The
experimenters then varied the internal and external cues available to the
subjects while they performed the task. Control group subjects were told
nothing additional about the task, whereas a second group of subjects
were promised money (an extrinsic reward) for their performance on the
task. Pittman *et al.* (1977) found that subjects who expected to earn
money for playing the game, subsequently acted as if they liked the game
less than subjects who did not expect to earn money. This is a phenomenon
known as the "overjustification effect" (Lepper, Greene, & Nisbett, 1973).

More importantly here, Pittman *et al.* (1977) tested two additional
groups of subjects. Subjects in these groups expected to earn money on
the basis of their performance on the task, just as had subjects in the
second group previously described. But these additional subjects were
stopped after performing five of the ten trials and were told that their
bodily readings from the electrodes indicated that they were "aroused."
Subjects from one group were told that the arousal signified their personal
involvement and interest in the *game*, whereas subjects from the other
group were told that the arousal reflected their interest in the *money*. That
is, some subjects were given bogus information about their level of
arousal that also pointed to intrinsic reasons for playing the game,
whereas other subjects were given bogus information about their arousal
that also highlighted the material reasons for playing the game. The
results are illustrated in Figure 5-4. What subjects were told about the
particular significance of their bogus physiological responses determined
whether or not the money undermined their interest in (and positive
attitude toward) the game. When the bodily reactions were said to reflect
interest in the game, intrinsic motivation to play the game was enhanced.
Conversely, when the bodily reactions were said to reflect interest in an
extrinsic cause (money), subjects' interest in the game waned. The Pittman
*et al.* study thus illustrates that situational information can have directive
effects on the nature of the inferences that follow discovery of physiological responses.

Thus far, we have illustrated only the phenomenological effects of
physiological reactions that are detected either by being felt or by being
discovered exteroceptively. In the next section, we turn to research on the
effects of undetected physiological responses.

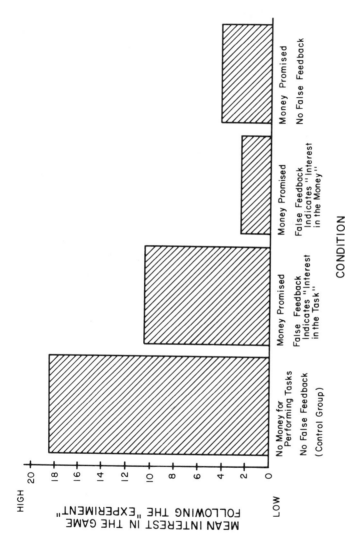

FIG. 5-4. Mean interest in a game as a function of extrinsic reward and false physiological feedback. Adapted from "Attribution of Causality and the Overjustification Effect," by T. S. Pittman, E. E. Cooper, and T. W. Smith, *Personality and Social Psychology Bulletin*, 1977, *3*, 280–283. Used with permission.

171

## PHYSIOLOGICAL RESPONSES THAT ARE UNDETECTED

The study of the attitudinal effects of actual but unperceived physiological reactions stands as the complement to the work on the role of detected physiological reactions. Elsewhere, we have emphasized the importance of the idiosyncratic thoughts and ideas, or "cognitive responses," generated by people (cf. Petty & Cacioppo, 1981, Chapters 8 and 9) in producing attitude change. The processes underlying these cognitive responses can vary from complete inattention or simple, effortless analyses to elaborate, associative analyses of incoming stimuli. The latter, but not the former, processes allow people to determine the implications of the event for themselves and for significant others (e.g., Cacioppo, Glass, & Merluzzi, 1979; Janis & Mann, 1977; Petty & Cacioppo, 1979; Rogers, Kuiper, & Kirker, 1977), and appear to be an important determinant of attitude development and change (cf. Cialdini *et al.,* 1981; Petty & Cacioppo, 1981; Petty, Ostrom, & Brock, 1981). Following these findings, we proposed that undetected changes in physiological activity may alter the likelihood that people would elaborate upon the arguments contained in a persuasive message and thereby alter their susceptibility or resistance to persuasion. Evidence for this mechanism has been obtained recently in an investigation of the effects of exogenous changes in heart rate on the facilitation of thought and the resistance to persuasion. Since the rationale for selecting heart rate and using the procedures that we did is based upon the germinatal work of the Laceys, we shall digress momentarily to review their formulation.

NEGATIVE AFFERENT FEEDBACK

The Laceys (e.g., B. C. Lacey & Lacey, 1974, 1978; J. I. Lacey, 1967) speculated that cardiovascular changes impact on the central nervous system via a modulating negative feedback system, with effects evident in sensorimotor behavior as well as in electrocortical activity:

> Scattered up and down the arterial tree are the baroreceptors, exquisitely responsive to blood pressure. The major concentrations of the baroreceptors are in the aortic arch and in the carotid sinus. . . . [The thin wall of the carotid sinus] is distended, stretched, and distorted by the pressure wave produced at each heartbeat. The resulting strain on the sinus is the adequate

stimulus for the baroreceptors. At each heart beat, then, a burst of impulses is produced in the baroreceptor afferents, which have their first synapse in the brain stem in *nucleus tractus solitarius,* close to reticular structures involved in cardiovascular control.

But activity of these baroreceptor afferents has widespread effects on other than cardiovascular activity. . . . Sensory and motor functions can be inhibited by increases in baroreceptor activity. (B. C. Lacey & Lacey, 1978, pp. 106–107)

The Laceys' model is consistent with what currently is known about the baroreceptor mechanism (cf. B. C. Lacey & Lacey, 1980) and accounts for a wide array of behavioral data, including: (1) cardiac deceleration accompanying the intention to note and detect external stimuli (e.g., viewing flashing lights), and cardiac acceleration accompanying "mental concentration" (e.g., sentence generation—J. I. Lacey, 1959; Lacey, Kagan, Lacey, & Moss, 1963; Obrist, 1963); (2) larger elevations in HR during the performance of intellective tasks by "efficient" rather than "inefficient" (i.e., successful vs. unsuccessful) problem solvers (Blatt, 1961; see also Kagan & Rosman, 1964); (3) larger cardiac accelerations during the performance of difficult rather than simple intellective tasks, and larger cardiac decelerations during the performance of difficult rather than simple sensorimotor tasks (e.g., Cacioppo & Sandman, 1978; B. C. Lacey & Lacey, 1974; Tursky, Schwartz, & Crider, 1970); (4) anticipatory cardiac deceleration in advance of subject-initiated key presses (J. I. Lacey & Lacey, 1970); and (5) enhanced visual detection during endogenous cardiac decelerations relative to acceleration (Sandman, McCanne, Kaiser, & Diamond, 1977). The Laceys' formulation and research from cardiovascular psychophysiology also seemed to suggest that normal fluctuations in heart rate can have differing effects on people's ability to perceive and elaborate upon incoming stimuli (see Chapter 6, this volume).

ACCELERATED HEART RATE AND ATTITUDE CHANGE

In an initial experiment, we operantly conditioned subjects to accelerate and decelerate HR (Cacioppo *et al.,* 1978). Subjects accumulated a monetary reward by surpassing the criteria set for cardiac speeding and slowing only when these HR responses were accompanied by little or no change in overt somatic and respiratory activity. At the end of the fifth day of training, recommendations with which undergraduates generally disagreed (e.g., not allowing undergraduates in graduate courses) were presented during periods of cardiac acceleration, cardiac deceleration, or basal HR trials. Attitudes toward the recommendations were obtained after each persuasive message, and retrospective reports of what subjects had thought about during each message were obtained immediately following the final message and attitude assessment.

The results of the study are displayed in Figure 5-5, which shows that cardiac acceleration was associated with increased counterargumentation

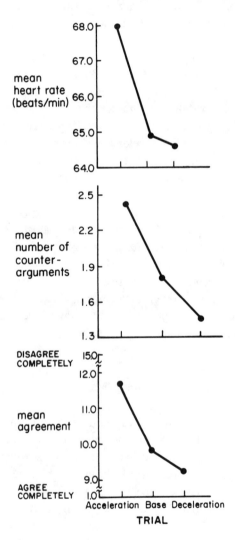

FIG. 5-5. The effects of cardiac conditioning on heart rate (top panel), counterargument production (middle panel), and resistance to persuasion (bottom panel). From "The Effects of Operant Heart Rate Conditioning on Cognitive Elaboration and Attitude Change," by J. T. Cacioppo, C. A. Sandman, and B. B. Walker, *Psychophysiology*, 1978, *15*, 330–338. Reprinted by permission.

and diminished attitude change. It is not clear from this study, of course, whether the conditioning led to the accelerated heart rate, which then facilitated information processing and resistance to persuasion, or some other causal sequence was operating. Moreover, subjects were aware that their heart rate changed since they received veridical feedback regarding whether or not they surpassed the set criterion level for HR during each trial. Nevertheless, the results of this initial study were encouraging with regard to the possible attitudinal effects of momentarily sustained fluctuations in HR.

Several design strategies might be adopted to provide information about the effects of undetected changes in HR on thinking and attitude change. We desired to vary HR exogenously without the individual's knowledge, to determine if such changes were sufficient for altering performance on difficult intellective tasks. In order to accomplish this, we used cardiac-pacing techniques to accelerate HR while subjects performed two difficult intellective tasks (i.e., sentence generation and college-level reading comprehension tests). The cardiac-pacing procedure involves placing a magnet over a reed of a subject's pacemaker to speed the heart beat. The research was conducted in a clinical setting under the supervision of a cardiologist (see Cacioppo, 1979). Unfortunately, this setting contained no resources for measuring any physiological process besides HR.[5]

The pacemaker worn by each subject had been implanted for at least 3 months and was necessary to maintain HR at 72 bpm. The pacemakers were "demand type," so called because they pace the heart at a constant rate when natural pacing produces a rate below the preset level of the cardiac pacemaker. To our knowledge, this is the only type of pacemaker that provides a nonsurgical means of altering HR simply, exogenously, and without the subject's awareness of the trials on which HR is or is not altered. The preset level of the pacemakers worn by our subjects was 72 bpm, whereas the level was accelerated to and maintained at a rate of 88 bpm when an uncapped magnet was placed appropriately over the pacemaker.

Importantly, subjects in this research have been unable to report accurately when and how frequently their pacemaker was pulsing their heart. Subjects instead have tended to report that they thought we were

---

5. Existing evidence suggests that paced changes in HR within the range of rates employed in our research—that is, 72–88 bpm—are unaccompanied by noticeable changes in visceral, somatic, or cardiac output responses (Gill, Jakobi, Morton, & Wechsler, 1975; Karloff, Bevegard, & Ovenfors, 1973).

altering their HR within each experimental trial, whereas we in fact manipulated the pacing of their HR between trials by placing either an uncapped (accelerated HR) or capped (basal HR) magnet over the pacemaker. Their inability to detect these exogenously induced changes in HR is consistent with the observations of Nowlin, Eisdorfer, Whalen, and Troyer (1971), who found that their patients were unaware of paced HR that exceeded 110 bpm. (We might note that subjects did not report feeling different sensations from their bodies during accelerated versus basal trials, but our measurement of these sensations was too informal to be confident there necessarily were no differences.)

In the first pacemaker study, we had subjects generate sentences and take a reading comprehension test under accelerated and basal HR trials. These effortful cognitive tasks were chosen because of the previous research that suggests that an accelerated HR might alter the performance of these tasks (e.g., J. I. Lacey, 1967; J. I. Lacey *et al.,* 1963; J. I. Lacey & Lacey, 1970). The sentence generation task had been used in previous research and was found to be associated with an accelerated HR (J. I. Lacey *et al.,* 1963). A task similar to reading comprehension was employed by Spence, Lugo, and Youdin (1972): Subjects were instructed to attend to, and were later asked to recall, sentences reflecting a certain theme while they listened to a 17-min passage from a clinical interview. Spence *et al.* found that subjects displayed a decelerated HR (presumably denoting sensory intake) followed by an accelerated HR (presumably denoting cognitive effort) during the presentation of thematic sentences that were subsequently recalled.[6]

The waveform associated with recalled thematic sentences in the Spence *et al.* (1972) study was distinct from those displayed in the absence

---

6. In a pair of recent experiments, we have found that the efficacy of encoding and the electromyographic activity of the lips covaried (Cacioppo & Petty, 1979b, 1981b), whereas HR did not vary as a function of the encoding task. In this research, we have varied the "level" at which stimuli are processed during encoding (cf. Cacioppo & Petty, 1981a), which can be varied orthogonally to the degree to which demands are placed upon the available processing capacity of the limited-capacity central processor (cf. Tyler, Hertel, McCallum, & Ellis, 1979). Generating thoughts and ideas about a stimulus and examining the relation of a stimulus to items stored in memory is cognitively effortful, can lead to cognitive overload, and has been associated with enhanced perioral EMG activity (Cacioppo & Petty, 1979a) and cardiac acceleration (e.g., Blaylock, 1972; Tursky *et al.*, 1970). We presently are conducting research to determine whether cardiac activity is related to a specific component of information processing termed "cognitive effort."

of thematic sentences and in the presence of unrecalled thematic sentences. Since the present procedure allowed the subject to take as long as he/she wished to read the passages (hence allowing subjects to control sensory intake by their allocation of reading time to items), we expected that an accelerated HR would facilitate the cognitive elaboration of the stimuli and thereby improve reading comprehension.

The findings of this experiment are illustrated in the upper two panels of Figure 5-6. We found that accelerated, relative to basal, HR significantly improved reading comprehension and tended (though not significantly) to improve performance of the sentence-generation task. The bottom panel of Figure 5-6 depicts the results of a small additional study we conducted. To gain some preliminary information about whether it was important that heart rate had been varied in the pacemaker study

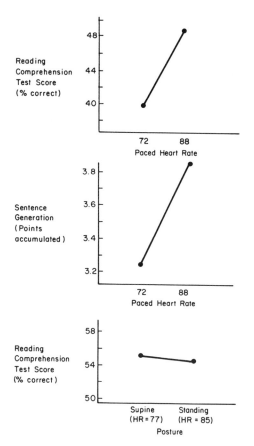

FIG. 5-6. The effects of pacemaker-induced heart rate changes on reading comprehension (top panel) and sentence generation (middle panel), and the effects of posture-induced changes on reading comprehension (bottom panel). Adapted from "The Effects of Exogenous Changes in Heart Rate on the Facilitation of Thought and Resistance to Persuasion," by J. T. Cacioppo, *Journal of Personality and Social Psychology*, 1979, *37*, 487–496. Used with permission.

within a fairly quiescent pattern of physiological activity in order to alter intellective performance, we replicated a portion of the study using healthy undergraduates who, of course, had no pacemakers. They either stood or lay down to perform a reading comprehension test. These postural variations cause not only HR to differ but also respiration, muscle tension, blood pressure, and so forth. As illustrated in the bottom panel of Figure 5-6, reading comprehension was not associated with HR in this study. These data are by no means definitive and are not intended as such. They are, however, consistent with the speculations by the Laceys (e.g., B. C. Lacey & Lacey, 1974) that altered cardiac activity influences attention/ cognition, particularly when the changes are relatively independent of other major changes in physiological activity.

A second experiment using the cardiac-pacing technique was conducted to determine whether an undetected increase in paced HR facilitates stimulus-relevant thinking and consequently influences attitudes. The procedures were identical to those already described except that a shortened version of the comprehension test was used for training and adaptation. During the experimental trials, subjects read two personally important messages, each of which was approximately 400 words long and recommended a highly counterattitudinal proposition (e.g., eliminate all Social Security and Medicare programs). The order in which HR was varied (basal–accelerated vs. accelerated–basal) served as a between-subjects factor, whereas paced HR (basal vs. accelerated) served as a within-subjects factor. The messages were always presented in the same order. Thus, half of the subjects read the first message while their HR was accelerated, whereas half read the second message while their HR was accelerated.

All subjects read the messages at their own speed. After reading each, subjects were given 2.5 min to verbally report everything about which they had thought while reading and were asked to indicate their agreement with each recommendation.

The retrospective reports of subjects' thoughts were transcribed by a judge who was unaware of the experimental hypotheses. Transcribed as a "cognitive response" was any phrase or sentence expressing a single thought or idea; although grammar was not a criterion, a subject's pauses and voice inflections were used in a few instances to determine whether a phrase or group of phrases formed a single thought or idea. The total number of cognitive responses was determined, as was the number of cognitive responses that were proarguments, counterarguments, and neither pro- nor counterarguments (i.e., neutral/irrelevant thoughts).

The results, which are displayed in Figure 5-7, indicated that more counterarguments were produced when HR was accelerated than when it was not accelerated. However, no treatment or interaction of treatments affected subjects' rating of agreement with the advocacies. An inspection of the raw data revealed that 59% of the subjects' responses to the attitude measure were "disagree completely"; thus, the attitude measure was probably insensitive to treatment effects. Subjects may have been able to counterargue and reject completely the advocacies, whether their HR was accelerated (thus facilitating cognitive responding) or not. Accordingly, we found that few thoughts other than counterarguments were generated during the entire experiment (cf. Cacioppo, 1979).

## The Mechanism of Attitude Change

We might note that although the results of the experiments just described cannot be considered definitive regarding the Laceys' negative feedback hypothesis (see Chapters 6 and 11, this volume) and are not dependent

FIG. 5-7. The effects of pacemaker-induced heart rate changes on counterargument production. Adapted from "The Effects of Exogenous Changes in Heart Rate on the Facilitation of Thought and Resistance to Persuasion," by J. T. Cacioppo, *Journal of Personality and Social Psychology*, 1979, *37*, 487–496. Used with permission.

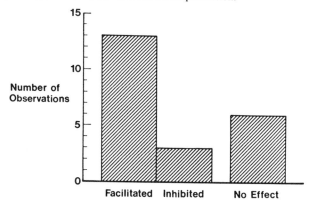

upon its veracity, the nature of the investigations owe much to the Laceys' work in cardiovascular psychophysiology. Moreover, the results of the pacemaker studies suggest a means by which undetected physiological responses can influence attitude change. Specifically, these data suggest that undetected physiological changes can alter the likelihood that people will elaborate cognitively upon information (see Figure 5-8). The likelihood of elaboration theoretically can be affected by changes either in a person's motivation or ability, though the pacemaker studies presumably altered only the ability factor. An alteration of the elaboration likelihood has effects on attitude change through its effects on stimulus-relevant thinking, such as cognitive responses to a persuasive message and labeling processes when searching for a plausible cause of a detected physiological response. In other words, undetected physiological responses (e.g., paced changes in HR) can have *indirect* effects on affect and attitudes. In Figure 5-8 we have outlined the full model and postulated the mechanisms by which felt, found, and undetected bodily responses can alter attitude change independently and in concert. It should be clear from viewing Figure 5-8 that physiological, phenomenological, and behavioral responses reflect independent though partially integrated systems that can influence attitude change. As the social psychophysiological research that we have surveyed in this chapter should also have made clear, cardiovascular psychophysiology has contributed greatly to advances in the study of biosocial factors and attitude change. Cardiovascular variables, because of their ease of measurement (see Chapter 2, this volume) and their psychological significance (see, for instance, Chapter 11, this volume), have served as the focus of initial and the majority of subsequent studies on the role of bodily processes in attitude change.

CONCLUSION

For decades research on attitude change has focused primarily on situations in which there are neither significant physiological reactions arising within one's body nor salient external information about one's physiological reactions. There has now accumulated, however, a surprisingly large data base with regards to bodily processes and attitude change. The following tripartite was used to organize this literature:

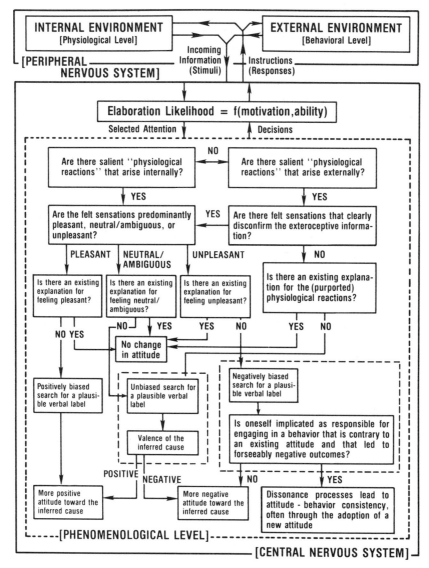

FIG. 5-8. Biosocial routes by which "bodily reactions" influence attitudes.

1. *Symptoms: physiological responses that are detected internally*—
   The subject becomes aware of internal (i.e., interoceptive, proprioceptive) sensations that influence attitude change.
2. *Signs: physiological responses that are detected externally*—The
   subject obtains information through exteroceptive channels regarding the status of his/her bodily reactions while the sensations
   obtained through internal channels are absent, weak, or ambiguous.
3. *Physiological responses that are undetected*—The attitudinal effects of actual bodily reactions of which the subject is unaware are
   investigated.

Cardiac activity has been among the most common foci on physiological
response in part because of its ease of measurement and quantification,
and its past association with emotion in the literature. The data reviewed
in the present chapter suggest that changes in cardiac activity should be
interpreted not only within the context of other physiological responses
(e.g., see also Schwartz, Chapter 11, this volume), but also within the
phenomenological context involving whether or not the changes in cardiac
and physiological activity were detected and, if detected, by what means
(e.g., felt vs. discovered through external sources of information). Mechanisms are suggested by which these distinct types of bodily response might
influence attitude change.

## ACKNOWLEDGMENT

The authors would like to thank Charlotte Lowell and Barbara Andersen for their
helpful comments on an earlier draft.

This work was supported by National Science Foundation Grant BNS 80-23589 and a
University Faculty Scholar Award.

## REFERENCES

Acker, L. E., & Edwards, A. E. Transfer of vasoconstriction over a bipolar meaning
    dimension. *Journal of Experimental Psychology,* 1964, *67,* 1–6.
Allport, G. W. Attitudes. In C. Murchinson (Ed.), *A handbook of social psychology.*
    Worcester, Mass.: Clark University Press, 1935.
Aronson, E. The theory of cognitive dissonance: A current perspective. In L. Berkowitz
    (Ed.), *Advances in experimental social psychology* (Vol. 4). New York: Academic
    Press, 1969.
Bem, D. J. Self-perception theory. *Advanced Experimental Social Psychology,* 1972, *6,* 1–62.

Blascovich, J., Nash, R. F., & Ginsburg, G. P. Heart rate and competitive decision making. *Personality and Social Psychology Bulletin,* 1978, *4,* 115-118.

Blatt, S. J. Patterns of cardiac arousal during complex mental activity. *Journal of Abnormal and Social Psychology,* 1961, *63,* 272-282.

Blaylock, B. Some antecedents of directional fractionation: Effects of "intake-rejection," verbalization requirements, and threat of shock on heart rate and skin conductance. *Psychophysiology,* 1972, *9,* 40-52.

Brener, J., & Jones, J. M. Interoceptive discrimination in intact humans: Detection of cardiac activity. *Physiology and Behavior,* 1974, *13,* 763-767.

Buckhout, R. Changes in heart rate accompanying attitude change. *Journal of Personality and Social Psychology,* 1966, *4,* 695-699.

Cacioppo, J. T. The effects of exogenous changes in heart rate on the facilitation of thought and resistance to persuasion. *Journal of Personality and Social Psychology,* 1979, *37,* 487-496.

Cacioppo, J. T., Glass, C. R., & Merluzzi, T. V. Self-statements and self-evaluations: A cognitive-response analysis of heterosocial anxiety. *Cognitive Therapy and Research,* 1979, *3,* 249-262.

Cacioppo, J. T., Harkins, S. G., & Petty, R. E. The nature of attitudes and cognitive responses and their relationships to behavior. In R. E. Petty, T. M. Ostrom, & T. C. Brock (Eds.), *Cognitive responses in persuasion.* Hillsdale, N.J.: Erlbaum, 1981.

Cacioppo, J. T., & Petty, R. E. Attitudes and cognitive response: An electrophysiological approach. *Journal of Personality and Social Psychology,* 1979, *37,* 2181-2199. (a)

Cacioppo, J. T., & Petty, R. E. Lip and nonpreferred forearm EMG activity as a function of orienting task. *Journal of Biological Psychology,* 1979, *9,* 103-113. (b)

Cacioppo, J. T., & Petty, R. E. Electromyograms as measures of extent and affectivity of information processing. *American Psychologist,* 1981, *36,* 441-456. (a)

Cacioppo, J. T., & Petty, R. E. Electromyographic specificity during covert information processing. *Psychophysiology,* 1981, *18,* 518-523. (b)

Cacioppo, J. T., & Petty, R. E. (Eds.). *Social psychophysiology: A sourcebook.* New York: Guilford Press, in press.

Cacioppo, J. T., Petty, R. E., & Snyder, C. W. Cognitive and affective response as a function of relative hemispheric involvement. *International Journal of Neuroscience,* 1979, *9,* 81-89.

Cacioppo, J. T., & Sandman, C. A. Physiological differentiation of sensory and cognitive tasks as a function of warning, processing demands, and unpleasantness. *Journal of Biological Psychology,* 1978, *6,* 181-192.

Cacioppo, J. T., & Sandman, C. A. Psychophysiological functioning, cognitive responding, and attitudes. In R. E. Petty, T. M. Ostrom, & T. C. Brock (Eds.), *Cognitive responses in persuasion.* Hillsdale, N. J.: Erlbaum, 1981.

Cacioppo, J. T., Sandman, C. A., & Walker, B. B. The effects of operant heart rate conditioning on cognitive elaboration and attitude change. *Psychophysiology,* 1978, *15,* 330-338.

Cannon, W. B. The James–Lange theory of emotions: A critical examination and an alternative theory. *American Journal of Psychology,* 1927, *39,* 106-124.

Cantor, J. R., Zillmann, D., & Bryant, J. Enhancement of experienced sexual arousal in response to erotic stimuli through misattribution of unrelated residual excitation. *Journal of Personality and Social Psychology,* 1975, *32,* 69-75.

Carver, C. S. Self-awareness, perception of threat, and the expression of reactance through attitude change. *Journal of Personality,* 1977, *45,* 501-512.

Cialdini, R. B., Petty, R. E., & Cacioppo, J. T. Attitudes and attitude changes. In M. R. Rosenweig & L. W. Porter (Eds.), *Annual review of psychology* (Vol. 32). Palo Alto, Calif.: Annual Reviews, 1981.

Collins, B. E., Ellsworth, P. C., & Helmreich, R. L. Correlations between pupil size and the semantic differential: An experimental paradigm and pilot study. *Psychonomic Science*, 1967, *9*, 627–628.

Comer, R., & Rhodewalt, F. Cue utilization in the self-attributions of emotions and attitudes. *Personality and Social Psychology Bulletin*, 1979, *5*, 320–324.

Cooper, J., Fazio, R. H., & Rhodewalt, F. Dissonance and humor: Evidence for the undifferentiated nature of dissonance arousal. *Journal of Personality and Social Psychology*, 1978, *36*, 280–285.

Cooper, J., Zanna, M. P., & Taves, P. A. Arousal as a necessary condition for attitude change following induced compliance. *Journal of Personality and Social Psychology*, 1978, *36*, 1101–1106.

Dabbs, J. M., Jr., & Moorer, J. P., Jr. Core body temperature and arousal. *Personality and Social Psychology Bulletin*, 1975, *1*, 517–520.

Dunlap, K. (Ed.). *The emotions*. Baltimore: Williams & Wilkins, 1922.

Fazio, R. H., Zanna, M. P., & Cooper, J. Dissonance and self-perception: An integrative view of each theory's proper domain of application. *Journal of Experimental Social Psychology*, 1977, *13*, 464–479.

Fazio, R. H., Zanna, M. P., & Cooper, J. On the relationship of data to theory: A reply to Ronis and Greenwald. *Journal of Experimental Social Psychology*, 1979, *15*, 70–76.

Festinger, L. *A theory of cognitive dissonance*. Stanford, Calif.: Stanford University Press, 1957.

Fishbein, M., & Ajzen, I. *Belief, attitude, intention, and behavior: An introduction to theory and research*. Reading, Mass.: Addison-Wesley, 1975.

Fries, A., & Frey, D. Misattribution of arousal and the effects of self-threatening information. *Journal of Experimental Social Psychology*, 1980, *16*, 405–416.

Geen, R. G., & Gange, J. J. Drive theory of social facilitation: Twelve years of theory and research. *Psychological Bulletin*, 1977, *84*, 1267–1288.

Gerard, H. B. Choice difficulty, dissonance, and the decision sequence. *Journal of Personality*, 1967, *35*, 91–108.

Gill, G., Jakobi, W., Morton, T., & Wechsler, A. *The cardiovascular system as it relates to heart pacing: Medtronics currents* (Vol. 1, 2nd ed.). Minneapolis, Minn.: Medtronics, 1975.

Greenwald, A. H., & Ronis, D. L. Twenty years of cognitive dissonance: A case study of the evolution of a theory. *Psychological Review*, 1978, *85*, 53–57.

Grings, W. W., & Dawson, M. E. *Emotions and bodily responses*. New York: Academic Press, 1978.

Harlow, H. F., & Stagner, R. Psychology of feelings and emotions: II. Theory of emotions. *Psychological Review*, 1933, *40*, 184–195.

Harris, V. A., & Katkin, E. S. Primary and secondary emotional feedback: An analysis of the role of autonomic feedback on affect, arousal, and attribution. *Psychological Bulletin*, 1975, *82*, 904–916.

Higgins, E. T., Rhodewalt, F., & Zanna, M. P. Dissonance motivation: Its nature, persistence, and reinstatement. *Journal of Experimental Social Psychology*, 1979, *15*, 16–34.

Hirschman, R. Cross-modal effects of anticipatory bogus heart rate feedback in a negative emotional context. *Journal of Personality and Social Psychology*, 1975, *31*, 13–19.

Hirschman, R., & Hawk, G. Emotional responsivity to nonveridical heart rate feedback as a function of anxiety. *Journal of Research in Personality*, 1978, *12*, 235–242.

Izard, C. E. *Human emotions*. New York: Plenum Press, 1976.

James, W. *The principles of psychology* (Vol. 2). New York: Henry Holt & Co., 1905. (Originally published, 1890.)

Janis, I. L., & Mann, L. *Decision making: A psychological analysis of conflict, choice, and commitment*. New York: Free Press, 1977.

Kagan, J., & Rosman, B. L. Cardiac and respiratory correlates of attention and an analytic attitude. *Journal of Experimental Child Psychology*, 1964, *1*, 50–63.

Karloff, I., Bevegard, S., & Ovenfors, C. O. Adaptation of the left ventricle to sudden changes in heart rate in patients with artificial pacemakers. *Cardiovascular Research*, 1973, *7*, 322–330.

Kelley, K., & Byrne, D. Psychophysiology of sexual behavior. In J. T. Cacioppo & R. E. Petty (Eds.), *Social psychophysiology*. New York: Guilford Press, in press.

Kerber, K. W., & Coles, M. G. The role of perceived physiological activity in affective judgments. *Journal of Experimental Social Psychology*, 1978, *14*, 419–433.

Kiesler, C. A., & Pallak, M. S. Arousal properties of dissonance manipulations. *Psychological Bulletin*, 1976, *83*, 1014–1025.

Lacey, B. C., & Lacey, J. I. Studies of heart rate and other bodily processes in sensorimotor behavior. In P. A. Obrist, A. H. Black, J. Brener, & L. V. DiCara (Eds.), *Cardiovascular psychophysiology*, Chicago: Aldine, 1974.

Lacey, B. C., & Lacey, J. I. Two-way communication between the heart and the brain: Significance of time within the cardiac cycle. *American Psychologist*, 1978, *33*, 99–113.

Lacey, B. C., & Lacey, J. I. Cognitive modulation of time-dependent primary bradycardia. *Psychophysiology*, 1980, *17*, 209–221.

Lacey, J. I. Psychophysiological approaches to the evaluation of psychotherapeutic process and outcome. In E. A. Rubinstein & M. B. Parloff (Eds.), *Research in psychotherapy*. Washington, D.C.: American Psychological Association, 1959.

Lacey, J. I. Somatic response patterning and stress: Some revisions of activation theory. In M. H. Appley & R. Trumbull (Eds.), *Psychological stress: Issues in research*. New York: Appleton-Century-Crofts, 1967.

Lacey, J. I., Kagan, J., Lacey, B. C., & Moss, H. A. The visceral level: Situational determinants and behavioral correlates of autonomic response patterns. In P. H. Knapp (Ed.), *Expression of the emotions in man*. New York: International Universities Press, 1963.

Lacey, J. I., & Lacey, B. C. Verification and extension of the principle of autonomic response stereotypy. *American Journal of Psychology*, 1958, *71*, 50–73.

Lacey, J. I., & Lacey, B. C. Some autonomic–central nervous system interrelationships. In P. Black (Ed.), *Physiological correlates of emotion*. New York: Academic Press, 1970.

Lang, P. J. The application of psychophysiological methods to the study of psychotherapy and behavior modification. In A. E. Bergin & S. L. Garfield (Eds.), *Handbook of psychotherapy and behavior change: An empirical analysis*. New York: John Wiley & Sons, 1971.

Lazarus, R. S. *Psychological stress and the coping process*. New York: McGraw-Hill, 1966.

Lazarus, R. S., Averill, J. R., & Opton, E. M. Towards a cognitive theory of emotion. In M. Arnold (Ed.), *Feelings and emotion*. New York: Academic Press, 1970.

Lepper, M. R., Greene, D., & Nisbett, R. E. Undermining children's intrinsic interest with extrinsic reward. *Journal of Personality and Social Psychology*, 1973, *28*, 129–137.

Liebhart, E. H. Information search and attribution: Cognitive processes mediating the effect of false autonomic feedback. *European Journal of Social Psychology*, 1979, *9*, 19–37.

Linder, D. E., Cooper, J., & Jones, E. E. Decision freedom as a determinant of the role of incentive magnitude in attitude change. *Journal of Personality and Social Psychology*, 1967, *6*, 245–254.

MacBryde, C. M., & Blacklow, R. S. *Signs and symptoms: Applied pathologic physiology and clinical interpretation* (5th ed.). Philadelphia: J. B. Lippincott, 1970.

Mackay, C. J. The measurement of mood and psychophysiological activity using self-report techniques. In I. Martin & P. H. Venables (Eds.), *Techniques in psychophysiology*. Chichester, England: John Wiley & Sons, 1980.

Mandler, G., Mandler, J. M., & Uviller, E. T. Autonomic feedback: The perception of autonomic activity. *Journal of Abnormal and Social Psychology*, 1958, *56*, 367–373.

Marshall, G. D., & Zimbardo, R. P. Affective consequences of inadequately explained physiological arousal. *Journal of Personality and Social Psychology*, 1979, *37*, 970–988.

Maslach, C. Negative emotional biasing of unexplained arousal. *Journal of Personality and Social Psychology*, 1979, *37*, 953–969.

Matthews, K. A., Scheier, M. F., Brunson, B. I., & Carducci, B. Attention, unpredictability, and reports of physical symptoms: Eliminating the benefits of predictability. *Journal of Personality and Social Psychology*, 1980, *38*, 525–537.

Mewborn, C. R., & Rogers, R. W. Effects of threatening and reassuring components of fear appeals on physiological and verbal measures of emotion and attitudes. *Journal of Experimental Social Psychology*, 1979, *15*, 242–253.

Newman, P. P. *Visceral afferent functions of the nervous system.* London: Edward Arnold, 1974.

Norman, R. When what is said is important: A comparison of expert and attractive sources. *Journal of Experimental Social Psychology*, 1976, *12*, 294–300.

Nowlin, J. B., Eisdorfer, C., Whalen, R., & Troyer, W. G. The effect of exogenous changes in heart rate and rhythm upon reaction time performance. *Psychophysiology*, 1971, *7*, 186–193.

Obrist, P. A. Cardiovascular differentiation of sensory stimuli. *Psychosomatic Medicine*, 1963, *25*, 450–459.

Obrist, P. A. The cardiovascular–behavioral interaction—As it appears today. *Psychophysiology*, 1976, *13*, 95–107.

Oskamp, S. *Attitudes and opinions.* Englewood Cliffs, N.J.: Prentice-Hall, 1977.

Ostrom, T. M. The relationship between the affective, behavioral, and cognitive components of attitude. *Journal of Experimental Social Psychology*, 1969, *5*, 12–30.

Pennebaker, J. W. *Self-perception of emotion and specificity of physical sensations.* Paper presented at the annual meeting of the American Psychological Association, New York, 1979.

Petty, R. E., & Cacioppo, J. T. Issue-involvement can increase or decrease persuasion by enhancing message-relevant cognitive responses. *Journal of Personality and Social Psychology*, 1979, *37*, 1915–1926.

Petty, R. E., & Cacioppo, J. T. *Attitudes and persuasion: Classic and contemporary approaches.* Dubuque, Iowa: Wm. C. Brown, 1981.

Petty, R. E., Ostrom, T. M., & Brock, T. C. Historical foundations of the cognitive response approach to attitudes and persuasion. In R. E. Petty, T. M. Ostrom, & T. C. Brock (Eds.), *Cognitive responses in persuasion*. Hillsdale, N.J.: Erlbaum, 1981.

Pittman, T. S., Cooper, E. E., & Smith, T. W. Attribution of causality and the overjustification effect. *Personality and Social Psychology Bulletin*, 1977, *3*, 280–283.

Quanty, M. B., & Becker, L. A. *Physiological indices of dissonance arousal and reduction in a stressful situation.* Unpublished manuscript, University of Missouri, Columbia, 1974.

Rhodewalt, F., & Comer, R. Induced-compliance attitude change: Once more with feeling. *Journal of Experimental Social Psychology*, 1979, *15*, 35–47.

Rogers, T. B., Kuiper, N. A., & Kirker, W. S. Self-reference and the encoding of personal information. *Journal of Personality and Social Psychology*, 1977, *35*, 677–688.

Ronis, D. L., & Greenwald, A. G. Dissonance theory revised again: Comment on the paper by Fazio, Zanna, and Cooper. *Journal of Experimental Social Psychology*, 1979, *15*, 62–69.

Sandman, C. A., McCanne, T. R., Kaiser, D. N., & Diamond, B. Heart rate and cardiac phase influences on visual perception. *Journal of Comparative and Physiological Psychology*, 1977, *91*, 189–202.

Schachter, S. *Emotion, obesity, and crime*. New York: Academic Press, 1971.

Schachter, S., & Singer, J. E. Cognitive, social and physiological determinants of emotional state. *Psychological Review*, 1962, *69*, 379–399.

Schachter, S., & Singer, J. E. Comments on the Maslach and Marshall–Zimbardo experiments. *Journal of Personality and Social Psychology*, 1979, *37*, 989–995.

Scheier, M. F., & Carver, C. S. Self-focused attention and the experience of emotion: Attraction, repulsion, elation, and depression. *Journal of Personality and Social Psychology*, 1977, *35*, 625–636.

Scheier, M. F., Carver, C. S., & Gibbons, R. X. Self-directed attention, awareness of bodily states, and suggestibility. *Journal of Personality and Social Psychology*, 1979, *37*, 1576–1588.

Scheier, M. F., Carver, C. S., & Matthews, K. Focus of attention and awareness of bodily sensations. In J. T. Cacioppo & R. E. Petty (Eds.), *Social psychophysiology*. New York: Guilford Press, in press.

Schwartz, G. E., & Shapiro, D. Social psychophysiology. In W. F. Prokasy & D. C. Raskin (Eds.), *Electrodermal activity in psychological research*. New York: Academic Press, 1973.

Shaffer, D. R. Some effects of consonant and dissonant attitudinal advocacy on initial attitude salience and attitude change. *Journal of Personality and Social Psychology*, 1975, *32*, 160–168.

Shapiro, D., & Crider, A. Psychophysiological approaches in social psychology. In G. Lindzey & E. Aronson (Eds.), *The handbook of social psychology* (Vol. 3, 3rd ed.). Reading, Mass.: Addison-Wesley, 1969.

Shapiro, D., & Schwartz, G. E. Psychophysiological contributions to social psychology. *Annual Review of Psychology*, 1970, *21*, 87–112.

Shields, S. A., & Stern, R. M. Emotion: The perception of bodily change. In P. Pliner, K. R. Blankstein, & I. M. Spiegel, (Eds.), *Perception of emotion in self and others*. New York: Plenum Press, 1979.

Spence, D. P., Lugo, M., & Youdin, R. Cardiac change as a function of attention to and awareness of continuous verbal text. *Science*, 1972, *176*, 1344–1346.

Stagner, R. *Psychology of personality*. New York: McGraw-Hill, 1948.

Stern, R. M., Botto, R. W., & Herrick, C. D. Behavioral and physiological effects of false heart rate feedback: A replication and extension. *Psychophysiology*, 1972, *9*, 21–29.

Strongman, K. T. *The psychology of emotion*. London: John Wiley & Sons, 1973.

Tesser, A. Self-generated attitude change. *Advanced Experimental Social Psychology*, 1978, *11*, 289–338.

Thurstone, L. L. The measurement of attitudes. *Journal of Abnormal and Social Psychology*, 1931, *26*, 249–269.

Triandis, H. C. *Attitude and attitude change*. New York: John Wiley & Sons, 1971.

Tursky, B., Schwartz, G., & Crider, A. Differential patterns of heart rate and skin resistance during a digit-transformation task. *Journal of Experimental Psychology*, 1970, *83*, 451–457.

Tyler, S. W., Hertel, P. T., McCallum, M. C., & Ellis, H. C. Cognitive effort and memory. *Journal of Experimental Psychology: Human Learning and Memory*, 1979, *5*, 607–617.

Valins, S. Cognitive effects of false heart-rate feedback. *Journal of Personality and Social Psychology*, 1966, *4*, 400–408.

Valins, S. Emotionality and information concerning internal reactions. *Journal of Personality and Social Psychology*, 1967, *6*, 458–463.

Van Toller, C. *The nervous body*. Chichester, England: John Wiley & Sons, 1979.

Wicklund, R. A., & Brehm, J. W. *Perspectives on cognitive dissonance*. Hillsdale, N.J.: Erlbaum, 1976.

Zajonc, R. B. Feeling and thinking: Preferences need no inferences. *American Psychologist*, 1980, *35*, 151–175.

Zanna, M. P., & Cooper, J. Dissonance and the pill: An attribution approach to studying the arousal properties of dissonance. *Journal of Personality and Social Psychology*, 1974, *29*, 703–709.

Zanna, M. P., & Cooper, J. Dissonance and the attribution process. In J. H. Harvey, W. Ickes, & R. F. Kidd (Eds.), *New directions in attribution research* (Vol. 1). Hillsdale, N.J.: Erlbaum, 1976.

Zillmann, D. Attribution and misattribution of excitatory reactions. In J. H. Harvey, W. Ickes, & R. F. Kidd (Eds.), *New directions in attribution research* (Vol. 2). Hillsdale, N.J.: Erlbaum, 1978.

Zillmann, D., Johnson, R. C., & Day, K. D. Attribution of apparent arousal and proficiency of recovery from sympathetic activation affecting excitation transfer to aggressive behavior. *Journal of Experimental Social Psychology*, 1974, *10*, 503–515.

# 6

# *Influence of Afferent Cardiovascular Feedback on Behavior and the Cortical Evoked Potential*

CURT A. SANDMAN
BARBARA B. WALKER
CHRIS BERKA

## INTRODUCTION

The Cartesian dichotomy separating the brain and the body is rooted deeply in the history of psychology and physiology. Manifestations of this dichotomy are evident from the classical "debate" of William James and Walter Cannon. James (1892) suggested that perception (especially of emotional experience) was a product of visceral and autonomic input to the brain. He proposed that sensations developed perceptual qualities as a result of the context in which they were experienced, and that the peripheral nervous system provided this context. Thus, perceptions acquired unique qualities which corresponded to distinctive patterns of physiological response.

Curt A. Sandman. Departments of Psychiatry and Psychobiology, University of California Irvine Medical Center, Orange, California; and Fairview Hospital, Costa Mesa, California.
Barbara B. Walker. Ann Arbor VA Medical Center, University of Michigan, Ann Arbor, Michigan.
Chris Berka. Department of Neurosciences, University of California, San Diego, California.

However, a more popular viewpoint was proposed by Cannon (1929). He maintained that the peripheral nervous system was a "passive" executor of commands received from the central nervous system. Cannon suggested that the "fight-or-flight" response, critical for survival, was associated with a unidimensional nervous system response. It was assumed that since the peripheral nervous system response was controlled solely by the brain, all of the peripheral systems responded in unison. It was assumed further that only quantitative changes in physiological responses differentiated experience. This assumption suggested that larger physiological responses were related with more intense experiences, and that qualitative differences in physiological responding may be inconsequential. A practical outcome of acceptance of this view was the reliance on a single response system for studying behavior.

The view expressed by Cannon still guides the biological study of behavior. Even though the validity of this view has been questioned in recent years, the study of the relationship between the brain and behavior has flourished. Resolution of the differences between the views of Cannon and James has awaited methodological refinements and the proper *zeitgeist* for nurturing theoretical synthesis. The *zeitgeist*, due largely to the poineering efforts of Davis (1957), Miller (1969), and the Laceys (B. C. Lacey & Lacey, 1974), and evidenced by escalating interests in psychosomatic and behavioral medicine, appears to be appropriate. This chapter presents a view of behavioral relations with cardiovascular events and introduces a strategy for refined analysis of brain–body relationships.

## CARDIOVASCULAR AND BARORECEPTOR PHYSIOLOGY

Physiologists have studied homeostatic functions of the cardiovascular afferent fibers for years, and the existence of pressure-sensitive receptors (baroreceptors) in the carotid sinus and aortic arch is well established. The baroreceptors increase their firing rates during transient blood pressure increases and decrease their rate of discharge as blood pressure falls. Nerves from the carotid sinus and aortic arch join the vagus and the glossopharyngeal nerves, which terminate in the lower brainstem and assist in providing homeostatic control of blood pressure to ensure survival of the organism.

Quite interestingly, it appears that baroreceptors have functions in addition to those classified as homeostatic. In 1929 Tournade and

Malmejac found that stimulating the carotid sinus nerve led to diminished muscle tone in anesthetized animals. Shortly thereafter, Koch (1932) increased the pressure in the carotid sinus of a dog and found that it led to decreased motor activity and even prolonged sleep. These two reports were among the first to suggest that baroreceptor activity influenced higher levels of the nervous system than those needed to maintain cardiovascular homeostasis, and that these influences were inhibitory rather than excitatory.

In a compelling study, Bonvallet, Dell, and Hiebel (1954) mechanically distended the carotid sinus of cats in order to produce an experimental analogue of increased pressure. They discovered that increased pressure shifted electrocortical activity from low-voltage fast activity to high-voltage slow activity. Thus, when the baroreceptors in the wall of the carotid sinus detected increases in pressure, the electrocortical activity was inhibited. Decreased blood pressure released the cortex from this inhibitory influence. Indeed, Bonvallet *et al.* (1954) discovered that by severing the vagus and glossopharyngeal nerves, the inhibitory influence dissipated.

More recent experiments have demonstrated significant baroreceptor input to areas of the brain remote from those previously associated with cardiovascular control. In fact, contemporary cardiovascular physiologists have suggested that the concept of the "vasomotor center" be expanded to include a number of areas superior to the brainstem (Joy, 1975). In an investigation of baroreceptor input to the hypothalamus, Adair and Manning (1975) illustrated the importance of these supramedullary connections by recording evoked potentials in the posterior hypothalamus as early as 10 msec following stimulation of the carotid sinus. Moreover, when these hypothalamic areas were stimulated, a 65% reduction in single-unit firing occurred in medullary neurons known to be responsive to baroreceptor activation. Thus, even before reaching the vasomotor center, baroreceptor activity was detected by the hypothalamus and subsequently channelled to a number of supramedullary structures.

One supramedullary structure which is responsive to vasomotor activity is the locus coeruleus. Baroreceptor activation, by blood-volume loading, resulted in a significant reduction in single-unit firing in this area (Svensson & Thoren, 1979). Coleridge, Coleridge, and Rosenthal (1976) found that distension of the carotid sinus causes prolonged depression of activity of pyramidal tract cells in the motor cortex. This depression ranged from a 15% reduction in firing to complete cessation of activity and lasted approximately 85 sec after the distension ceased. Similarly, human spinal cord excitability has been shown to vary directly with the cardiac pulse. Forster and Stone (1976) demonstrated that the "physiological tremor" of normal skeletal muscles is a function of cardiovascular modulation, presumably via $\gamma$-motorneurons.

Sensory processes are also influenced by baroreceptor activity. Gahery and Vigier (1974) showed that stimulation of baroreceptor afferents depressed the responses of single cells in the nucleus cuneatus after stimulation of the skin. These data emphasize that baroreceptors play an important role in sensory and motor functions as well as in the control of blood pressure.

Thus, neurophysiological evidence has suggested that blood pressure increases detected by baroreceptors are transmitted via the vagus and the glossopharyngeal nerves to the area of the brainstem maintaining homeostasis and to other areas which may serve to *inhibit* cortical, autonomic (except cardiovascular), and muscular activity. Accordingly, increased blood pressure is part of an inhibitory or restraining process rather than an activating process. Conversely, decreased blood pressure releases this inhibition, resulting in lowering of sensory thresholds and a prolongation of stimulus impact.

The importance of the cortical inhibitory influence of the baroreceptors may have adaptive significance for the organism. For instance, the heart and even the baroreceptors (Obrist, Light, McCubbin, Hutcheson, & Hoffer, 1979) respond to environmental stimulation. These changes are detected in bulbar structures of the brain. Thus, cardiovascular responses to external events generate a direct inhibitory influence on the central nervous system. Further, cells firing with a cardiac rhythm have been recorded in the bulbar areas (Humphrey, 1967; Smith & Pearce, 1961), and coagulation in this region prolongs the effects of a stimulus. J. I. Lacey (1967) has suggested that the functions of this area, rich with cardiovascular representation, may be to "control the duration of an episode of stimulus produced in the brain" (p. 27).

The complexities and problems associated with this explanation have not gone unrecognized (J. I. Lacey & Lacey, 1970). One problem arises as a result of the fact that the carotid sinus is not purely passive. It has its own properties, and Peterson (1962) has shown that the stiffness of the carotid sinus wall, one determinant of baroreceptor sensitivity, is affected by acetylcholine and norepinephrine. It seems clear that other nervous system activity may alter the stiffness of the wall and the sensitivity of the baroreceptors. Thus, the inhibition thought to be determined solely by baroreceptor activity may, in part, be determined by other activity of the nervous system affecting the wall of the carotid sinus.

In view of this, it is not surprising that inhibitory effects do not occur every time blood pressure increases. It is clear that other processes modify the cardiovascular–central nervous system relationship. Exercise, for example, will not necessarily lead to inhibitory effects on the organism. The inhibition is subject to modification by higher levels of the central nervous system, not only from the level of the wall of the carotid sinus itself to the area of the brain it ultimately reaches, but also from the area of the brain back to the effector processes where inhibition is observed.

Another limitation is the fact that there are many baroreceptors throughout the body in addition to those in the aortic arch and carotid sinus. It would be naïve to assert that only those in the aortic arch and carotid sinus bear any relationship to the central nervous system and behavior. Undoubtedly, there are complex interactions at many levels of the nervous system, among various baroreceptor systems that are scattered throughout the body. Virtually nothing is known at this point regarding these possible interactions.

The temporal sequence of baroreceptor discharge poses another problem. Frequency of baroreceptor firing may be slightly out of phase with changes in blood pressure. Furthermore, little is reported concerning the interaction between tonic levels of blood pressure and phasic changes in blood pressure even at the level of the baroreceptors.

Finally, the significance of cerebral blood flow in this inhibitory process in unclear. When carotid baroreceptors are stimulated, there is a decrease in arterial blood pressure which may lead to a significant fall in cerebral blood flow (Purves, 1972). Diminished cerebral blood flow causes a decrease in oxygen available to the tissues, which might account for neuronal inhibition. While the widely accepted view is that cerebral blood flow is autoregulatory and not subject to any significant neurogenic control (see Purves, 1972, for a review), there are data to indicate that cerebral vasoconstriction occurs when systemic blood pressure is raised, and that this vasoconstriction is related specifically to baroreceptor activity (Ponte & Purves, 1974). It is possible, therefore, that increases in baroreceptor firing lead to cerebral vasoconstriction, which in turn leads to neuronal inhibition. The situation is complicated, however, since Ingvar (1972) has emphasized that cerebral blood flow is regulated by the metabolic activity of neuronal tissue. Decreases in neuronal activity lead to a decrease in carbon dioxide output and an increase in extracellular pH, giving rise to cerebral vasoconstriction. Thus, while it is certain that neuronal activity and cerebral blood flow are closely coupled, the precise nature of the relationship is unknown.

The complexity of cardiovascular events and the proposed relationship with behavior are simplified in Figure 6-1. Each ventricular contraction of the heart (the R wave) propogates a bolus of blood through the vascular system which is detected as a resonating pulse. As evident in Figure 6-1, the peak of the carotid pulse wave begins to ascend at about the R wave and reaches a peak value (systolic pressure) several milliseconds later. The firing rate of the baroreceptors is related to both the peak of the carotid pulse and to heart rate. Thus, as heart rate increases, the firing rate of the baroreceptors increases during each pulse. The Laceys (J. I. Lacey, 1959; J. I. Lacey, Kagan, Lacey, & Moss, 1963; J. I. Lacey & Lacey, 1970) were among the first to recognize the significance of these neurophysiological relationships for the study of behavior.

Recent evidence suggests that stress-induced changes in baroreceptor activity modulates sensory threshold. Dworkin, Filewich, Miller, Craigmyle, and Pickering (1979) reported that animals deprived of baroreceptor modulation were more responsive to aversive stimulation, exhibited lower thresholds to stress-evoking situations, and were unable to respond appropriately to reinforcement. The authors suggest that "baroreceptor activation reduces the aversiveness or motivational consequences of noxious stimulation" (p. 1300). Although these data could be interpreted as an influence of baroreceptors on perceptual threshold, evidence supportive of a role for the cardiovascular system in emotional behavior has been generated by Angyan (1978). Self-stimulation in the septum, thalamus, hypothalamus, and midbrain elicted reliable, transient increases in arterial pressure in cats. Moreover, the frequency of stimulation varied directly as a function of pressure responses. Since nonrewarding sites produced no pressure responses, measurement of pressure responses was sufficient to determine if a stimulation site was pleasurable or aversive.

## CARDIOVASCULAR RELATIONS WITH BEHAVIOR

In a series of tasks ranging from those requiring attention to the external environment (i.e., detection of flashes) to those in which attention to the

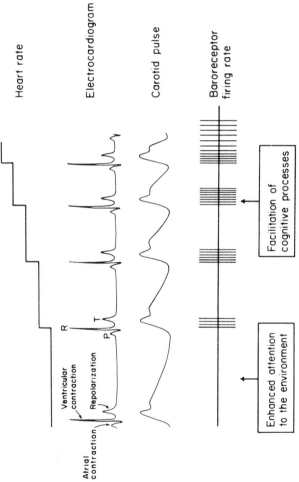

FIG. 6-1. Proposed relationships among heart rate, the electrocardiogram, the carotid pulse, baroreceptor activity, and psychological processes.

environment interfered with performance of the task (i.e., mental arithmetic), it was discovered that heart rate and blood pressure were the physiological responses which best differentiated the cognitive–perceptual processes (J. I. Lacey et al., 1963; J. I. Lacey, 1967). Heart rate decreased during tasks requiring environmental attention, whereas tasks demanding "mental concentration" or "rejection of the environment" were related with heart rate acceleration. These findings were related to the neurophysiological evidence which indicated that decelerating heart rate would release the cortex from inhibitory control of the baroreceptors. Thus, during decelerating heart rate, fast-frequency electroencephalographic activity may result, and this activity has been related consistently with vigilant behavior (Lindsley, 1969). Conversely, increased heart rate may stimulate the baroreceptors and thereby inhibit cortical activity in this case. Slow wave formations of the EEG would develop which have been related to problem-solving behavior.

Studies from our laboratory (Sandman, 1971, 1975; Walker & Sandman, 1977) and others (Hare, 1973; Libby, Lacey, & Lacey, 1973) indicated that subjects responded with decelerated heart rate while viewing unpleasant stimuli. This response was surprising since heart rate acceleration was commonly believed to be an aspect of the overall sympathetic nervous system response to stressful stimuli. The findings were interpreted as indicating that stressful stimuli can involve a strong attentional component, and that viewing these stimuli also involves "morbid fascination."

In a refined analysis of this issue, Cacioppo and Sandman (1978) presented subjects with stressful visual stimuli (pictures of accident victims) and stimuli which were equated with the pictures of accident victims on the dimension of unpleasantness but required "cognitive effort." These latter stimuli included arithmetic problems, anagrams, and strings of digits to be memorized. Thus two sets of stressful stimuli were generated, one set depicting gruesome material and involving emotional reactions, and another set reflecting cognitive stress. Consistent with previous studies, heart rate decelerated during viewing of the accident victims but increased for the equally unpleasant stimuli which required "mental effort." Thus it appeared that heart rate reflected the type of processing required by the task but not its affective components. Specifically, heart rate decelerated during processing which required only "attention to the environment," whereas tasks requiring "cognitive elaboration" or "rejection of the environment" resulted in heart rate acceleration.

## INFLUENCE OF THE HEART ON ATTENTION

In a recent set of experiments (Sandman, McCanne, Kaiser, & Diamond, 1977), the influence of heart rate and cardiac phase on detection of stimuli was examined. As illustrated in Figure 6-2, subjects' fluctuating heart rates were detected by a computer, and when a fast beat (upper decile of a subject's resting heart rate), slow beat (lower decile of resting heart rate), or a midrange beat (average of fast and low) was emitted spontaneously, a digit of extremely brief exposure (6, 10, 20 msec) was flashed on a screen in front of the individual. The subjects were required to report the digit (single digits from 0 to 9) that they perceived. If attention to the external environment is related to low heart rate, better performance would be expected during low rather than during high heart rate.

The results of this experiment provided support for the bradycardia of attention. When heart rate was low, subjects perceived the stimuli which were presented for the briefest exposure significantly better than when heart rate was fast. This influence of the heart on behavior is

FIG. 6-2. The paradigm designed and employed to permit the ECG, heart rate, or pulse pressure waves to initiate the stimulus. The subjects' physiological responses are recorded by a polygraph and compared by a computer with a criterion. If the criterion is met or exceeded, the stimulus is automatically delivered.

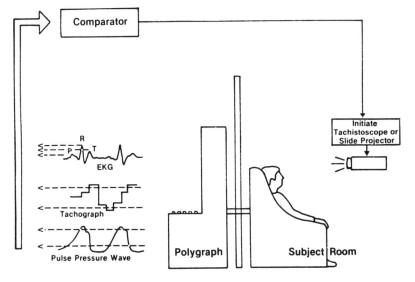

illustrated in Figure 6-3. In addition to the enhancement of perception, increased cerebral perfusion was also related to decelerating heart rate.

Since similar influences on the baroreceptors may be expected during low heart rate and during the P wave of the cardiac cycle, and during fast heart rate and the R-T interval of the cardiac cycle (Figure 6-1), the behavioral significance of the discrete waves during each cardiac cycle also was examined. Previous investigations yielded equivocal results; some studies reported greater attention to the environment during the early components of the cycle (Birren, Cardon, & Phillips, 1963; Callaway & Layne, 1964), while other studies found no significant influence of the cardiac cycle on behavior (Delfini & Campos, 1972; Elliott & Graf, 1972; Thompson &

FIG. 6-3. Accuracy during a tachistoscopic perception task. Performance was enhanced when stimuli were synchronized with low heart rate. From "Heart Rate and Cardiac Phase Influences on Visual Perception," by C. A. Sandman, T. R. McCanne, D. N. Kaiser, and B. Diamond, *Journal of Comparative and Physiological Psychology*, 1977, *91*, 189–202. Reprinted by permission.

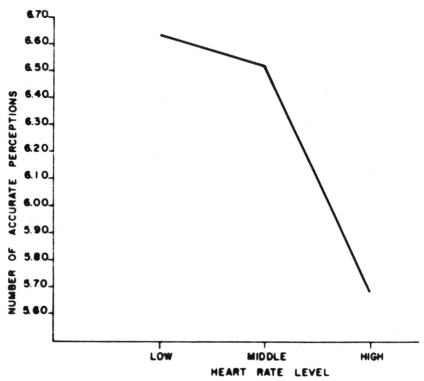

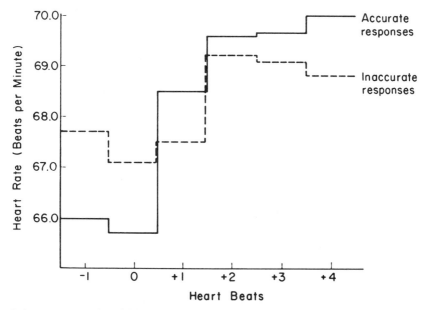

FIG. 6-4. When subjects initiated their own stimulus, a pervasive deceleration was observed (heart beat 0). Greater heart rate deceleration was related to accurate perceptual performance.

Botwinick, 1970). Just as in the previous study, and as illustrated in Figure 6-2, digits were presented for brief periods of time but were synchronized with the waves of the cardiac cycle. Consistent with the findings of the first study, stimuli presented during the P wave were perceived more accurately than stimuli presented during the T wave, just ½ sec later.

We reasoned further that if heart rate has an important or adaptive influence on attention or perception, the cardiovascular system should reflect the intention to receive information. A study was designed in which subjects were instructed to depress a telegraphic key whenever they "felt ready to perceive a stimulus." The stimuli, as before, were digits presented for just an instant. As Figure 6-4 indicates, the depression of the key indicating intention to perceive was associated with heart rate deceleration, and, further, accurate perception was related to greater deceleration than inaccurate perception. These data suggested that changes in the cardiovascular system were coupled with intention to receive information (J. I. Lacey & Lacey, 1970). Further, the extent of the deceleratory response was related to accuracy of the subjects' perception.

INFLUENCE OF THE HEART ON COGNITIVE ACTIVITY

As already suggested, the Laceys have related increases in heart rate to "rejection of the environment" or to tasks requiring cognitive processing. They and others (Tursky, Schwartz, & Crider, 1970) have found that tasks requiring mental concentration or cognitive elaboration were related consistently to increases in heart rate. For instance, Kaiser and Sandman (1975) found that solution of anagrams was related to heart rate increase such that the most difficult problems (reflecting more processing) produced the greatest acceleration and the easiest problem produced the least acceleration. Further, the rate of problem solution was positively correlated with heart rate.

In another study (Baker, Sandman, & Pepinsky, 1975) subjects were required to prepare, "mentally," a two-minute speech. One "speech" was to be about a visible object (to which they could attend and then describe) or about "someone they disliked very much." Heart rate (and other responses) was measured during the preparation interval, during the speech, and then several minutes after the speech. Increases in heart rate were recorded only during the rehearsal period for the nonvisible object (requiring imagery and fantasizing). Further, a significant relationship between heart rate increases and verbal output was observed. While no casual link can be developed from these studies, a clear relationship between the magnitude of heart rate increases and an objective measure of underlying thought was developed.

Decrease of simple reaction time (when the subject does not have to make a decision but only responds during the presentation of a stimulus) is related to decelerating heart rate and facilitation of attention. However, Duncan-Johnson and Coles (1974) have illustrated that the heart rate deceleration can be attenuated if the subject is required to perform a decision before responding. Utilizing the same design employed for assessing the impact of the heart on perception (Figure 6-2), the relationship between heart rate and cognitive processing was elaborated. Stimuli were presented during either fast, slow, or midrange heart rate (as described earlier). The subjects were shown either a circle or a square; when a circle was presented, the subjects were to depress a telegraphic key as rapidly as they could. During the second stimulus, a square, they withheld their response. The latency to respond to the circle is one measure of the time required to make a decision. It was found that increases of heart rate related to faster reaction time. The clear influence of heart rate on a reaction time task which reflected cognitive processing or decision making is illustrated in Figure 6-5. During elevated heart rate, reaction time decreased; and conversely, during lower heart rate, reaction time increased. Since many earlier studies had shown a disassociation between behavior (reaction time) and arousal using a simple task, it could be assumed that the relationship found in this study supports the notion that cognitive processing is facilitated during elevated heart rate.

FIG. 6-5. Faster choice reaction time (requiring cognitive processing) was related to accelerating heart rate.

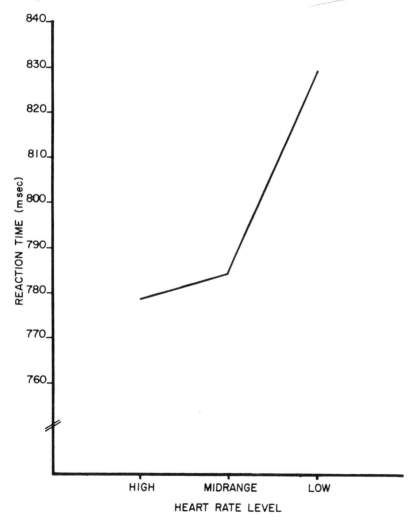

In a second part of this experiment, the influence of cardiac phase on this task was examined. Unlike the results for studies fo perception, no effect of cardiac phase upon reaction time was observed. This could be due to two factors: (1) the comparative insensitivity of the reaction time task compared with the test of perception and (2) the reliably robust influence of heart rate compared with the seemingly delicate impact of events during the cardiac cycle.

## INFLUENCE OF CONTROL OF HEART RATE ON BEHAVIOR

The focus of our studies was not the demonstration that procedures such as biofeedback might alleviate clinical symptoms, at least not initially. Instead, our approach was to attempt to examine the possibility that behaviors which had been linked to discrete physiological responses could be liberated by altering the physiology of the organism. In our initial experiment (McCanne & Sandman, 1974), we attempted to link control of heart rate to changes in attention or perception of environmental stimuli. In this study, subjects were shown tachistoscopic stimuli during periods of conditioned heart rate acceleration and deceleration.

During the first five sessions, the subjects were "shaped" to produce increases or decreases in their heart rate on cue. The shaping procedure was designed to make the criterion more and more difficult as the subjects improved, and, conversely, easier to accommodate slower learners. The subjects received both visual and auditory feedback regarding their performance by means of a real-time clock. The technique was very successful, producing differences in heart rate of 8-12 beats with three sessions (see McCanne & Sandman, 1975, for a complete description of the conditioning procedures).

To test the effects of learned speeding and slowing of the heart on perception, tachistoscopic stimuli were flashed at the subject during trials of reinforced heart rate. The findings indicated that subjects perceived stimuli more accurately during trials of reinforced heart rate deceleration than during acceleration.

In a subsequent study (McCanne & Sandman, 1976), we examined the influence of autonomic nervous system conditioning procedures on performance of the Rod and Frame Test. Accuracy of performance of this task requires the ability of the subject to ignore distracting information in order to align a rod to a true vertical position. Subjects were given either heart rate training as described earlier, false heart rate feedback, galvanic skin response (GSR) conditioning, or no feedback at all. All of the subjects receiving contingent feedback performed better on the Rod and Frame Test. However, a dramatic difference was observed in the comparison between contingent and noncontingent heart rate feedback.

A similar paradigm was employed to examine the influence of learned heart rate control on cognitive activity (Cacioppo, Sandman, & Walker, 1978). Resistance to persuasion is, in part, a function of the number of counterarguments subjects can generate to rebut an issue. The greater the number of reasons (counterarguments) subjects develop to reject a message, the less likely they will be persuaded by the message (Petty & Cacioppo, 1977). We hypothesized that controlled increases in heart rate would enhance cognitive activity. During elevated heart rate, subjects should generate more counterarguments and be less susceptible to persuasion. Conversely, subjects should become more susceptible to persuasion during low heart rate since their critical "thinking" ability is compromised. As in the previous experiments, subjects were trained to control their heart rate for several days with operant procedures prior to behavioral testing.

Messages differing in persuasiveness were presented to subjects as they were reinforced for heart rate increases and decreases. The subjects were instructed to report their opinion of the message by giving a number corresponding to a continuum of agree–disagree. At the end of the presentation, the subjects were asked to list their thoughts.

The results indicated that during reinforced heart rate acceleration, subjects generated more counterarguments (assessed after presentation of the message) and were less willing to endorse the persuasive message. However, during reinforced heart rate deceleration, the subjects provided fewer counterarguments and were much more susceptible to persuasion. This may have occurred because during high heart rate, cognitive elaboration tends to be facilitated, and self-convincing arguments may be generated against a persuasive message. However, during lowered heart rate, our cognitive functioning gives way to environmental attention, and the demands of the environment may prevail.

There is substantial evidence linking discrete behavior (and presumably the brain) to dimensions of cardiovascular activity. These data, though mostly "correlative" in nature, are difficult to reconcile with views which ascribe all intellectual abilities, such as perception and attention, solely to the brain. Few studies exist in intact human subjects which illustrate the impact of the heart on the brain. The following group of studies are among the first which describe the influence of the heart on aspects of brain function.

## CARDIOVASCULAR RELATIONS WITH THE CORTICAL EVOKED POTENTIAL

### VISUAL EVOKED POTENTIALS

In order to probe the influence of the heart on the brain, we chose to study the cortical averaged evoked potential (AEP). As in earlier experiments (Figure 6-2), stimuli were synchronized with fast, slow, and midrange heart rates (Walker & Sandman, 1979). Sixteen right-handed men who met several criteria (absence of drug use, 20/20 vision, etc.) volunteered to participate. Bright flashes of light were presented for 20 msec to each subject. The AEPs were averaged for 50 stimuli at each heart rate from EEGs recorded from the right and the left hemispheres of the brain ($O_1$ and $O_2$ to ipsilateral mastoids).

The results were subjected to several analyses. A discriminant function analysis indicated that the major influence of high and low heart rate was evident in the right but not the left hemisphere of the brain (Figure 6-6). In the right hemisphere, 81.3% of the AEPs recorded during low and midrange heart rate were classified correctly. Only 50% were classified correctly during high heart rate. The stepwise procedure was unable to discriminate better than chance, AEPs during high and low heart rate in the left hemisphere.

The amplitude of the secondary characteristics of the AEP ($P_1$ and $P_2$) in the right hemisphere was largest when elicited during low heart rate. These components were not different when recordings were made from the left hemisphere. Thus, characteristics, which reflect relatively simple perceptual processing, appeared to be discretely coupled with cardiovascular dynamics.

Although it may be peculiar to the paradigm we employed, it was apparent that the influence of the heart on the brain was lateralized. These findings are consistent with the growing body of literature which suggests that tasks requiring attention to the environment are associated with AEPs recorded from the right hemisphere (Dustman, Schenkenberg, & Beck, 1976) and with low heart rate (B. C. Lacey & Lacey, 1974;

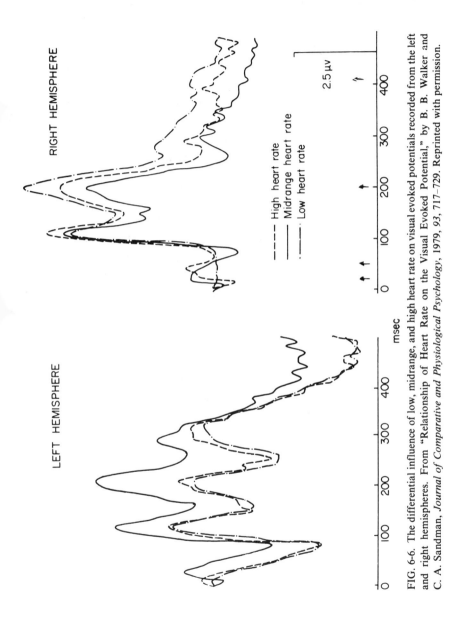

FIG. 6-6. The differential influence of low, midrange, and high heart rate on visual evoked potentials recorded from the left and right hemispheres. From "Relationship of Heart Rate on the Visual Evoked Potential," by B. B. Walker and C. A. Sandman, *Journal of Comparative and Physiological Psychology,* 1979, *93,* 717–729. Reprinted with permission.

205

Sandman *et al.*, 1977). Thus, the heart may influence attentional/perceptual functioning by uniquely affecting the right hemisphere of the brain. Further tests of the lateralized influence of cardiovascular dynamics on the brain have confirmed our initial finding.

In the second study of the influence of the cardiovascular system on the brain, stimuli were synchronized with pulse pressure components recorded above the carotid, cephalic, and digital arteries. As reviewed earlier, each ventricular pulse of the heart sends a bolus of blood rushing through the arteries which is detected by baroreceptors as a transient shift in pressure. At the peak of the wave (systolic pressure), pressure is the greatest and the baroreceptors increase their firing rate. During the lowest point of the wave (diastolic pressure), the baroreceptors are relatively quiescent. As illustrated in Figure 6-2, these transient shifts in pressure are roughly analogous to the spontaneous changes in heart rate.

It was presumed that stimuli synchronized with the diastolic component of the cephalic and carotid pulse wave would produce AEPs similar to that observed during low heart rate. However, the impact of stimuli synchronized with digital pulse pressure changes, significantly out of phase with central measures, was unknown. Eighteen (nine male and nine female) right-handed subjects were recruited to participate in this study. Carotid pulse pressure was measured by placing a photoplethysmograph (especially designed by Robert Isenhart) directly over the carotid artery. Cephalic pulse pressure was monitored by placing the transducer over the supraorbital artery. This pulse is only slightly out of phase (20–30 msec) with the carotid pulse and thus provides a functional replication. The peripheral measure of pulse pressure was achieved by placing the transducer on the third flange of the ring finger. A considerable shift in phase from carotid pulse pressure (150–200 msec) was observed.

Discriminant function analysis indicated that AEPs synchronized with pulse pressure waves recorded from the carotid and cephalic placements were differentiated only in the right hemisphere. For both the carotid and cephalic placements, stimuli presented during diastolic phases of the pulse pressure wave were augmented only in the right hemisphere. This finding is illustrated in Figure 6-7. Accuracy of classification with discriminant analysis reflected this finding since between 77.8% (systolic–carotid) and 100% (systolic, diastolic–cephalic) AEPs were sorted correctly with jackknifing procedures. Surprisingly, AEPs elicited by presentation during cephalic pulse pressure waves were sorted more accurately than AEPs stimulated by stimuli triggered during carotid waves. No

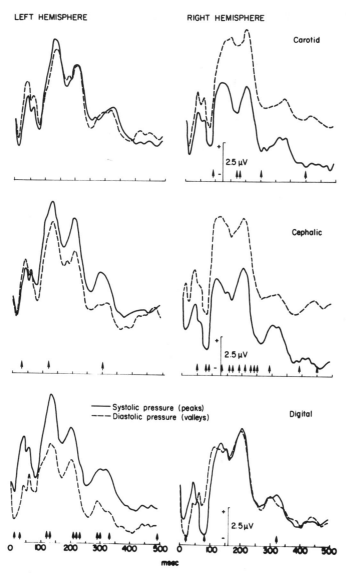

FIG. 6-7. Visual evoked potentials recorded from the left and right hemispheres when stimuli were synchronized with systolic and diastolic pressure recorded from the area of the carotid, ophthalmic, and digital arteries.

significant findings were detected in the left hemisphere with stimulus presentation during carotid waves, and only a few points were significant when triggered by cephalic pulse waves.

Presentation of stimuli synchronized with digital placements (about 150–200 msec after carotid and cephalic waves) produced dramatically different results. Not only was the major effect of stimulus synchronization observed in the left hemisphere, but the augmentation of the AEP occurred during the systolic pulse. Accuracy of classification of the AEPs in the left hemisphere was 100% for both systole and diastole.

The results of the discriminant function analysis was dissected with other procedures. The amplitude and latencies of major components were subjected to analysis of variance. The major finding was that the $P_1$ component was enhanced in the right hemisphere during diastole of both the carotid and cephalic waves. There were no significant effects for either the digital placement or for any of the latencies measurements of the major components of the AEP.

The data of this experiment provided partial support for the proposed relationship between the transient pressure changes during heart rate and each beat of the heart. In both experiments, events that related to decreased pressure resulted in augmented AEPs only in the right hemisphere. The effect observed during diastole in the cephalic placement was the most robust finding. Further, the fact that the nature of the phenomenon is dramatically altered when stimuli are phase shifted argues for the importance of the temporal relations between cardiovascular events and the brain. Thus, cardiovascular changes which are detected by pressure receptors in the carotid artery, and possibly the vasculature of the brain, appear to sensitize the brain to environmental stimulation. Further, with the paradigm employed, this sensitization appears to be particular to the right hemisphere of the brain.

The remarkable similarity between the findings of the heart rate and pulse pressure experiments prompted a third study. The aim of this study was to examine the effects on the AEP of the interaction of heart rate and pulse pressure waves. In this study, 15 right-handed males volunteered to participate. Essentially, the methods for this experiment were identical to the previous experiment except that presentation of the stimulus was contingent upon changes of heart rate *and* changes of the pulse pressure wave.

As in the previous experiments, the major effects of stimuli synchronized with heart rate and pulse pressure changes were observed in the right hemisphere of the brain. Between 80% and 100% of the AEPs were sorted accurately with discrimiant function analysis. In the left hemisphere the percentage of accurate classification ranged from 60% to 73%. Analyses of variance indicated that only during accelerating heart rate, in the right hemisphere, was the difference between systole and diastole reflected in the AEP. The most significant difference during accelerating heart rate was enhancement of $P_1$ during stimuli synchronized with diastole. A similar trend was apparent during low heart rate but failed to achieve an acceptable level of statistical significance.

The results of this study indicated that complex relations exist between heart rate and the pulse pressure wave. These components do not appear to be simply additive. Indeed, if they were additive, the AEP would be maximally enhanced during stimuli presented during low heart rate and diastole. This result was not forthcoming although the converse was; that is, maximal suppression was observed during high heart rate and systole (however, only in the right hemisphere). The major finding which did emerge was that maximal separation between the influence of systole and diastole was observed only during elevated heart rate. These findings may suggest that during high heart rate the impact of transient changes in pulse pressure is discriminated by the baroreceptors with greater precision than during low heart rate. The mechanisms involved in producing these findings are not known. It is inviting to speculate that during elevated heart rate, maximal (or near maximal) activity of the baroreceptors is achieved during each beat (ventricular pulse) of the heart. It is conceivable that this barrage "exhausts" the cells temporarily, resulting in significant quiescence during diastole. Thus, the greatest contrast between systole and diastole may be during elevated heart rate. A revised, and perhaps more accurate, illustration of cardiovascular relations (compared to that portrayed in Figure 6-1) is presented in Figure 6-8.

These findings provide a basis for understanding discrepancies in the behavioral literature. Studies attempting to relate cardiac phase with behavior have yielded equivocal results; some studies (Thompson & Botwinick, 1970; Delfini & Campos, 1972) reported no effect, whereas others (Sandman et al., 1977; Saari & Pappas, 1976) generated predictable relations. The former studies employed tasks which included a warning signal, a technique which generally results in heart rate deceleration. From the current studies it was found that the impact of intracardiac events is not clearly discriminable (as evidenced by the AEP) during lowered heart rate. The two later studies, which found predictable re-

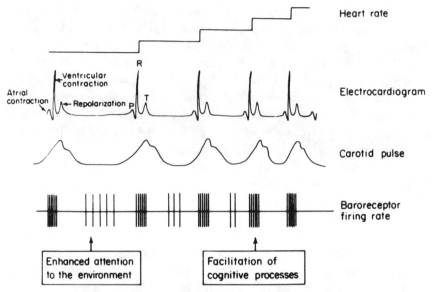

FIG. 6-8. Revised model of the proposed relationship among cardiovascular events.

lations between the heart and behavior, did not use a warning signal. Although direct tests of this possibility should be conducted, the often neglected interaction of cardiovascular variables may account for some of the discrepancies in the behavioral literature.

## AUDITORY EVOKED POTENTIALS

In a parallel study, utilizing an identical design as for the visual evoked potentials, the impact of cardiovascular changes on the auditory evoked potential was examined. Fifteen right-handed males, ranging in age from 18 to 24, served as subjects. Monopolar AEPs to pure tones were recorded from EEG leads $C_3$ and $C_4$ to ipsilateral mastoids. Fifty tones were synchronized with systole and diastole from three different plethysmograph placements (cephalic, carotid, and digital). A major difference between the study of auditory responses and the studies of visual evoked potentials was that the subjects were instructed to keep their eyes closed and to count the number of tones they heard.

The results of this procedure, illustrated in Figure 6-9, are somewhat different than those with the visual AEP paradigm. First, although the impact of the cardiovascular system on the AEP is lateralized, there is a differential effect in each hemisphere (as compared to an effect only in the right hemisphere previously). Perhaps the fact that the subjects counted stimuli in the current procedure accounted for this difference. Second, the impact of the different plethysmograph placements is considerably less significant than observed during the visual AEP studies. Although significant differences between diastole and systole were observed with the carotid and cephalic placements, the digital placement produced similar findings. Visual AEPs synchronized with digital placement were reversed for diastole and systole when compared with the more central placements. It is not known if this difference is a result of the nature of stimulus (auditory) or of the differing procedures (counting stimuli). Studies underway in our laboratory do not resolve this issue but to indicate that the $P_3$ wave which distinguishes the more central from the distal placements is a result of the attention (i.e., counting) directed toward the stimuli. However, further research is required to clarify these phenomena.

When the results were subjected to analysis of variance, they were complementary to the results observed with the visual AEP procedure. The $N_1$ response, typically reflecting the attentional state of the organism, was larger during systolically induced AEPs only in the right hemisphere.

The $P_2$ component was clearly enhanced during diastole in the right hemisphere, especially for stimuli synchronized with the carotid artery (Figure 6-9, peak-to-valley measurements). Thus, two components of the AEP, which are related to attention to environmental stimulation, appeared to be discretely synchronized with characteristics of the cardiovascular system and also appeared to be lateralized in hemispheres of the brain. However, these findings must be considered preliminary until definitive studies are completed which bridge the hiatus among the various designs.

STUDIES IN PATIENT GROUPS

Several preliminary studies have been conducted with clinical groups including patients diagnosed with essential hypertension, depression, and attentional deficits. The findings with the auditory evoked potential ob-

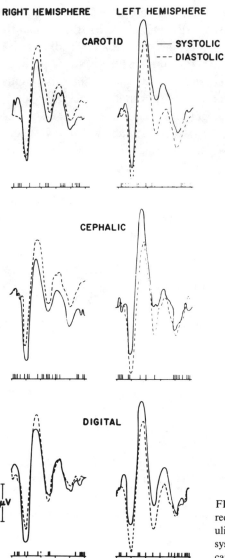

FIG. 6-9. Auditory evoked potentials recorded while subjects counted stimuli. The stimuli were synchronized with systolic and diastolic pulses of the carotid, ophthalmic, and digital arteries.

tained with hypertensives and hyperactive children are presented in Figures 6-10 and 6-11. As is apparent from Figure 6-10, there is a virtual absence of an evoked potential during systole in both hemispheres in the patient suffering essential hypertension. The evoked potential in this patient (age 65) is fairly normal during diastole, although it is somewhat dampened and the latencies are longer than normal. Further, there is no obvious difference between the hemispheres of the brain. Perhaps the "resetting" of baroreceptors, a common mechanism proposed for the maintenance of hypertension, is reflected by this finding. It is conceivable that the anomolous response during systole is due to saturation of the baroreceptors. Thus, maximal inhibition of cortical activity may result. The findings that cognitive/perceptual difficulties accompany the symptoms of hypertension are consistent with the AEP data (Friedman & Bennett, 1977). It may be presumed that information from the external environment simply does not register during the systolic phase of the carotid artery. Thus, approximately one-half of the time, information may not be properly processed in patients suffering from essential hypertension. Although the data presented in Figure 6-10 are an extreme example of this phenomenon, other patients displaying lesser, but clinically significant, symptoms of hypertension also evidence similar re-

FIG. 6-10. Auditory evoked potentials from the right and left hemispheres in a patient suffering essential hypertension. The stimuli were synchronized with systole and diastole of the carotid artery. Note the virtual absence of an AEP during systole.

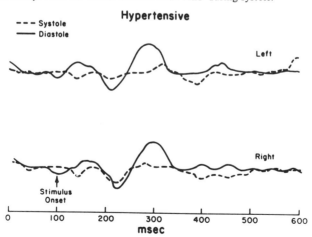

214  /  SANDMAN, WALKER, AND BERKA

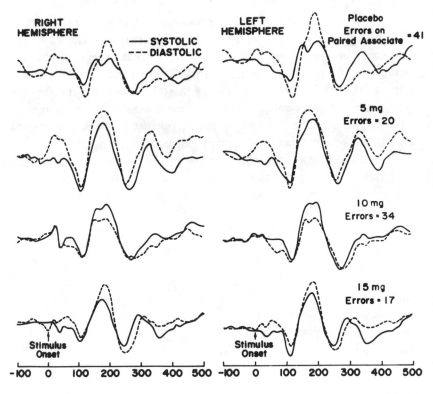

FIG. 6-11. Auditory AEP recorded from a hyperactive child given three doses of Ritalin and placed in a double-blind procedure. Even though the response to medication was unconventional, the relationship between learning, drug, and the AEP was consistent.

sponses. In one fully studied patient (age 32), remission of the deviant blood pressure symptoms (by use of biofeedback) was associated with "normalizing" of the evoked potential.

The findings with hyperactive children are illustrated by one case in Figure 6-11. In collaboration with James Swanson, the relationships between cognitive performance, drugs, and cardiovascular influences on the auditory AEP have been examined. Essentially, we observed no hemispheric differences in any children (normal or patients) examined to date. This is reflected in Figure 6-11. However, the interesting finding is the extent to which the relationships in the AEP related to dosage of drug and the performance of a paired-associated learning test. When untreated by stimulant medication (Ritalin), the patient made a large number of errors on the test of learning. The evoked potential had a very distinctive form, characterized by a dampening of $N_1$ and $P_2$ during systole in both hemispheres. Further, during systole the $P_2$ component was biphasic, and a clear $P_3$ component emerged. Response to medication was unconventionally quadratic, with 5 mg and 15 mg of Ritalin eliciting a positive response (fewer errors on the test of learning), and 10 mg producing essentially no change from placebo. Surprisingly, the AEP reflected this response to medication. The two beneficial doses functionally normalized the AEP, especially during systole. The dosage which produced the adverse response considerably diminished the AEP during diastole. Further, the relationship between systole and diastole was reversed in both hemispheres when the patient received the dosage to which he exhibited an adverse response. Thus, it appears that this procedure is exquisitely sensitive to the effects of medication and may reflect, in a very precise way, the cognitive integrity of the patient.

THE "NO-STIMULUS" PARADIGM

In order to examine the possible contaminating influences of the ECG on the AEP, trials were averaged with the stimulus turned off. The strategy employed was identical to the conventional AEP; the sampling was initiated by the detection of systolic and diastolic pulses of the carotid or cerebral arteries. Forty trials were averaged, each for systole and diastole. This procedure was construed as a control for possible contaminants we observed of the ECG on the AEP. This was of primary concern since some of the effects occurred very early (in the first 100 msec) in the developing AEP.

The typical response from $C_3$-$C_4$ to linked mastoids is illustrated in Figure 6-12. These data were collected from a normal subject, and they are representative of the responses we have observed. The resulting response is the *averaged* EEG phase locked to the cerebral pulse pressure wave. Complementary responses are locked to systole and diastole, and appear about 50 msec after the pulse. This response may account for some of the differences observed very early in the AEP and may reflect ECG artifact. However, the response is apparent even when the electrodes are placed more laterally and appears to be exacerbated when subjects close

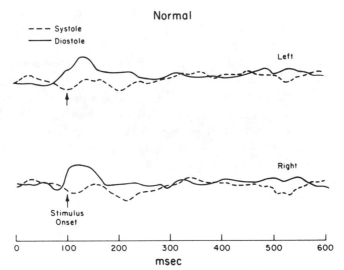

FIG. 6-12. Sampling of episodes of the EEG in a normal subject during systolic and diastolic pulses of the carotid artery with the external stimulus turned off. The resulting response is the average EEG phase locked to the pulse pressure wave. The complementary response of 50 msec after the pulse may be an ECG artifact.

their eyes. The data do indicate very clearly that the major components of the AEP (100+ msec) are not paralleled by any "artifact" after the 50-msec period.

We have applied this procedure in depressed patients and children. Figure 6-13 illustrates a dramatic example of a phenomenon seen in three depressed patients and, to a lesser degree, in children. This figure illustrates a phase-locked cyclicity of the EEG to the cerebral pulse pressure wave. The reliability of this phase relationship is considerable since the tracing is the result of 40 samples. Roughly 4 to 4½ cycles are observed in the 500-msec sampled, indicating a signal in the alpha range (8–9 Hz). There is a striking 180-degree phase relationship between pulse samples initiated at systole and those initiated at diastole.

These observations are preliminary and their significance is uncertain They may reflect relatively primitive processing capacity, as reflected in children or depressed patients. This pattern may suggest that for certain groups of subjects an inviolable relationship exists between the brain and the cardiovascular system.

These data may relate to the suggestions that brain activity in the alpha range is an artifact of "square wave" (the ventricular pulse of the heart) stimulation applied to a gelatinous mass (the brain) in a limited, closed container (the skull) (Bering, 1955; Kennedy, 1959). Figure 6-14 illustrates the relationships among several electromechanical events in the body which may initiate and sustain such activity (Bering, 1955). This figure illustrates the transfer of mechanical energy from the ventricular contraction of the heart to the cerebrospinal fluid. Kennedy assumes that the pumping action of choroid plexuses in this process may also mechanically drive the surrounding brain tissue. The frequency of oscillation depends on the consistency of the brain (gel). During states of attention, the brain may be engorged with blood, thereby "detuning" the "gel oscillators," resulting in alpha blocking. Kennedy's (1959) conclusion is that alpha rhythms, as well as the anterior temporal rhythm, "arise from mechanical oscillation of the gel of the living brain, not necessarily from synchronization of neural activity directly" (p. 352).

It is inviting to speculate that psychological states such as depression result in both inattention and an abundance of alpha activity. It is possible that states of synchrony between the heart and brain reflect the relative slavish control of the brain by afferent input from the body. As such, certain states (i.e., depression) may be associated with an absence of

FIG. 6-13. This illustrates the time-locked cyclicity of the EEG to the pulse pressure wave. This tracing is the average of 40 samples and is thus considered reliable. The frequency is roughly in the alpha range (8–9 Hz).

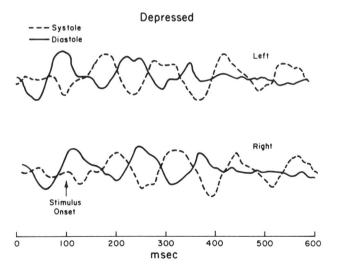

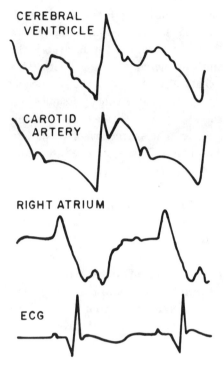

CEREBRAL
VENTRICLE

CAROTID
ARTERY

RIGHT ATRIUM

ECG

FIG. 6-14. Illustration of the relationships between cardiovascular events and the pulse measured in the cerebral ventricle. From "Choroid Plexus and Arterial Pulsation of Cerebrospinal Fluid," by E. A. Bering, *Archives of Neurology and Psychiatry*, 1955, *73*, 165–172. Reprinted by permission.

spontaneous (i.e., "independent" from body) brain activity. The very preliminary data we have collected lend tentative credibility to some of the provocative speculations of Kennedy and deserve meticulous study.

## CONCLUSIONS

From several different laboratories reliable relationships between the cardiovascular system and behavior have been reported. Although there is debate about the independence of the heart's influence on the brain (Obrist, Howard, Lawler, Galosy, Meyers, & Gaebelein, 1974), the consensus is that attention to the environment relates to bradycardia. Conversely, rejection of the environment, associated with thinking, relates to increases in heart rate. Further, recent findings indicate that events occurring within a cardiac cycle (which reflect transient changes in pressure) are associated also with acceptance or rejection of the environment. The most parsimonious explanation for these findings is that the transient pressure increases detected by baroreceptors, inhibit cortical activity. During quiescent periods, the cortex is released from inhibition, and processing of external events is facilitated.

The relationship between cardiovascular events and the cortical evoked response supports and extends the behavioral findings. These studies suggest that the afferent input from the heart to the brain is very specific. Generally, stimuli synchronized with diastole or with low heart rate resulted in larger cortical evoked responses than stimuli synchronized with systole or high heart rate. Further, it is clear that the effects of the cardiovascular system are most apparent in the right hemisphere of the brain with the paradigms employed. Thus, the influence of the heart on the brain is not diffuse, but specific, and results in a unique influence on perception. Fascinating support for the notion that the heart may "pulse" perception derives from a report by Oswald (1959).

Oswald was intrigued by anecdotal reports that schizophrenics often indicated that their hallucinations "pulsed." However, since reliable testing of this phenomenon was quite difficult, Oswald developed an ingenious procedure for evaluating an analogue of hallucinations. A bright light was flashed to normal subjects which resulted in vivid afterimages, persisting for about 5 sec. The subjects reported that the afterimage "pulsed." In an effort to determine the frequency of the pulsing image, the subjects were instructed to depress a telegraphic key as the afterimage waxed and waned. The pulsing image was perfectly synchronized with the ventricular contraction of the heart.

From the early studies of the relationship between the heart and behavior, to studies indicating that the autonomic nervous system could be conditioned, to studies of the impact (or covariation) of the cardiovascular system and the brain, and the intriguing report of Oswald, it can be concluded that the heart exerts a dynamic influence on the brain and behavior. The recent studies with the AEP suggest that the influence of the heart fluctuates between liberating and suppressing the left and right hemispheres of the brain. If such a possibility exists, the time frame for such an important effect is very precise. Even subtle responses within a cardiac cycle, occurring within milliseconds, exert profound effects. Thus the historical and political separation of the brain and the body is being reevaluated with the tools of modern technology. The significance of the data reviewed suggests that the sea of consciousness (once thought the private domain of the brain) has many components, including the oscillating waves of the cardiovascular system.

# REFERENCES

Adair, J. R., & Manning, J. W. Hypothalamic modulation of baroreceptor afferent unit activity. *American Journal of Physiology*, 1975, *229*, 1357–1364.

Angyan, L. Cardiovascular effects of septal, thalamic, hypothalamic and midbrain self-stimulation. *Physiology and Behavior*, 1978, *20*, 217–226.

Baker, W. M., Sandman, C. A., & Pepinsky, H. P. Affectivity of task rehearsal time and physiological response. *Journal of Abnormal Psychology*, 1975, *84*, 539.

Bering, E. A. Choroid plexus and arterial pulsation of cerebrospinal fluid. *Archives of Neurology and Psychiatry*, 1955, *73*, 165–172.

Birren, J., Cardon, P., & Phillips, S. Reaction time as a function of the cardiac cycle in young adults. *Science*, 1963, *140*, 195–196.

Bonvallet, M., Dell, P., & Hiebel, G. Tonus sympathétique et activité électrique corticale. *Electroencephalography and Clinical Neurophysiology*, 1954, *6*, 119.

Cacioppo, J. T., & Sandman, C. A. Physiological differentiation of sensory and cognitive tasks as a function of warning, processing demands and reported unpleasantness. *Biological Psychology*, 1978, *6*, 181.

Cacioppo, J. T., Sandman, C. A., & Walker, B. B. The effects of operant heart rate conditioning on cognitive elaboration and attitude change. *Psychophysiology*, 1978, *15*, 330–338.

Callaway, E., & Layne, R. Interaction between the visual evoked response and two spontaneous biological rhythms: The EEG alpha cycle and the cardiac arousal cycle. *Annals of the New York Academy of Sciences*, 1964, *112*, 424–431.

Cannon, W. B. *Bodily changes in pain, hunger, fear and rage: An account of recent researches into the function of emotional excitement.* New York: Appleton, 1929.

Coleridge, H. M., Coleridge, J. C. G., & Rosenthal, F. Prolonged inactivation of cortical pyramidal tract neurons in cats by distension of the carotid sinus. *Journal of Physiology*, 1976, *256*, 635–649.

Davis, R. C. Response patterns. *Transactions of the New York Academy of Sciences*, 1957, *19*, 731.

Delfini, L., & Campos, J. Signal detection and the "cardiac arousal cycle." *Psychophysiology*, 1972, *9*, 484–491.

Duncan-Johnson, C., & Coles, M. Heart rate and disjunctive reaction time: The effects of discrimination requirements. *Journal of Experimental Psychology*, 1974, *103*, 1160–1168.

Dustman, R. E., Schenkenberg, T., & Beck, E. C. The development of the evoked response as a diagnostic and evaluative procedure. In R. Karrer (Ed.), *Developmental psychophysiology of mental retardation.* Springfield, Ill.: Charles C. Thomas, 1976.

Dworkin, D. R., Filewich, R. N., Miller, N. E., Craigmyle, N., & Pickering, T. G. Baroreceptor activation reduces reactivity to noxious stimulation: Implications for hypertension. *Science*, 1979, *205*, 1299–1301.

Elliott, R., & Graf, V. Visual sensitivity as a function of phase of cardiac cycle. *Psychophysiology*, 1972, *9*, 357.

Forster, A., & Stone, T. W. Evidence for a cardiovascular modulation of central neuronal activity in man. *Experimental Neurology*, 1976, *51*, 141–149.

Friedman, M., & Bennett, P. L. Depression and hypertension. *Psychosomatic Medicine*, 1977, *39*, 134–141.

Gahery, Y., & Vigier, D. Inhibitory effects in the cuneate nucleus produced by vago-aortic afferent fibers. *Brain Research*, 1974, *75*, 241–246.

Hare, R. D. Orienting and defensive responses to visual stimuli. *Psychophysiology*, 1973, *10*, 453-464.

Humphrey, D. R. Neuronal activity in the medulla oblongata of cat evoked by stimulation of the carotid sinus nerve. In P. Kezdi (Ed.), *Baroreceptors and hypertension.* New York: Pergamon Press, 1967.

Ingvar, D. H. Patterns of thought recorded in the brain. *Totus Homo*, 1972, *4*, 98-103.

James, W. *Psychology.* New York: Henry Holt, 1892.

Joy, M. D. The vasomotor center and its afferent pathways. *Clinical Science and Molecular Medicine*, 1975, *48*, 253s-256s.

Kaiser, D. N., & Sandman, C. A. Physiological patterns accompanying complex problem solving during warning and nonwarning conditions. *Journal of Comparative and Physiological Psychology*, 1975, *89*, 357-363.

Kennedy, J. L. A possible artifact in electroencephalography. *Psychological Review*, 1959, *66*, 347-352.

Koch, E. Die Irradiation der pressoreceptorischen Krieslaufreflexe. *Klinische Wochenschrift*, 1932, *11*, 225-227.

Lacey, B. C., & Lacey, J. I. Studies of heart rate and other bodily processes in sensorimotor behavior. In P. A. Obrist, A. H. Black, J. Brener, & L. V. DiCara (Eds.), *Cardiovascular psychophysiology.* Chicago: Aldine, 1974.

Lacey, J. I. Psychophysiological approaches to the evaluation of psychotherapeutic process and outcome. In E. A. Rubinstein & M. B. Parloff (Eds.), *Research in psychotherapy.* Washington, D.C.: American Psychological Association, 1959.

Lacey, J. I. Somatic response patterning and stress: Some revisions of activation theory. In M. H. Appley & R. Trumbull (Eds.), *Psychological stress: Issues in research.* New York: Appleton, 1967.

Lacey, J. I., Kagan, J., Lacey, B. C., & Moss, H. The visceral level: Situational determinants and behavioral correlates of autonomic response patterns. In P. H. Knapp (Ed.), *Expression of the emotions in man.* New York: International Universities Press, 1963.

Lacey, J. I., & Lacey, B. C. Some autonomic-central nervous system interrelationships. In P. Black (Ed.), *Physiological correlates of emotion.* New York: Academic Press, 1970.

Libby, W. L., Lacey, B. C., & Lacey, J. I. Pupillary and cardiac activity during visual attention. *Psychophysiology*, 1973, *10*, 270.

Lindsley, D. Average evoked potentials—Achievements, failures and prospects. In E. Donchin & D. Lindsley (Eds.), *Average evoked potentials: Methods, results and evaluations* (NASA Sp-191). Washington, D.C.: NASA, 1969.

McCanne, T. R., & Sandman, C. A. Instrumental heart rate responses and visual perception: A preliminary study. *Psychophysiology*, 1974, *11*, 283-287.

McCanne, T. R., & Sandman, C. A. Determinants of human operant heart-rate conditioning: A systematic investigation of several methodological issues. *Journal of Comparative and Physiological Psychology*, 1975, *88*, 609.

McCanne, T. R., & Sandman, C. A. Operant autonomic conditioning and Rod-and-Frame Test performance. *Journal of Personality and Social Psychology*, 1976, *34*, 821.

Miller, N. E. Learning of visceral and glandular responses. *Science*, 1969, *163*, 434.

Obrist, P. A., Howard, J. L., Lawler, J. E., Galosy, R. A., Meyers, K. A., & Gaebelein, C. J. The cardiac-somatic interaction. In P. A. Obrist, A. H. Black, J. Brener, & L. V. DiCara (Eds.), *Cardiovascular psychophysiology.* Chicago: Aldine, 1974.

Obrist, P. A., Light, K. C., McCubbin, J. A., Hutcheson, J. S., & Hoffer, J. L. Pulse transit time: Relationship to blood pressure and myocardial performance. *Psychophysiology*, 1979, *16*, 292.

Oswald, I. A case of fluctuation of awareness with the pulse. *Quarterly Journal of Experimental Psychology*, 1959, *11*, 45.

Peterson, L. H. The mechanical properties of the blood vessels and hypertension. In J. G. Cort, V. Fencl, Z. Hejl, & J. Jirka (Eds.), *The pathogenesis of essential hypertension*. Prague: State Medical Publishing House, 1962.

Petty, R. E., & Cacioppo, J. T. Forewarning, cognitive responding and resistance to persuasion. *Journal of Personality and Social Psychology*, 1977, *35*, 645–655.

Ponte, J., & Purves, M. J. The role of the carotid body chemoreceptors and carotid sinus baroreceptors in the control of cerebral blood vessels. *Journal of Physiology*, 1974, *237*, 315–340.

Purves, M. J. The neural control of cerebral blood vessels. In *The physiology of the cerebral circulation*. London: Cambridge University Press, 1972.

Saari, M., & Pappas, B. Cardiac cycle phase and movement and reaction times. *Perceptual and Motor Skills*, 1976, *42*, 767–770.

Sandman, C. A. *Psychophysiological parameters of emotion*. Unpublished doctoral dissertation, Louisiana State University, 1971.

Sandman, C. A. Physiological responses during escape and non-escape from stress in field independent and field dependent subjects. *Biological Psychology*, 1975, *2*, 205–216.

Sandman, C. A., McCanne, T. R., Kaiser, D. N., & Diamond, B. Heart rate and cardiac phase influences on visual perception. *Journal of Comparative and Physiological Psychology*, 1977, *91*, 189–202.

Smith, R. E., & Pearce, J. W. Microelectrode recordings from the region of the nucleus solitarius in the cat. *Canadian Journal of Biochemical Physiology*, 1961, *39*, 933.

Svensson, T. H., & Thoren, P. Brain noradrenergic neurons in the locus coeruleus: Inhibition by blood volume load through vagae afferents. *Brain Research*, 1979, *172*, 174–178.

Thompson, L. W., & Botwinick, J. Stimulation in different phases of the cardiac cycle and reaction time. *Psychophysiology*, 1970, *7*, 57.

Tournade, A., & Malmejac, J. Diversité des action réflexes qui déclenche l'excitation du sinus carotidien et de son nerf. *Comptes Rendus des Séances de la Société de Biologie*, 1929, *100*, 708–711.

Tursky, B., Schwartz, G. E., & Crider, A. Differential patterns of heart rate and skin resistance during a digit transformation task. *Journal of Experimental Psychology*, 1970, *83*, 451.

Walker, B. B., & Sandman, C. A. Physiological response patterns in ulcer patients: Phasic and tonic components of the electrogastrogram. *Psychophysiology*, 1977, *14*, 393–400.

Walker, B. B., & Sandman, C. A. Relationship of heart rate on the visual evoked potential. *Journal of Comparative and Physiological Psychology*, 1979, *93*, 717–729.

# 7

# Respiratory–Heart Rate Interactions: Psychophysiological Implications for Pathophysiology and Behavior

STEPHEN W. PORGES
PHILIP M. MCCABE
BRANDON G. YONGUE

## INTRODUCTION

It is commonly acknowledged that respiratory influences on the cardio-vascular system may confound the measurement of heart rate responses in psychophysiological research. There is the omnipresent observation that oscillations in heart rate covary with respiration (Siddle & Turpin, 1980). Operant control of heart rate is often confounded by respiratory mediation (Katkin & Murray, 1968). Moreover, event-related heart rate responses are related to respiratory phase (Coles, Pellegrini, & Wilson, 1980).

To deal with these problems researchers have treated respiration as a *nuisance* variable and have attempted to remove its influence with two distinct strategies: manipulation and statistical evaluation. Respiratory parameters have been manipulated to experimentally assess the relationship between characteristics of respiratory activity and responses such as the event-related heart rate response. Techniques such as paced breathing

Stephen W. Porges, Philip M. McCabe, and Brandon G. Yongue. Department of Psychology, University of Illinois, Champaign–Urbana, Illinois.

have been used to stabilize respiratory patterns to isolate the biofeedback effects on heart rate (Brener & Hothersall, 1967). Stimulation during specific phases of the respiratory cycle has been used to control the influence of inspiration and expiration on the characteristics of the heart rate response (Riege & Peacock, 1968). Alternatively, the spontaneous characteristics of respiration have been assessed and related to the heart rate response (Cheung & Porges, 1977; B. C. Lacey & Lacey, 1978; Porges & Raskin, 1969).

Psychophysiological research has attempted to partition the *true* heart rate response from potentially confounding variables. Attempts have been made to remove the variance due to the respiration–heart rate interaction in order to describe lawful relationships between manipulations external to the subject (e.g., auditory or visual stimulation) and responses within the subject (e.g., heart rate response). Unfortunately, given the interest in the description of stimulus–response relationships in cardiovascular psychophysiology, measures of within-organism function such as the *degree* of respiratory mediation of heart rate have been neglected within the domain of psychophysiological research.

This chapter focuses on respiratory sinus arrhythmia (RSA), a respiratory–heart rate interaction, characterized by a parallel between phases of respiration and heart rate increases and decreases. To understand the unique information conveyed by individual and state differences in RSA this chapter focuses on three areas: (1) the physiological mechanisms underlying respiration–heart rate interactions, (2) a quantitative method to describe RSA, and (3) the application of the quantification of RSA as a psychophysiological variable.

The interest in RSA may be theoretically justified by the *continuity model* (see Porges & Smith, 1980), which assumes that the patterning of autonomic activity is under constant control by the central nervous system (CNS). The precise description of a component of this patterning may provide important information regarding CNS function. To clarify this point, two individuals may exhibit a mean heart rate of 72 beats per minute (bpm) over a 1-hour period. However, one individual may exhibit a relatively constant heart rate while the other individual may exhibit a large amplitude RSA. Over the hour, both individuals may pump the same quantity of blood and maintain the same metabolic rate. However, since RSA is primarily neurally mediated, the measurement of RSA may provide information regarding the CNS.

The continuity model assumes that the centrally mediated autonomic control system is a complex homeostatic system consisting of peripheral and central afferent–efferent feedback mechanisms. The model makes no inference regarding afferent feedback on perceptual sensitivity, the underlying basis of J. I. Lacey's (1967) intake–rejection hypothesis. Moreover, the model acknowledges that small shifts in autonomic activity, mediated by the CNS, may be insignificant in terms of the effector organ's contribution to biological survival, the underlying thesis of Obrist (Obrist, Webb, Sutterer, & Howard, 1970). Physiological survival may be a function of the rate the heart beats, while the patterning of heart rate (e.g., RSA) may represent varying neural influences and thus reflect CNS status.

Although seldom explicitly stated, the prevalence of heart rate as a variable in psychophysiological research is a function of an *assumed* relationship between the CNS and the heart. The impact of this assumption has been to shift the role of heart rate monitoring from that of a global index of arousal or emotion to a sensitive index of cognitive processing. This assumption underlies the burgeoning field of cognitive psychophysiology. Ironically, psychophysiological research evaluating neural influences on the heart is scant. This chapter has been written to partially fill this void. The chapter focuses on RSA as a psychophysiological variable that conveys information regarding the neural mediation of heart rate.

## RESPIRATORY SINUS ARRHYTHMIA: PHYSIOLOGICAL BASIS

Respiratory sinus arrhythmia was first described by Ludwig in 1847 (see Anrep, Pascual, & Rossler, 1936*a*). Although the phenomenon was described immediately following Ludwig's report, the first extensive study of the respiratory influences on heart rate was reported by Anrep, Pascual, and Rossler (1936*a*, 1936*b*). Anrep and his colleagues investigated several characteristics of the interaction between respiration and heart rate, including: the influence of the respiratory rate and amplitude on heart rate, the influence of blood gas tensions on the extent of RSA, the relative contributions of central and peripheral reflexive actions on the cardioregulatory nerves, and an assessment of the efferent neural pathways involved in this relationship. These characteristics define the foci of past and present research on RSA. Subsequently other investigators have elaborated on each of these points. In the following paragraphs, we discuss research dealing with: (1) the development of RSA, (2) the influence of respiratory parameters on steady-state sinus arrhythmia, (3) the use of respiratory maneuvers to elucidate the mechanisms underlying RSA, (4) the efferent neural pathways involved in the respiratory modulation of heart rate, and (5) the possible influences of higher CNS processes on the amplitude of RSA.

## DEVELOPMENT OF RESPIRATORY SINUS ARRHYTHMIA

In most of the population, RSA increases during childhood to a level which persists throughout most of adulthood and then decreases in the aged. In an early investigation of RSA, McKenzie (see Anrep *et al.*, 1936*a*) labeled RSA as "juvenile arrhythmia" because of its prevalence in children and young adults. Jennet and McKillop (1971) measured the amplitude of RSA in five age groups of male subjects from 5 to 69 years of age. The mean amplitude of RSA in each of the three lowest age groups (5–7, 12–14, and 21–25 years) was significantly higher than for each of the two older age groups (41–48 and 59–69 years). These differences were not related to either respiratory frequency or mean pulse rate. Davies (1975) studied eight elderly subjects between the ages of 71 and 94. Six subjects showed a small but detectable RSA which was much smaller than young adults. Even in this select sample there was a tendency for an age effect; two of the three oldest subjects (83 and 94) exhibited no detectable RSA. In a longitudinal study of 199 male and female subjects, Reeve and De Boer (1960) assessed the changes in the amplitude of RSA from 1 month to 27 years of age. He reported that low-amplitude RSA was present from the early months following birth. There was a monotonic increase in the range of RSA which reached a peak between 8 and 12 years of age and was maintained throughout young adulthood. The possible mechanism underlying the early developmental changes in RSA is discussed later in this chapter.

## THE INFLUENCE OF RESPIRATION ON STEADY-STATE SINUS ARRHYTHMIA

Although the amplitude of RSA exhibits a characteristic developmental trend, there are short-term fluctuations in RSA that can be attributed to phasic changes in respiratory parameters. It appears that the amplitude of RSA in resting human subjects is primarily determined by the frequency of respiration. Changes in tidal volume seem to exert some influence on RSA when these changes are consciously made. However, alterations in tidal volume either through involuntary manipulations (Anrep *et al.*, 1936*a*) or in spontaneous breathing (Sroufe, 1971) do not seem to be effective in changing RSA. In addition, the degree of the respiratory influence on heart rate is affected by blood gas tensions, primarily $Pco_2$. Hypercapnia is associated with increased RSA. This leads to the hypothesis that a system which couples heart rate activity (a major determinant of blood flow) and respiration (the gas exchange mechanism) would be sensitive to circulating gas tensions.

Sroufe (1971) assessed the effects of respiratory rate and depth (i.e., tidal volume) on heart rate levels and heart rate variability (HRV). Sroufe found an inverse relationship between respiratory rate (rates of 14, 16, and 18 cycles per minute [cpm]) and HRV independent of heart rate level. The effects of depth of respiration on heart rate were assessed by splitting subjects into two groups, one that increased tidal volume by at least 50% and one that did not. Heart rate levels were elevated with increased tidal volume although HRV did not change. In a second experiment, Sroufe (1971) had subjects voluntarily breathe at fast or normal rates, while controlling tidal volume at 50%, 100%, or 200% of normal. Heart rate variability increased with increasing tidal volume and decreasing rate. Supporting data come from Melcher (1976), who also described a positive relationship between tidal volume and amplitude of RSA.

Angelone and Coulter (1964) studied the effects of respiratory rate in human subjects on both the amplitude and phase lag of RSA. They found that as respiratory rate is systematically increased from 1 to 40 breaths per minute, the amplitude of RSA changes in a triphasic manner (see Figure 7-1). The amplitude of RSA decreases in a linear fashion from 22 to 14 bpm as respiratory rate is increased to 3 cpm. As respiratory rate is increased to 5-6 cpm, RSA reaches a peak of approximately 25 bpm. Further increases in respiratory rate result in a rapid nonlinear decrease in the amplitude of RSA to a low of 3 bpm when respiration is 40 cpm. At the low respiratory frequencies, 1-4 cpm, maximum expiration temporally coincides with maximum HR (i.e., a phase angle approaching zero between expiration and HR). As respiratory rate increases from 4 cpm, a phase lag between peak HR and peak expiration appears which increases rapidly with respiratory rate. It is interesting to note that the phase lag from 0° to 90° seems to monotonically parallel the amplitude of RSA. The peak amplitude of RSA occurs with a phase lag of about 90°,

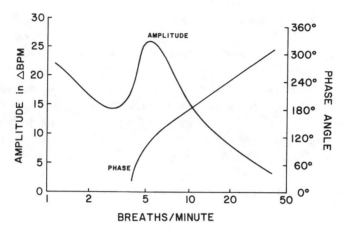

FIG. 7-1. Amplitude of RSA and its phase relationship with respiration as a function of respiratory frequency (breaths per minute). Redrawn from "Respiratory-Sinus Arrhythmia: A Frequency Dependent Phenomenon," by A. Angelone and N. A. Coulter, *Journal of Applied Physiology*, 1964, *19*, 479–482. Used with permission.

whereas a phase lag greater than 90° is associated with a decrease in RSA amplitude. At normal respiratory rates of 8–10 cpm, this phase relationship is reversed and represents the typical description of RSA.

Angelone and Coulter interpreted their results as evidence that RSA is a frequency-dependent system. In such a system, respiration acts as a driving function, and heart rate responds monotonically for a limited band of frequencies. When the critical respiratory frequency band is exceeded, a lag develops between the driving and responding functions, and the amplitude of the response is attenuated. Similar findings have been reported by other investigators. Manzotti (1958), in a study of the effects of transient respiratory maneuvers on heart rate, noted that in some human subjects, RSA lagged behind respiration one complete cycle when these subjects began or ended a period of voluntary apnea. Manzotti, however, did not manipulate respiration rate in a systematic manner in these experiments.

Clynes (1960) found that during normal respiration, biphasic heart rate transients in response to inspiration and expiration were superimposed and resulted in a sinusoidal heart rate pattern. The phase relationship of heart rate and respiration is determined by the degree of overlap between the inspiratory and expiratory transients, which is determined by the respiratory rate. Davies and Neilson (1967a) also studied the respiratory modulation of heart rate in terms of transient responses to respiration. They found a biphasic heart rate transient of constant latency to inspiration but not to expiration. Davies and Neilson interpreted the phase characteristics of heart rate and respiration in a manner similar to Clynes. At slow respiratory frequencies, inspiratory onset elicits a biphasic increase and decrease in heart rate, followed by the expiratory period in which heart rate is constant. As the respiratory rate increases, the inspiratory transients occur more closely in time, approximating a sinusoidal pattern that is phasic with respiration. With further increases in respiration rate, the transients begin to overlap, relocating the peak of the response and attenuating its amplitude. Davies and Neilson proposed that RSA could be explained in terms of a single inspiratory transient of constant latency, rather than a true phasic modulation of heart rate by respiration.

Observations by several researchers indicate that RSA may be related to blood gas tensions, particularly hypercapnia. Anrep *et al.* (1936*a*) found that in an innervated canine heart–lung preparation, perfusion of the head with hypercapnic blood resulted in an enhancement of the respiratory modulation of heart rate. Other reports (Kollai & Koizumi, 1979; Kunze, 1972; Levy, DeGeest, & Zieske, 1966) have described an increased amplitude of RSA in response to chemoreceptor stimulation in animal preparations.

RESPIRATORY MANEUVERS IN THE STUDY OF THE
MECHANISMS OF RSA

Three mechanisms may be responsible for RSA: (1) central influences, via a direct brainstem projection from respiratory to cardiac centers; (2) afferent feedback from stretch receptors in the lungs; and (3) volume receptor and baroreceptor reflexes elicited by alterations in blood flow from changing intrathoracic pressure. Each of these mechanisms has been described either in human or infrahuman preparations; each is functional under certain conditions. Central respiratory influences have been demonstrated in animal preparations when peripheral influences have been eliminated. These mechanisms have not been clearly demonstrated in humans, primarily due to methodological problems. The existence and function of pulmonary stretch afferents have been demonstrated in acute animal preparations, and there is no doubt that this is a viable mechanism for RSA. It is difficult to assess the influence of stretch receptors on RSA in humans, since any movements of the lungs are also associated with alterations in blood flow. Therefore, pulmonary afferent feedback may not be totally eliminated as a possible mechanism controlling RSA. Davies and Neilson (1967a) have indicated that this type of model cannot account for all of the changes in RSA amplitude, such as those related to posture, and the influences of hypocapnia. The influences of blood flow and blood pressure have been the most extensively studied of the three models in man. It has been claimed (Bainbridge, 1920; Melcher, 1976) that increased pulmonary return to the heart results in reflexive increases in heart rate via stimulation of cardiac volume receptors. Others have proposed that the mediating receptors are in the systemic arterial circulation (Davies & Neilson, 1967a). Under resting conditions in man, it seems that the primary respiratory influence on RSA is due to the peripheral influences from pulmonary and circulatory receptors.

## The Baroreceptor Reflex as a Controlling Mechanism of RSA

Studies as early as Bainbridge (1920) have attempted to explain RSA mechanisms in terms of alterations in baroreceptor and volume receptor responses to changes in blood flow caused by changes in thoracic pressure associated with respiration. Manzotti (1958) used respiratory maneuvers such as positive- and negative-pressure breath holding to assess the effects of expiration and inspiration on heart rate. He found that the heart rate response to positive intrathoracic pressure was a slow increase in heart rate that was related to the degree of pressure exerted. The response to sustained negative pressure was a heart rate deceleration that was related to the positive intrathoracic pressure immediately before the negative-pressure maneuver. These findings, together with the observation of the rapid rate at which vagally mediated heart rate responses could occur suggest that: (1) heart rate, due to its capacity for rapid change, is an instantaneous reflection of its controlling factors (i.e., any delay in the manifestation of respiratory influences on heart rate is due to the controlling rather than the efferent end of the system); (2) the heart rate responses to the respiratory manipulations are of a latency which precludes a central respiratory projection or stretch receptor reflex as an acceptable mechanism for the mediation of the respiratory influence on heart rate; and (3) the relationship between heart rate and positive intrathoracic pressure indicates that the heart rate responses, and possibly

RSA, are due to disruptions of the pulmonary return of blood to the heart, which affects left ventricular output and systemic blood pressure. The receptor site in such a model would be the aortic baroreceptors.

Davies and Neilson (1967a) also proposed a blood flow mechanism that mediates RSA. Using maneuvers similar to those of Manzotti (1958), they found heart rate responses of a much shorter latency than those reported by Manzotti. The shape and amplitude of the transient heart rate response to inspiration could be modified by postural changes. Davies and Neilson interpreted the results as support for a mechanism in which alterations in left ventricular output, due to increased venus return during inspiration, affects heart rate via the baroreceptor reflex. However, Jennet and McKillop (1971) measured arterial blood pressure in resting human subjects and found that heart rate and blood pressure fluctuated together, increasing during inspiration and decreasing during expiration. Since the baroreceptor reflex is characterized by a heart rate decrease in the presence of increased blood pressure, they claim that this reflex is not a reasonable candidate for the mechanism of RSA.

Melcher (1976) reported a positive relationship between mean heart rate and blood pressure during respiration in resting human subjects. He noted that arterial *pulse* pressure was negatively correlated with heart rate, and that heart rate was positively correlated with right-ventricular filling pressure. Melcher proposed that RSA was the result of a central integration of reflexive heart rate adjustments to stimulation of both low-pressure receptors in the right atrium and high-pressure receptors in the systemic circulation.

## Pulmonary Afferents and Central Control of RSA

It has been proposed (Hering, 1871, cited in Anrep *et al.*, 1936a) that reflex modulation of the cardioregulatory centers by pulmonary afferent feedback may be the physiological mechanism underlying RSA. Clynes (1960) used computer modeling to simulate heart rate activity from respiratory information. The best-fitting model described a biphasic heart rate transient, acceleration followed by deceleration, to both inspiration and expiration. Clynes speculated that the inspiratory and expiratory transients were caused by afferent feedback from pulmonary stretch receptors to medullary cardiac control systems. This argument was based upon the following observations: (1) The time course of the heart rate transient is independent of blood flow rate; (2) the heart rate transient to impulse breathing (rapid out–in) is greater than the transient to normal inspiration, and is of the same shape (note that this is not consistent with a blood flow model like Manzotti's [1958] since the impulse breath would result in less disruption of blood flow); and (3) inspiratory and expiratory transients are similar biphasic patterns but are caused by respiratory movements in opposite directions. Davies and Neilson (1967a) argued that the close fit of Clynes's simulation suggests, but does not prove, a contribution of stretch afferent input to RSA. Based upon their research they claimed that the modification of the shape and amplitude of the heart rate transient by posture cannot be explained in terms of pulmonary afferent input.

In 1865 Traube (cited in Anrep et al., 1936a) proposed that the brainstem nuclei controlling heart rate might be phasically influenced by direct irradiations from the medullary respiratory centers. Some investigators have concluded that central mechanisms have little influence on RSA in the human. This is based upon the following points: (1) Heart rate is not phasically modulated during periods of voluntary apnea (Davies & Neilson, 1967a), (2) the latency from the respiratory movement to the heart rate response is too long (Manzotti, 1958), and (3) the extent of RSA is not altered by assisting voluntary respiration with the application of negative extrathoracic pressure (Melcher, 1976). In view of the powerful voluntary influences on respiration which may be capable of inhibiting the medullary respiratory drive, it seems premature to rule out central influences on RSA.

In animal studies, the data indicate that central respiratory influences can exert an influence on heart rate when peripheral feedback is eliminated. Joels and Samueloff (1956) studied heart rate activity under conditions of diffusion respiration in dogs. In one condition, peripheral respiratory movements and afferent feedback were eliminated by injection of succinylcholine. Heart rate fluctuated in a rhythmic pattern similar to the prior respiratory rate. When centrally generated respiratory impulses were eliminated by deepening the level of anesthesia, RSA disappeared. Levy et al. (1966) studied the centrally mediated respiratory modulation of heart rate and contractility in the innervated canine left-ventricle preparation. In this preparation, the possibility of confounding peripheral influences was eliminated when the chest of the subject was open and the hili of the lungs ligated. They observed heart rate fluctuations of 26½ bpm which were phasic with contractions of the intercostal musculature. Other investigators (Anrep et al., 1936b; Hamlin, Smith, &

Smetzer, 1966; Lopes & Palmer, 1976) have also demonstrated that a central modulation of heart rate persists after the pulmonary afferent and barosensory feedback to the brainstem are eliminated.

Anrep *et al.* (1936*b*) carried out extensive experiments on the role of both central and peripheral (reflexive) influences in the mediation of RSA in an innervated canine heart–lung preparation. Central respiratory influences were eliminated by perfusing the head with hypocapnic blood. In the absence of central respiratory activity: (1) Heart rate accelerated in response to either positive or negative pressure inflation of the lungs; (2) sustained inflation or deflation of the lungs resulted in equally sustained heart rate accelerations or decelerations, respectively; (3) inflation of the lungs past a moderate tidal volume failed to increase the size of the tachycardia; and (4) sectioning vagal afferents from the lungs resulted in a heart rate increase. They also reported that sudden deflations of the lungs occasionally resulted in a 2:1 heart rhythm or complete AV block that could be eliminated by lung inflation. In normocapnic preparations, they eliminated stretch receptor influences on heart rate by sectioning the vagal afferents above the lungs but below the heart. This left only central influences to modulate heart rate since in an open-chest preparation, there are no thoracic pressure changes to elicit baroreceptor or Bainbridge reflexes. With this preparation, they found that heart rate fluctuations were in phase with phrenic nerve activity. Tachycardia was associated with phrenic nerve firing, and bradycardia was associated with the absence of activity. Although heart rate did not always fluctuate in the presence of phrenic activity, it never fluctuated in its absence.

In the past decade researchers have investigated the respiratory modifications of reflexive heart rate responses, providing interesting insights into the mechanisms of RSA. Haymet and McCloskey (1975) found that neither baroreceptor nor chemoreceptor stimulation in the carotid sinus region elicited a bradycardia if the stimuli were delivered during inspiration. If delivered during expiration, baroreceptor or chemoreceptor stimulation resulted in a prompt heart rate deceleration. Moreover, these stimuli were effective if presented during periods of sustained end-inspiratory apnea (Hering–Breuer inflation apnea), a period in which central inspiratory efferents are silent and the lungs are immobile. Inflation apnea represents a period in which neither central nor peripheral respiratory activity exerts an influence on heart rate responses. To further test the central respiratory influences on heart rate, the lungs were denervated to eliminate stretch receptor afferent projections to the medulla. Baroreceptor and chemoreceptor reflexive heart rate responses were blocked or attenuated during inspiration, while typical bradycardias were elicited during expiration.

Lopes and Palmer (1976) and Angell-James and Daly (1978) used stimulation of the superior laryngeal nerve (SLN) to inhibit central inspiratory activity and its associated lung movements. Lopes and Palmer found that SLN stimulation resulted in a bradycardia which could be terminated by section of the barosensory nerves. Angell-James and Daly reported that during the inspiratory inhibition of SLN stimulation, chemoreceptor stimuli at the carotid sinus elicited a greatly enhanced bradycardia which occasionally stopped the heart. In both studies, sudden inflation of the lungs reversed the bradycardia and restarted the heart in cases in which it had stopped. It has been demonstrated that central inspiratory activity, assessed by phrenic nerve recordings, modulates both resting heart rate and evoked heart rate responses in the absence of lung movement (Angell-James & Daly, 1978; Davidson, Goldner, & McCloskey, 1976; Davis, McCloskey, & Potter, 1977; Gandevia, McCloskey, & Potter, 1978a; Kordy, Neil, & Palmer, 1975; Lopes & Palmer, 1976). In addition, these studies reported that lung inflation, independent of phrenic activity, results in an increase in heart rate or an inhibition of the reflex bradycardia associated with baroreceptor or chemoreceptor stimulation. Lung inflation also inhibits the bradycardia normally elicited by ocular pressure and nasopharyngeal stimulation (Gandevia, McCloskey, & Potter, 1978b).

## EFFERENT NEURAL PATHWAYS IN RSA

### Parasympathetic Influences

Parasympathetic influences have been shown to play a major role in RSA. Although the precise mechanism is unknown, respiratory activity influences vagal control of the heart. Investigators have described a respiratory periodicity in the firing of cardiac vagal efferents. This periodicity arises from both central sources and pulmonary afferent feedback, and it can be manipulated by artificially ventilating the lungs. Furthermore, it has been reported that the amplitude of RSA is related to background vagal tone, and RSA can be virtually eliminated by atropine administration or vagotomy.

Several investigators have reported that cardiac vagal efferents are spontaneously active only during the expiratory phase of respiration (Iriuchijima & Kumada, 1964; Jewett, 1964; Katona, Poitras, Barnett, & Terry, 1970; Kollai & Koizumi, 1979; Kordy et al., 1975; Kunze, 1972; Neil & Palmer, 1975), and that this neural activity is accompanied by cardiac slowing (Iriuchijima & Kumada, 1964; Jewett, 1964; Katona et al., 1970; Kollai & Koizumi, 1979; Neil & Palmer 1975). These fibers increase their activity following catecholamine infusion (Jewett, 1964; Kollai & Koizumi, 1979; Kunze, 1972), electrical stimulation of the carotid sinus nerve (Iriuchijima & Kumada, 1964), pressure manipulations of the isolated carotid sinus (Neil & Palmer, 1975), and chemoreceptor stimulation with cyanide (Jewett, 1964; Kollai & Koizumi, 1979). All increases in firing were observed only during expiration except during asphyxia (Jewett, 1964), which causes continuous firing of vagal efferents.

During normal respiration inspiration inhibits cardiac vagal activity (Iriuchijima & Kumada, 1964; Jewett, 1964; Katona et al., 1970), whereas artificial ventilation seems to disrupt this effect. Iriuchijima and Kumada (1964) reported that positive pressure ventilation at a tidal volume just large enough to suppress spontaneous respiratory movements eliminates the firing of vagal efferents mediated by respiration. However, if tidal volume is increased, cardiac vagal activity follows the respiratory rhythm. This respiratory rhythm in vagal efferent activity persists following bilateral vagotomy but is abolished after denervation of the carotid sinus. This demonstrates that pulmonary stretch afferents are not essential for the respiratory rhythmicity in vagal efferents. During positive pressure ventilation this rhythmicity can be attributed to blood pressure fluctuations, due to intrathoracic pressure changes, which lead to phasic baroreceptor reflexes through the carotid sinus baroreceptor. These findings have been replicated by Katona and associates (Katona et al., 1970).

Cardiac vagal efferent activity has been reported to change during manipulations of artificial ventilation. Jewett (1964) found that decreasing tidal volume leads to increased vagal efferent activity and cardiac slowing, whereas increasing tidal volume produces the opposite results. Kollai and Koizumi (1979) reported increased vagal activity and enhanced RSA by decreasing tidal volume and elevating end-expired $CO_2$.

Central influences, as well as reflex mechanisms, appear to play a role in the respiratory modulation of vagal efferent activity. Several researchers reported a persistence of vagal efferent respiratory rhythmicity following bilateral section of the vagus (Iriuchijima & Kumada, 1964; Jewett, 1964; Kunze, 1972) or pneumothorax (Jewett, 1964). One may conclude that pulmonary stretch afferents are not necessary for the respiratory discharge of cardiac vagal efferents. Kunze (1972) reported that after vagotomy the central source for the modulation of vagal efferent firing can be manipulated by decreasing end-expired $CO_2$ through hyperventilation. During this period, phrenic nerve activity is suppressed. As the end-expired $CO_2$ level rises, phrenic activity returns and the efferent vagal fibers fire in reciprocal fashion to the phrenic discharge.

The amplitude of RSA is related to vagal tone. Anrep (Anrep et al., 1936a) found that increasing vagal tone by elevating blood pressure leads to an accentuated RSA, whereas low arterial blood pressure causes the heart to beat at a uniformly fast rate. Similarly, section of the aortic depressor nerves and occlusion of the common carotid arteries reduces vagal tone and RSA amplitude. Under these conditions vagal tone is increased with mild asphyxia, and an accompanying increase in RSA amplitude occurs. Anrep et al. (1936a) reported that bilateral section of the cervical vagus eliminates RSA. Levy et al. (1966) also mentioned that the amplitude of RSA varies with the extent of vagal tone. Enhanced RSA occurs during hypoxic stimulation of the carotid sinus. After the vagus is cut, only a small amount of RSA is seen, which the authors attribute to sympathetic influences. McCrady, Vallbona, and Hoff (1966) reported attenuated RSA amplitude following vagotomy, emphasizing the importance of tonic background vagal activity. They suggested that during inspiration this vagal activity is centrally suppressed. Hamlin et al. (1966) studied RSA in the dog and reported unchanged RSA following cardiac sympathetic blockade with propranolol. They concluded that RSA could be explained solely from changes in vagal efferent activity.

Katona and Jih (1975) suggested that since RSA is tightly linked to vagal activity, it can be used to estimate parasympathetic control of the heart. These investigators examined RSA amplitude during various autonomic manipulations. They correlated changes in RSA amplitude with the degree of parasympathetic control, which was defined as the heart rate change after reversibly cooling the vagus. Greater parasympathetic control occurred with increased heart period and larger amplitude RSA. In addition, RSA amplitude correlated highly (.969) with the degree of parasympathetic control.

Chess, Tam, and Calaresu (1975) utilized spectral analysis to describe an oscillation in heart period that occurred at the respiratory frequency. The amplitude of this oscillation, a measure of RSA, was greatly reduced with administration of atropine. This finding has been supported by other investigators (Davies & Neilson, 1967*b*; Hamlin *et al.*, 1966; Katona & Jih, 1975). However, Chess *et al.* (1975) suggested that sympathetic and nonneural factors probably contribute to the genesis of RSA.

## Sympathetic Influences

Sympathetic influences have been proposed to play a role in RSA. Several investigators have suggested that opposing action of the sympathetic and parasympathetic nervous systems generates RSA (Anrep *et al.*, 1936*b*; Kollai & Koizumi, 1979; Levy *et al.*, 1966; McCrady *et al.*, 1966). It has been demonstrated that sympathetic fibers fire synchronously with inspiration (Adrian, Bronk, & Phillips, 1932; Gootman & Cohen, 1974; Kollai & Koizumi, 1979; Mannard & Polosa, 1973; Priess, Kirchner, & Polosa, 1975). In this explanation of RSA, sympathetic fibers would accelerate the heart during inspiration and during expiration vagal activity would slow the heart. McCrady and associates (McCrady *et al.*, 1966) noted that it would not be likely in the CNS that action in one autonomic branch should occur without central inhibition of the other system. Support for sympathetic involvement comes from Davis and associates (Davis, McCloskey, & Potter, 1977), who reported that following section of both vagi, baroreceptor and chemoreceptor stimuli produced bradycardia during expiration only. This response is smaller than the vagal response and it is mediated through the sympathetics. However, Anrep (Anrep *et al.*, 1936*b*) reported that sympathetics play a role only in centrally generated RSA but not in reflex RSA.

Kollai and Koizumi (1979) proposed that only under certain conditions do vagal and sympathetic influences act reciprocally. This action occurs during baroreceptor stimulation. The reciprocal neural activity can be accentuated by increasing end-expired $CO_2$ level and decreasing tidal volume. The net result is an enhanced RSA. However, during chemoreceptor stimulation nonreciprocal activity is observed. Although the vagus is still gated by inspiration, sympathetics fire continuously without being interrupted by respiration. One might expect RSA to be smaller in this case, although RSA has been reported during prolonged chemoreceptor stimulation (Levy *et al.*, 1966). Levy *et al.* mentioned that sympathetic firing is more variable during the respiratory cycle than vagal activity. In addition, they noted that following stimulation of efferent fibers there is a greater latency to the cardiac response in sympathetics than in the vagus. Due to these factors it is possible that the sympathetic firing may drift out of phase and therefore overlap with vagal activity. Given the present knowledge of sympathetic–parasympathetic interactions (see Levy, 1971), such overlap may produce an unpredictable response.

## Nonneural Influences

Nonneural influences of respiration on heart rate appear to play a small role in RSA. Some investigators have reported that removal of neural influences on the heart eliminates RSA (Anrep et al., 1936a; Hamlin et al., 1966). However, it has also been reported that very small respiratory oscillations in heart rate can be detected following complete denervation or pharmacological blockade of the heart (Chess et al., 1975; Katona & Jih, 1975). Observations from our laboratory suggest that this nonneural RSA can be eliminated by pneumothorax and therefore may be a direct effect of thoracic pressure on the heart.

The evidence seems to indicate a role for parasympathetic and sympathetic influences in RSA, although parasympathetic effects appear to be dominant (Anrep et al., 1936b; Chess et al., 1975; Katona & Jih, 1975; Levy et al., 1966). Vagal predominance is not surprising since the vagus exerts the major control over cardiac chronotropic effects. The rhythmic sympathetic influence may be less evident because it is more variable within the respiratory cycle and it is sluggish in its response characteristics.

## Proposed Respiratory Gate of Neural Influences on the Heart

It has been proposed that respiratory neurons may gate cardiovascular efferents producing respiratory oscillations in heart rate. Lopes and Palmer (1976) stated: "A vagal bradycardia unrelated to respiration can in fact only be induced by stimulation of the cells of origin [of the vagus] in the nucleus ambiguus" (p. 455). The authors further proposed that the $R\beta$ respiratory neurons which lie near the nucleus ambiguus are strong candidates to be involved in the gating of the cardiac vagal preganglionics.

Jordan and Spyer (1978) have demonstrated that the respiratory gating of baroreceptor and chemoreceptor reflexes does not occur at the primary afferent terminal in the nucleus tractus solitarius. Although this is not conclusive proof that the gate is in the vagal cells of origin, it does support the notion that respiratory gating occurs at some point after the initial afferent synapse. Spyer (1979) has reported that since cardiac vagal cells receive barosensory input during both inspiration and expiration, effectiveness of the baroreceptor reflex must be modulated at the vagal cells of origin. He further suggested that inspiratory neurons provide powerful inhibitory control over the cardiac vagal cells and that this influence involves a cholinergic mechanism.

Although sympathetic preganglionics are also influenced by respiration, the site of the respiratory influence is unknown (Koizumi, Seller, Kaufman, & Brooks, 1971; Polosa, Mannard, & Laskey, 1979; Priess et al., 1975). It has been mentioned that transection of the spinal cord below the medulla eliminates all background rhythmic sympathetic activity (Koizumi et al., 1971; Tang, Maire, & Amassian, 1957). Tang (Tang et al., 1957) suggested that the sympathetic activity occurring with respiratory rhythmicity is due to two major influences on the medullary vasomotor center: First, central respiratory neurons affect the vasomotor area; and second, blood pressure fluctuations due to respiratory intrathoracic pressure changes feed back on the vasomotor control mechanisms. These influences were eliminated by hyperventilation and pneumothorax, respectively, and hence, respiratorily related sympathetic discharges disappeared.

## CENTRALLY MEDIATED INFLUENCES ON RSA

Although higher CNS regions can modulate RSA, they are not necessary for RSA to exist. Brainstem transections have been performed without loss of RSA. McCrady et al. (1966) suggested that the most caudal transection that can be made without loss of RSA is in the pons just anterior to the medulla. Chess et al. (1975) found a respiratory component of heart period variability in the decerebrate cat with a transection at the midcollicular level. Therefore, it appears that the respiratory influence on heart rate occurs in the caudal brainstem.

Vallbona, Cardus, Spencer, and Hoff (1965) observed RSA in patients with CNS damage. These authors describe a peculiar respiratory–heart rate interaction in patients who presented a clinical syndrome of decerebration. During breathing epochs a large tachycardia was seen which was followed by overshoot deceleration of heart rate during apneic periods. The authors suggested that high cortical and subcortical influences on brainstem autonomic regions are disrupted by decerebration, leaving the cardiovascular control centers uninhibited and at a heightened level of activity. They also reported that comatose patients have no fluctuations in spontaneous heart rate. According to Vallbona et al., fixed heart rate in unanesthetized patients invariably preceeds a fatal outcome. Kero, Antilla, Ylitalo, and Valimaki (1978) reported diminished heart rate variability in brain death newborn infants. They speculated that this is a vagal phenomenon and that the brain death infant has damaged brain-stem vagal nuclei.

Stimulation of supramedullary regions can augment the amplitude of RSA. Kaufman, Hamilton, Wallach, Petrik, and Schneiderman (1979) found that stimulation of the lateral zona incerta in the rabbit produced a primary vagal bradycardia of approximately 100 bpm. Although it was not stated, it appears from the figures that RSA increased dramatically during stimulation.

Klevans and Gebber (1970) reported that stimulation of the area preoptica, area septalis, or anterior hypothalamus facilitates the cardiac vagal component of the baroreceptor reflex. Stimulation of these sites alone fails to produce significant blood pressure or heart rate changes. It can be seen from their figures that combined forebrain and barosensory stimulation produced an enhanced bradycardia and an increased ampli-tude of RSA above the level for either stimulus alone. This effect was abolished by the administration of atropine. It is apparent that enhanced background vagal tone, produced by increasing blood pressure or inducing hypercapnia, is needed for the stimulation effects to be seen.

Supramedullary facilitation of RSA amplitude can be explained if it is assumed that the higher structures enhance vagal tone through the vagal cells of origin in the medulla. This heightened vagal activity would still be gated by respiratory influences, and the net effect would be greater respiratory fluctuations in heart rate. This mechanism could be viewed metaphorically as a pipe through which water flows. In the middle of the pipe is a valve which is phasically opened and closed. The net amount of water flowing from the pipe (vagal efferent activity) at any given time is dependent on the water flowing through the pipe (supra-medullary facilitation of vagal tone) and the state of the valve (respiratory gate of vagal activity). It is possible that similar gating mechanisms regulate sympathetic outflow.


## QUANTIFICATION OF RESPIRATORY SINUS ARRHYTHMIA

Heart period variability (HPV) is the change in sequential beat-to-beat intervals over time. Some of the influences on the heart period have *direct* neural mediation and others do not. In the preceding section a number of physiological studies are reviewed which have demonstrated that the respiratory influence on heart period is primarily mediated through the vagus. Thus, it may be possible to develop an estimate of the influence of the vagus on the heart by quantifying the amplitude of RSA. This variability may be quantitatively assessed by calculating descriptive statistics of variability, including variance, standard deviation, range, and mean squared successive differences.

There are numerous physiological mechanisms which result in the variation in the time intervals between successive heartbeats. If HPV were only influenced by respiration, HPV would be equivalent to RSA and would, hypothetically, covary with vagal tone. However, since HPV is influenced by other factors, including nonneural and sympathetic influences, HPV would only be sensitive to vagal manipulations if it were assumed that the nonvagal influences were constant across conditions and individuals. This assumption is untenable. It is, therefore, necessary to partition from the total HPV a measure of RSA by quantifying the component mediated by breathing. This component may be described in terms of the amplitude of the RSA, the temporal coupling between respiration and heart period, the phase relationship between respiration and heart period, and the periodicities of the respiratory and heart period oscillations. The task of describing these dimensions requires unique and complex methods.

Since respiration and heart period are inherently rhythmic, spectral analysis is the natural tool to study oscillations in heart period such as RSA. Spectral analysis is a method of quantifying and partitioning the variance associated with each underlying rhythm. Although respiratory frequencies may be easily identified by observing a polygraph record, the frequency components of heart period activity are more difficult to identify.

Spectral analysis may be used to study rhythmic activity of heart period and respiration by decomposing both series of sequential observations into sinusoidal functions of different frequencies. The frequencies of interest in the study of RSA are the frequencies associated with normal spontaneous respiratory activity. If breathing were occurring at a rate of 12 times a minute, each breath would take approximately 5 sec and would have a frequency of .2 Hz (since one-fifth of the period would occur within 1 sec).

Power density is an estimate of the variance attributed to a specific frequency. In Figures 7-2 and 7-3 the power densities for each frequency

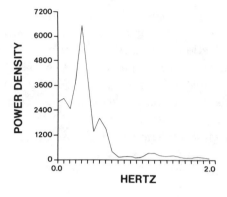

FIG. 7-2. Spectral density function of the heart period data pictured in Figure 7-4.

of heart period and respiration are plotted. The spectral analysis of heart period was conducted on the data described in Figure 7-4. Note that the spectral analyses of heart period and respiration exhibit a peak at the same frequency, representing the most characteristic respiratory frequency.

It is important to note that even though the spectral decomposition of both respiration and heart period processes results in similar dominant frequencies, the heart period process exhibits other prominent frequencies independent of respiration. Other investigators have identified and studied heart period rhythms which are outside the band of respiratory frequencies. Some of these rhythms have been theoretically associated with physiological processes such as temperature and blood pressure fluctuations (Chess *et al.*, 1975; Sayers, 1973).

To calculate the component of heart period variability *associated* with respiratory activity, the spectral densities for each frequency asso-

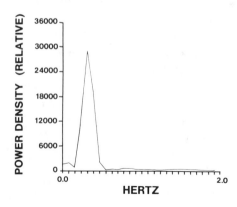

FIG. 7-3. Spectral density function of respiration data.

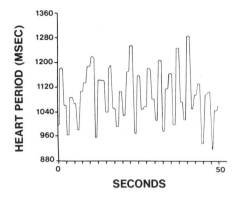

FIG. 7-4. Second-by-second heart period values (time intervals between sequential heart beats).

ciated with normal spontaneous breathing are summed. In adults this is about 8 to 25 breaths a minute; in children, approximately 15 to 30; in neonates, approximately 30 to 90; in mature rats, 48 to 120; and in rat pups, 120 to 240. The accumulation of spectral density estimates of heart period activity associated with the respiratory frequency band $(\hat{V})$ provides an accurate measure of RSA amplitude. Physiologically, $\hat{V}$ is the spectral representation of the amplitude of periodic heart period activity associated with the "gating" of the vagal efferents to the heart and thus should be a sensitive index of vagal tone. This is physiologically justified since the respiratory rhythms in heart period, independent of source (e.g., peripheral feedback from stretch receptors and central influences), that are manifested in heart period activity are primarily mediated through the vagus. Thus, by quantifying the amplitude of RSA, spectral analysis provides a noninvasive estimate of vagal tone, $\hat{V}$. Spectral analysis enables the description of other parameters of RSA such as phase, coherence, and the dominant periodicities of respiratory and heart period oscillations (e.g., Harper, Walter, Leake, Hoffman, Sieck, Sterman, Hoppenbrouwers, & Hodgman, 1978). These parameters are not discussed in this chapter.

## RESPIRATORY SINUS ARRHYTHMIA: CURRENT RESEARCH

The research in our laboratory is directed toward the quantification and interpretation of two parameters of RSA: the amplitude of RSA and the coupling between respiration and heart rate. Other characteristics such as the dominant frequency of RSA and the phase angle between respiration and RSA may be quantified but at present are not the focus of extensive research. This chapter deals solely with the amplitude of RSA, $\hat{V}$. For information regarding a statistic to describe the temporal coupling between respiration and heart period, the weighted coherence, the reader is referred to Porges, Bohrer, Cheung, Drasgow, McCabe, and Keren (1980).

The preceding sections provide the necessary foundation for the hypothesis that the spectral estimate of the amplitude of RSA, $\hat{V}$, is related to vagal tone. This hypothesis underlies much of the research conducted in our laboratory. On the surface this hypothesis appears viable and easily testable. However, because there is no readily measured criterion variable of vagal tone, the hypothesis is difficult to test. Moreover, treatments assumed to manipulate solely vagal activity may affect sympathetics, since the sympathetic and vagal influences on the heart are interactive.

Vagal tone cannot be accurately indexed by heart rate level or amount of heart rate variability. Use of either of these measures as an index of vagal tone is based upon the simplistic view that the sympathetics and the nonneural influences on the heart remain relatively constant.

An accepted experimental procedure to evaluate vagal tone is the administration of atropine. The change in heart rate in response to atropine is used as an index of the pretreatment vagal tone. Again, it is assumed that atropine blocks the vagal influence without a resulting change in the sympathetics. The dynamic characteristics of the autonomic nervous system (ANS) often result in a "reciprocal excitation" of one branch of the ANS when the other is inhibited (see Gellhorn, 1957). Therefore, the change in heart rate in response to atropine may not be an accurate measure of vagal tone if the sympathetic response to this manipulation is variable. Similarly, excitation or inhibition of sympathetic innervation to the heart may change heart rate and indirectly influence blood pressure. The shifts in blood pressure may stimulate baroreceptor mechanisms which contribute to vagal tone. Even if these pharmacological techniques provide a method to accurately measure vagal tone, the procedure is intrusive and the researcher forfeits the possibility of continuous assessment.

It has been suggested that direct recording from the vagus nerve would provide a criterion variable which could be compared to $\hat{V}$. However, recording from the vagus as an intact nerve is not sufficient, since the vagus contains not only efferent fibers to organs other than the heart but many afferent fibers as well. Moreover, if it were feasible to identify only the efferent vagal fibers to the heart, the pulse train paralleling apparent vagal tone may be a complicated code. Thus, if the time and technology were invested to measure directly off the vagus, the information gained might not aid in the evaluation of the hypothesis relating $\hat{V}$ to vagal tone.

By using known physiological relationships it may be possible to develop measurement techniques which approximate the underlying construct of vagal tone to the heart. The basis for much of our research is the strong relationship between vagal activity and RSA which is described in the preceding sections. Our research program does not intend to rediscover RSA but to accurately quantify it and employ it in psychophysiological research. The research program is characterized by three aspects: (1) quantitative methods to accurately describe RSA, (2) experimentation with manipulations which have primary sites of action on either the sympathetic or vagal control of the heart, and (3) assessment of developmental changes and individual differences in $\hat{V}$.

Most manipulations that are thought to solely influence vagal activity may indirectly influence the sympathetics. This is the very nature of the regulation of the cardiovascular system. The vagi and sympathetics form a dynamic interactive control system reciprocally responding and continuously adjusting as a function of afferent feedback from the periphery to the medullary sites of control. The control of heart rate is a function of both the additive components of the vagal and sympathetic systems plus an interactive component. The interaction between the two systems is often observed as a reciprocal inhibition of one system when the other is stimulated (see Gellhorn, 1957). The ability to evaluate the interaction is also dependent upon criterion measures of neural influences. Thus, if the interaction cannot be quantified, the ability to accurately estimate the contribution of either the sympathetic or vagal systems on the heart would be difficult. An acceptable option would be the convergence of descriptive and manipulative approaches. The descriptive approach is based upon the accurate quantification of RSA during the development of the vagal system. The manipulative approach is dependent upon treatments which have primary sites of action on the vagal system.

MANIPULATIONS OF CARDIOVAGAL TONE

If $\hat{V}$ is an accurate estimate of cardiovagal tone, then manipulations of vagal activity should be reflected as changes in $\hat{V}$. Vagal tone can be altered by manipulations of barosensory information, which can be achieved by electrical stimulation of barosensory fibers or by elevation of blood pressure. Vagal activity can be eliminated by administration of atropine.

In the first experiment, vagal tone was manipulated in the anesthetized rabbit by stimulation of the aortic depressor nerve (ADN) (McCabe, Porges, & Yongue, 1979), an afferent nerve which contains predominantly barosensory fibers. Stimulation of this nerve produces a reflex bradycardia which is mediated by both divisions of the autonomic nervous system (Kardon, Peterson, & Bishop, 1973).

The ADN was stimulated with monophasic rectangular pulses for 45 sec at current intensities ranging between 10 $\mu$A and 1 mA (.1-msec pulse duration, 100 pulses/sec). Stimulation of the ADN increased the amplitude of oscillations in heart period associated with respiration (Figure 7-5). Cholinergic blockade (atropine methyl nitrate, i.v., 5 mg/kg) eliminated the increase in $\hat{V}$ produced during stimulation. In summary, ADN stimulation increased the spectral estimate of the amplitude of RSA, $\hat{V}$, in all animals at all currents tested. In addition, the elimination of vagal tone resulted in near zero values for $\hat{V}$. This supports the hypothesis that $\hat{V}$ is sensitive to manipulations of cardiovagal tone.

In the previous study, RSA accounted for nearly all of the heart period variance since the subjects were anesthetized. However, in a freely moving preparation there are sources of HPV other than those associated with respiration. It is therefore necessary to partition the respiratory influence on HPV from the total HPV through the use of spectral analysis.

In a subsequent study (Yongue, McCabe, Kelley, Rivera, & Porges, 1980) the relationship between $\hat{V}$ and vagal influences on the heart was assessed in a freely moving preparation. Vagal tone was manipulated by pharmacological treatments which are known to either enhance (phenylephrine) or block (atropine) cardiovagal activity. Phenylephrine, an $\alpha$-adrenergic agonist, produces an elevation in arterial blood pressure through vasoconstriction, which leads to a secondary bradycardia of predominantly vagal origin (Glick & Braunwald, 1965).

Nine adult male Long–Evans hooded rats were tested under three conditions (order counterbalanced across subjects): phenylephrine (1 mg/kg), saline (1 ml/kg .9%), and atropine methyl nitrate (5 mg/kg). Heart period and respiration data were collected in 60-sec samples every 10 min starting 30 min before drug injection and continuing for 180 min posttreatment. Data were collapsed into blocks of three trials representing sequential

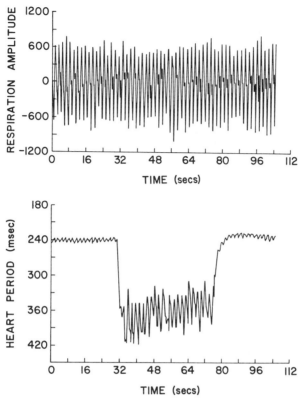

FIG. 7-5. Respiration amplitude and heart period as a function of time during aortic depressor nerve stimulation. A 45-sec stimulus instituted at second 30. Note amplitude of heart period oscillations, rhythmic with respiration, during stimulation.

30-min segments (one baseline and six posttreatment segments). In Figure 7-6, the time-by-drug plot of $\hat{V}$ is presented. Note the clear enhancement of $\hat{V}$ during the phenylephrine treatment, which peaks between 60 min and 90 min posttreatment. This follows the predicted time course of phenylephrine when administered subcutaneously. The elimination of vagal tone to the heart via atropine administration is reflected in the near zero values for $\hat{V}$ which occur immediately after the injection and persist throughout the session. Although there were significant drug effects and drug by trial block interactions reflected in the mean heart period and heart period variability measure, they did not follow the reported time course effects of the drugs as clearly as $\hat{V}$. This could be due to extravagal

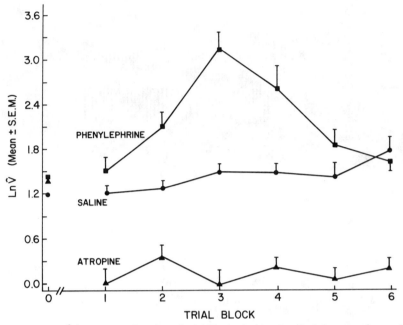

FIG. 7-6. Ln $\hat{V}$ in rats as a function of trial blocks during phenylephrine, atropine, and saline. Trial blocks consist of the average of three trials taken 10 min apart ($n=9$).

influences affecting mean heart period and total heart period variability. Therefore, $\hat{V}$ seems to be a sensitive measure of vagal control of the heart in the freely behaving animal.

The logic underlying these experiments is that the amplitude of RSA reflects background vagal tone to the heart. This argument is based upon the physiological experiments reviewed in the preceding sections of this chapter. We are presenting a quantification strategy which would provide a measure of the amplitude of RSA at times when heart period is influenced by factors in addition to respiration. In all our studies we have measured, concurrent with $\hat{V}$, heart period variability and heart period. These measures also exhibit reliable effects due to potent manipulations of vagal control of the heart. This is not surprising since the level of heart rate is primarily a function of the balance between sympathetic and vagal influences. Heart period, like $\hat{V}$, should be related monotonically to changes in vagal tone produced by the enhancement or blocking of vagal efferent activity to the heart. However, from our data it appears at present that the $\hat{V}$ measure is less sensitive to the extravagal influences than heart period or heart period variability. This is easily demonstrated in the acute rabbit preparation during the propranolol condition. Sympathetic blockade increased the mean heart period but failed to eliminate the evoked increase in $\hat{V}$.

## $\hat{V}$ AND DEVELOPMENT

Within obstetrics and neonatology it has been assumed that the vagal influence on the heart reflects the general well-being of the fetus or infant (see Porges, 1979). Thus, measures of vagal tone have been of interest to these disciplines. The two most common methods of vagal assessment rely on measuring the variability of heart rate or blocking the vagal influences to the heart with atropine and recording the change in heart rate. The basic criticisms of these methods are obvious. Heart rate variability is not solely influenced by the vagus, and atropine is invasive and may affect other components of the ANS. Even with these limitations, the monitoring of HRV and use of atropine have identified some important developmental trends.

When atropine is given to pregnant mothers, fetal heart rate increases and the magnitude of the change is correlated with gestational age (Schifferli & Caldeyro-Barcia, 1973). Similarly, one would expect that premature newborns without identifiable complications would exhibit a relationship between an estimate of vagal tone, $\hat{V}$, and gestational age. To evaluate possible early developmental trends in neural control of the heart, a preliminary study (Porges, Srinivasan, Cheung, Shanker, Pildes, & Bohrer, 1979) was conducted. To assess the relationship between $\hat{V}$ and gestational age, data were collected from term and preterm infants who were free from clinical complications. In Figure 7-7 the relationship between $\hat{V}$ and gestational age is plotted. The correlation between gestational age and $\hat{V}$ was .82; this is similar to the correlation of .74 between weeks of pregnancy and increase in fetal heart rate in response to atropine reported by Schifferli and Caldeyro-Barcia (1973).

The developmental trends in $\hat{V}$ may be studied more easily in an animal preparation in which the neural control of the autonomic nervous system matures rapidly. Researchers (e.g., Adolph, 1967; Ashida, 1972; Mills, 1978) have identified in rats, developmental trends in baseline and event-related heart rate responses which they have attributed to the changing control of the autonomic nervous system. Based upon this research, it has been hypothesized that the vagal control of the heart does not mature fully

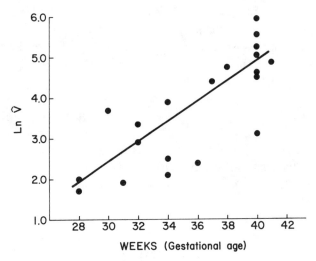

FIG. 7-7. Ln $\hat{V}$ in preterm and term infants.

until approximately 14–21 days postpartum. If $\hat{V}$ is a sensitive measure of vagal tone to the heart, measurement of heart rate patterns in the rat pup during the first few weeks postpartum should provide an experimental preparation to evaluate the development of $\hat{V}$. A study (Larson & Porges, 1980) was conducted to describe the ontogeny of $\hat{V}$ in rats from birth through 24 days postpartum. In Figure 7-8 the developmental trend of $\hat{V}$ is presented. Note the monotonic increase in $\hat{V}$ during the first 18 days postpartum, a period in which the development of vagal control of the heart is assumed to occur. Individually, each rat exhibited the greatest $\hat{V}$ on day 12, 15, or 18.

The data from the developmental studies just described clearly indicate that $\hat{V}$ increases with age during periods characterized by rapid maturation of neural control of the autonomic nervous system. These findings are consistent with the theorized development of the medullary control of the heart through the vagus.

## $\hat{V}$ AND PATHOPHYSIOLOGY

In our laboratory we have been interested in the relationship between pathophysiology and neural control of the heart. In this section we describe phenomena which relate RSA to two classes of pathophysiology.

Since it is assumed that vagal influences on the heart may reflect central pathologies, we have been investigating in neonates the relationship between individual differences in $\hat{V}$ and CNS dysfunction. Moreover, since a component of cardiovascular risk has been associated with neural control of the heart, we have been investigating factors which result in an exaggerated respiratory sinus arrhythmia (ERSA) which may be potentially dangerous, particularly in the presence of myocardial insults.

Perinatal Research

Monitoring of the fetus and newborn infant has established that several factors can affect heart rate variability (e.g., Porges, 1979). Persistent hypoxia *in utero* will reduce variability and result in a depressed central nervous system at birth. Any central nervous system depressant (e.g., narcotics, barbiturates, alcohol) given to the mother will reduce heart rate variability if given in doses high enough to produce any other detectable effect in the fetus. Anticholinergic drugs suppress HRV and increase heart

FIG. 7-8. Ln $\hat{V}$ as a function of age in rat pups ($n = 19$).

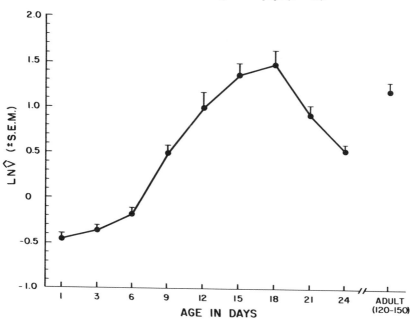

rate through vagal blockade. An increase in intracranial pressure will also decrease spontaneous HRV (Lowensohn, Weiss, & Hon, 1977). The return of normal HRV following a period of increased intracranial pressure is dependent on the restoration of cerebral function rather than the return of normal intracranial pressure. Heart rate variability has also been used to discriminate the severity of neonatal distress factors (see Kero, 1974). In general, these factors influence the medullary control of the cardiovascular system. The changes in HRV are viewed as a manifestation of dysfunction in the CNS. Thus, the quantification of HRV as an estimate of vagal influence has been useful in the obstetric management of labor and as a diagnostic during the first few days postpartum.

In pediatrics there is a great interest in the identification of CNS dysfunction. Since it may be easily and noninvasively monitored, HRV has been used by pediatricians and obstetricians as an index of CNS status (see Porges, 1979). The causal relationship between the neural influences on the heart and HRV has been the primary justification for employing measures of HRV as an assessment index. The primary neural contribution to HRV is vagal. Moreover, there is documentation that CNS dysfunction results in a suppression of vagal influence on the heart (Kero et al., 1978; Vallbona et al., 1965). Our research with neonates has focused on the parallel between $\hat{V}$ and clinical indices of CNS dysfunction.

Research projects initiated in our laboratory have attempted to demonstrate that it may be possible to identify, during the neonatal period, individual differences in physiological activity which may place the infant on a continuum of risk. This research centers on the measurement of $\hat{V}$ during the neonatal period and the relationship between this measure and individual differences in behavior and psychophysiological responsivity during subsequent development.

In the literature there is ample evidence to suggest that the heart rate response during conditioning and attention-demanding tasks differentiates normals from severely brain-damaged individuals (e.g., Karrer, 1976; Krupski, 1975). Overall, the findings have encouraged researchers to employ psychophysiological paradigms (e.g., orienting, habituation, and conditioning) as methods of identifying CNS dysfunction in the neonate.

In spite of its promising potential, a psychophysiological strategy to assess neonates would suffer from two major limitations: (1) It would be time consuming and would necessitate administration and interpretation by trained technicians; and (2) deficits (absence or low amplitude) in the physiological response may *not* be related to a higher-level cognitive process associated with central nervous system dysfunction, but could be a function of motivation or dysfunction in a specific sensory system.

If it were possible to assess the status of the neural control of the heart (i.e., the influence of the CNS on the heart), the same information might be obtained more efficiently and accurately than by evaluating heart rate responses to stimulus manipulations. Since central nervous system influences are encoded in the pattern of heart rate, it might be possible to use heart rate as an *indexing* variable of underlying physiological dysfunction. Pediatricians and obstetricians have frequently used the beat-to-beat variability as a clinical index of the general status of the CNS (Lowensohn et al., 1977; Nelson, 1976). For example, the extreme pathophysiological condition of a brain-death infant (Kero et al., 1978) produces a constant heart rate without beat-to-beat variability.

We are conducting research at Cook County Hospital in Chicago to address this problem. The research has as its goal the development of an assessment technique which could reliably be applied within the hospital setting. Our early research with newborns (Porges, 1974; Porges, Arnold, & Forbes, 1973; Porges, Stamps, & Walter, 1974; Stamps & Porges, 1975) identified a relationship between spontaneous autonomic activity and reactivity to visual and auditory stimuli. Consistent with the pediatric research, newborns with high HRV were more responsive to environmental stimuli. Our current research employs $\hat{V}$ as an index of CNS influence on the heart. The application of spectral analysis enables the detection and evaluation of a component of the heart rate pattern which is directly influenced by the CNS. In preliminary research (Porges et al., 1979) we evaluated $\hat{V}$ in a group of normal infants and a group containing a variety of clinical pathologies including severe brain damage. Heart period variability and heart period data were also collected. In Figure 7-9, $\hat{V}$ and HPV are presented for all the subjects.

There is an apparent monotonic relationship between $\hat{V}$ and severity of clinical dysfunction. The one hydrocephalic infant which appears to be misclassified by $\hat{V}$ was evaluated by the pediatrician to be functioning within the bounds of normal intellectual and social development. When the same infants were ranked in terms of HPV (see Figure 7-9), there was a clear distinction between those who died and all other infants. Heart period variability clearly distinguished between infants diagnosed as brain death, with their characteristic absence of neural influence on the heart, and all other infants. Heart period variability did not distinguish among the various neural tube defects, respiratory distress syndrome, and normal

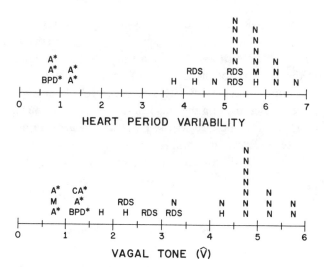

FIG. 7-9. The top scale represents Ln HPV for normal and pathological infants. The bottom scale represents Ln $\hat{V}$ for the same infants. The letters on the scales represent the diagnosis or insult associated with the individual infants (A = asphyxia, BPD = bronchiopulmonary dysplasia, CA = cardiac arrest, H = hydrocephalic, M = microcephalic, N = normal, and RDS = respiratory distress syndrome; * denotes infants who subsequently expired).

infants. Heart period did not reliably discriminate among the various pathologies although there was a tendency for the severely brain damaged to have shorter heart periods. Categorization with HPV partitioned the infants into two global categories, while $\hat{V}$ classified the infants along a continuum of severity of neuropathology. Thus, although HPV is sensitive to gross dysfunction, $\hat{V}$ is a more sensitive index to individual differences in central dysfunction.

## Exaggerated RSA

During the past few years it has become increasingly evident that the nervous system is a primary factor in the genesis of lethal arrhythmias. The mechanism of how the nervous system exerts its influence is unknown. The significance of the problem lies in the overwhelming importance of cardiac arrhythmias as a cause of death. Coronary death is the major medical catastrophe in the industrialized West. In the United States approximately 1,000,000 people experience acute myocardial infarction each year. Over 650,000 people die yearly of ischemic heart disease. Understanding of the mechanisms involved in neurally generated arrhythmias would have important implications for cardiovascular health.

It has been demonstrated that psychological stress can play an important role in the generation of cardiac arrhythmias (Matta, Lawler, & Lown, 1976). Several investigators have found that the ventricular fibrillation threshold is lowered after a stressful manipulation in the ischemic heart (Corbalan, Verrier, & Lown, 1974; Lown, Verrier, & Rabinowitz, 1977). Disturbances of the sinus rhythm may take the form of tachycardia, bradycardia, or rapid fluctuations between fast and slow rates. Bradycardia increases temporal dispersion of refractory periods and decreases the ventricular fibrillation threshold (Han, Millet, Chizzonitti, & Moe, 1966). James (1962) has described clinical reports which suggest that excess vagal discharge is the universal mechanism of sudden death during myocardial ischemia.

Although there has been casual observation of large fluctuations in sinus rhythm before ventricular fibrillation, research on this disturbance has been neglected. Engel (1978) mentioned this phenomenon and stated that "the temporal and spatial imbalances that might ensue from such fluctuations, especially in the presence of localized myocardial damage, are known to increase electrical instability of the heart" (p. 409). Moreover, cardiac arrhythmias during respiratory maneuvers have been reported. Lamb, Dermksian, and Sarnoff (1958) found sinus arrest with ventricular escape, AV block, ventricular premature beats, ventricular bigeminy, and paroxysmal nodal tachycardia during common respiratory maneuvers in humans. Therefore, respiratory–heart rate interactions play a major role in cardiac arrhythmias.

In an experiment dealing with cardiac rate adjustments during a period of recovery from stress in rats (Yongue, Porges, & McCabe, 1979), a small subgroup of the stressed animals exhibited an unusually large variation in heart period. Figure 7-10 is an example of this arrhythmia. This type of arrhythmia was present in 4 of 16 stressed animals, was always superimposed on a slow mean heart rate, and was transient in nature, lasting 1 to 20 min. The onset and offset of this arrhythmia were sudden. Cross-spectral analysis of the heart period and respiratory amplitude indicated that the oscillations in heart period were coupled (coherent) with respiration during these arrhythmias. Examination of the respiratory

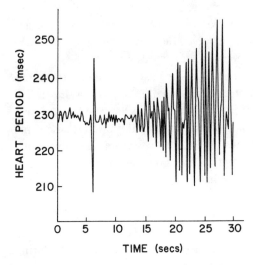

FIG. 7-10. Heart period as a function of time in a rat approximately 4 hours after unsignaled/ inescapable shock.

trace before and during these arrhythmias indicated that respiratory amplitude and frequency were not related to the occurrence or maintenance of the arrhythmia.

Certain characteristics of the exaggerated RSA (ERSA), such as slow heart rate and rhythmic oscillations in the respiratory frequency, suggest that strong vagal influences may be involved in its production. The inhibitory effects of the vagus on the heart would account for the slow mean HR, while the high coherence of the heart rate patterning with respiration may be due to inspiratory inhibition at the brainstem level of the strong vagal chronotrophic influences. The sudden appearance and disappearance of the arrhythmia in the absence of large respiratory changes suggests that state changes in the CNS which result in either an increase in vagal efferent tone or an inhibition of SNS antagonism may be involved.

In the phenylephrine study described earlier, similar arrhythmias were observed. This enhanced or exaggerated RSA was also superimposed on a slow mean HR and was coherent with respiration. Like the stress-induced arrhythmia, it was also of sudden onset and offset, and appeared in transient epochs of 1 to 20 min. The previously mentioned enhanced RSA is on the order of 10% of the mean HP, a value that is not abnormal but is relatively large. Occasionally following stress, under phenylephrine treatment and in an adult human, we have observed fluctuations between heart beats that were on the order of 20–50% of the mean heart period. For operational purposes we are considering respiratory-related fluctuations in heart period of 20% or more of the mean heart period to be exaggerated RSA. We are presently investigating the psychological and physiological factors involved in the production of neurally mediated arrhythmias of this type. We are interested in the relationship between ERSA and vulnerability to cardiovascular dysfunction.

## CONCLUSION

Based upon the literature reviewed in this chapter, one may conclude that the amplitude of RSA is related to vagal tone. Since vagal efferents to the heart are gated by respiration, under most conditions there is a parallel between background vagal tone and the amplitude of RSA. The amplitude of RSA reflects the change in heart rate primarily due to the transitory blocking of the vagal efferents with each breath. The phenomenon of respiratory gating of vagal efferent activity is well known (e.g., Haymet & McCloskey, 1975) and serves as a primary method of identifying cardioinhibitory units in electrophysiological studies of neural regulation of the heart.

Although RSA amplitude is related to vagal tone, the ability to accurately and precisely describe this component of the heart period pattern is dependent upon both the experimental preparation and the quantitative strategy. In many situations the primary contribution to HPV is respiratory. This is common in anesthetized preparations. In these situations a simple statistical description of HPV will be an accurate measure of RSA amplitude. In the unanesthetized preparation, movement and other physiological processes contribute to the total HPV. Under these conditions HPV is affected by more than respiratory gating of the vagus. Thus, to generate a good estimate of vagal tone, it is necessary to partition the variance associated with RSA from the total HPV. Spectral analysis provides the appropriate quantification strategy. Spectral analysis enables the partitioning of the HPV into frequency components. The component characteristic of the respiratory frequencies, $\hat{V}$, is thus an accurate description of the amplitude of RSA and should, theoretically, be sensitive to vagal tone. If one accepts the physiological relationship between respiration and the activity of vagal cardiac efferent, quantification of RSA amplitude is a logical approach to estimate vagal tone. Moreover, spectral analysis provides a quantitative method to accurately describe RSA amplitude when the heart period pattern is composed of numerous influences.

Cardiac parameters such as HPV and mean heart period are also related to vagal tone. In most situations the blocking of the vagal efferents to the heart is paralleled by decreases in heart period and HPV. These parameters appear to be more sensitive to extravagal influences than $\hat{V}$. This sensitivity to extravagal influences often distorts the parallel among these measures. For example, in our research $\hat{V}$ increased during the first 2 weeks postpartum in the rat pup, suggesting an increase in vagal influence on the heart. During this period of rapid increases in vagal control, heart period decreased, instead of the normally observed parallel between increased vagal tone and increased heart period. Similarly, in anesthetized rabbits propranolol increased heart period levels by blocking sympathetic influences on the heart but had no reliable influence on HPV or $\hat{V}$ during ADN stimulation. There are instances when HPV and $\hat{V}$ differ. In the rat pup, during the first week, HPV did not reliably rise but exhibited day-to-day oscillations of increases and decreases. In contrast, $\hat{V}$ exhibited monotonic increases. Moreover, in the study of brain-damaged newborns, $\hat{V}$ was more sensitive to CNS dysfunction than HPV.

The ramifications of a noninvasive index of vagal tone are far-reaching. Since the measurement of $\hat{V}$ is noninvasive and provides a relatively instantaneous assessment, the technology may have a variety of applications. $\hat{V}$ may provide a clinical tool for the study of neuropathology. In current research $\hat{V}$ is being assessed in the human fetus during labor. $\hat{V}$ has been observed to be suppressed during hypoxia. Continuous assessment of $\hat{V}$ during labor may provide the obstetrician with an index of fetal well-being to aid in the management of delivery. The neonatal research also provides evidence that CNS dysfunction is manifested in the patterning of neonatal heart rate.

The difficulties associated with the validation of $\hat{V}$ as a measure of vagal tone have been described at length in this chapter. The dynamic and interactive characteristics of the neural control of the heart preclude the possibility of a simple experimental procedure for validation. Our approach to this problem has been to develop a research program containing studies manipulating vagal efferent activity and describing the development of $\hat{V}$.

This chapter has attempted to stress three points: (1) that the amplitude of RSA is related to vagal tone; (2) that the spectral description of

RSA, $\hat{V}$, is an accurate estimate of the amplitude of RSA; and (3) that $\hat{V}$ is a useful and sensitive estimate of vagal tone. The chapter has provided the reader with both the physiological basis of RSA and a description of research being conducted in our laboratory to enable him/her to evaluate our thesis relating $\hat{V}$ to vagal tone. We believe that although sympathetic and thoracic pressure may influence RSA, $\hat{V}$ provides the psychophysiological community with a good measure of spontaneous vagal activity. Future research can now be directed to evaluate this measure of neural tone, not only as an individual difference but as a dependent variable in traditional psychophysiological paradigms.

## ACKNOWLEDGMENTS

The preparation of the manuscript and the research described in this chapter were supported in part by NIMH Research Scientist Development Award KO2-MH-0054 to Stephen W. Porges; NIMH Traineeship Award MH-15128 to Philip M. McCabe; NSF Graduate Fellowship Award SPI 80-19137 to Brandon G. Yongue; Biomedical Research Support Grant RR-07030; and a University of Illinois Research Board Grant.

## REFERENCES

Adolph, E. F. Ranges of heart rates and their regulation at various ages (rat). *American Journal of Physiology*, 1967, *212*, 595–602.

Adrian, E. D., Bronk, D. W., & Phillips, G. Discharges in mammalian sympathetic nerves. *Journal of Physiology*, 1932, *74*, 115–133.

Angell-James, J.E., & Daly, M.D.B. The effects of artificial lung inflation on reflexly induced bradycardia associated with apnea in the dog. *Journal of Physiology*, 1978, *274*, 349–366.

Angelone, A., & Coulter, N. A. Respiratory-sinus arrhythmia: A frequency dependent phenomenon. *Journal of Applied Physiology*, 1964, *19*, 479–482.

Anrep, G. V., Pascual, W., & Rossler, R. Respiratory variations of the heart rate: I. The reflex mechanism of respiratory arrhythmia. *Proceedings of the Royal Society*, 1936, *119*, 191–217. (a)

Anrep, G. V., Pascual, W., & Rossler, R. Respiratory variations of the heart rate: II. The central mechanism of the respiratory arrhythmia and the interrelations between the central and reflex mechanisms. *Proceedings of the Royal Society*, 1936, *119*, 218–230. (b)

Ashida, S. Developmental changes in the basal and evoked heart rate in neonatal rats. *Journal of Comparative and Physiological Psychology*, 1972, *78*(3), 368–374.

Bainbridge, F. A. The relation between respiration and the pulse rate. *Journal of Physiology*, 1920, *54*, 192–202.

Brener, J., & Hothersall, D. Paced respiration and heart rate control. *Psychophysiology*, 1967, *4*, 1–6.

Chess, G. F., Tam, R. M. K., & Calaresu, F. R. Influence of cardiac neural inputs on rhythmic variations of heart period in the cat. *American Journal of Physiology*, 1975, *228*, 775–780.

Cheung, M. N., & Porges, S. W. Respiratory influences on cardiac responses during attention. *Physiological Psychology*, 1977, *5*, 53–57.

Clynes, M. Respiratory sinus arrhythmia: Laws derived from computer simulation. *Journal of Applied Physiology*, 1960, *15*, 863–874.

Coles, M. G. H., Pellegrini, A., & Wilson, G. *The influences of respiration phase, heart rate, and information processing on the cardiac cycle time effect.* Paper presented at the meeting of the Society for Psychophysiological Research, Vancouver, B.C., 1980.

Corbalan, R., Verrier, R., & Lown, B. Psychological stress and ventricular arrhythmias during myocardial infarction in the conscious dog. *American Journal of Cardiology*, 1974, *34*, 692–696.

Davidson, N. S., Goldner, S., & McCloskey, D. I. Respiratory modulation of baroreceptor and chemoreceptor reflexes affecting heart rate and cardiac vagal efferent nerve activity. *Journal of Physiology*, 1976, *259*, 523–530.

Davies, C. T. M., & Neilson, J. M. M. Sinus arrhythmia in man at rest. *Journal of Applied Physiology*, 1967, *22*, 947–955. (a)

Davies, C. T. M., & Neilson, J. M. M. Disturbance of heart rhythm during recovery from exercise in man. *Journal of Applied Physiology*, 1967, *22*, 943–946. (b)

Davies, H. E. F. Respiratory changes in heart rate, sinus arrhythmia in the elderly. *Gerontologia Clinica*, 1975, *17*, 96–100.

Davis, A. L., McCloskey, D. I., & Potter, E. K. Respiratory modulation of baroreceptor and chemoreceptor reflexes affecting heart rate through the sympathetic nervous system. *Journal of Physiology*, 1977, *272*, 691–703.

Eckberg, D. L., & Orshan, C. R. Respiratory and baroreceptor reflex interactions in man. *Journal of Clinical Investigation*, 1977, *59*, 780–785.

Engel, G. L. Psychologic stress, vasodepressor (vasovagal) syncope, and sudden death. *Annals of Internal Medicine*, 1978, *89*, 403–412.

Gandevia, S. C., McCloskey, D. I., & Potter, E. K. Inhibition of baroreceptor and chemoreceptor reflexes on heart rate by afferents from the lungs. *Journal of Physiology*, 1978, *276*, 369–381. (a)

Gandevia, S. C., McCloskey, D. I., & Potter, E. K. Reflex bradycardia occurring in response to diving, nasopharyngeal stimulation and ocular pressure, and its modification by respiration and swallowing. *Journal of Physiology*, 1978, *276*, 383–394. (b)

Gellhorn, E. *Autonomic imbalance and the hypothalamus.* Minneapolis: University of Minnesota Press, 1957.

Glick, G., & Braunwald, E. Relative roles of the sympathetic and parasympathetic nervous systems in the reflex control of heart rate. *Circulation Research*, 1965, *16*, 363–375.

Gootman, P. M., & Cohen, M. I. The interrelationships between sympathetic discharge and central respiratory drive. In W. Umbach & H. P. Koepchen (Eds.), *Central rhythmic regulation: Circulation, respiration, and extra-pyramidal system.* Stuttgart: Hippokrates, 1974.

Hamlin, R. L., Smith, C. R., & Smetzer, D. C. Sinus arrhythmia in the dog. *American Journal of Physiology*, 1966, *210*, 321–328.

Han, J., Millet, D., Chizzonitti, B., & Moe, G. K. Temporal dispersion of recovery of excitability in atrium and ventricle as a function of heart rate. *American Heart Journal*, 1966, *71*(4), 481–487.

Harper, R. M., Walter, D. O., Leake, B., Hoffman, H. J., Sieck, G. C., Sterman, M. B.,

Hoppenbrouwers, T., & Hodgman, J. Development of sinus arrhythmia during sleeping and waking states in normal infants. *Sleep*, 1978, *1*, 33–48.

Haymet, B. T., & McCloskey, D. I. Baroreceptor and chemoreceptor influences on heart rate during the respiratory cycle in the dog. *Journal of Physiology*, 1975, *245*, 699–712.

Iriuchijima, J., & Kumada, M. Activity of single vagal fibers efferent to the heart. *Japanese Journal of Physiology*, 1964, *14*, 479–487.

James, T. N. Arrhythmias and conduction disturbances in acute myocardial infarction. *American Heart Journal*, 1962, *64*, 416–426.

Jennet, S., & McKillop, J. H. Observations on the incidence and mechanism of sinus arrhythmia in man at rest. *Journal of Physiology*, 1971, *213*, 58P–59P.

Jewett, D. L. Activity of single efferent fibers in the cervical vagus nerve of the dog, with special reference to possible cardio-inhibitory fibers. *Journal of Physiology*, 1964, *175*, 321–357.

Joels, N., & Samueloff, M. The activity of the medullary centers in diffusion respiration. *Journal of Physiology*, 1956, *133*, 360–372.

Jordan, D., & Spyer, K. M. The excitability of sinus nerve afferent terminals during the respiratory cycle. *Journal of Physiology*, 1978, *277*, 66.

Kardon, M. B., Peterson, D. F., & Bishop, V. S. Reflex bradycardia due to aortic nerve stimulation in the rabbit. *American Journal of Physiology*, 1973, *225*, 7–11.

Karrer, R. (Ed.). *Developmental psychophysiology of mental retardation: Concepts and studies.* Springfield, Ill.: Charles C Thomas, 1976.

Katkin, E. S., & Murray, E. N. Instrumental conditioning of autonomically mediated behavior: Theoretical and methodological issues. *Psychological Bulletin*, 1968, *1*, 52–58.

Katona, P. G., & Jih, F. Respiratory sinus arrhythmia: Noninvasive measure of parasympathetic cardiac control. *Journal of Applied Physiology*, 1975, *39*, 801–805.

Katona, P. G., Poitras, J. W., Barnett, G. O., & Terry, B. S. Cardiac vagal efferent activity and heart period in the carotid sinus reflex. *American Journal of Physiology*, 1970, *218*, 1030–1037.

Kaufman, M. P., Hamilton, R. B., Wallach, J. H., Petrik, G. K., & Schneiderman, N. Lateral subthalamic area as a mediator of bradycardia response in rabbits. *American Journal of Physiology*, 1979, *236*, H471–H479.

Kero, P. Heart rate variation in infants with the respiratory distress syndrome. *Acta Paediatrica Scandinavica*, 1974, Suppl. 250.

Kero, P., Antila, K., Ylitalo, V., & Valimaki, I. Decreased heart rate variation in decerebration syndrome: Quantitative clinical criterion of brain death. *Pediatrics*, 1978, *62*, 307–311.

Klevans, L. R., & Gebber, G. L. Facilitatory forebrain influence on cardiac component of baroreceptor reflexes. *American Journal of Physiology*, 1970, *219*, 1235–1241.

Koizumi, K., Seller, H., Kaufman, A., & Brooks, C. McC. Pattern of sympathetic discharges and their relation to baroreceptor and respiratory activities. *Brain Research*, 1971, *27*, 281–294.

Kollai, M., & Koizumi, K. Reciprocal and non-reciprocal action of the vagal and sympathetic nerves innervating the heart. *Journal of Autonomic Nervous System*, 1979, *1*, 33–52.

Kordy, M. T., Neil, E., & Palmer, J. F. The influence of laryngeal afferent stimulation on cardiac vagal responses to carotid chemoreceptor excitation. *Proceedings of the Physiological Society*, 1975, *247*, 24–25.

Krupski, A. Heart rate changes during a fixed reaction time task in normal and retarded adult males. *Psychophysiology*, 1975, *12*, 262–267.

Kunze, D. L. Reflex discharge patterns of cardiac vagal afferent fibers. *Journal of Physiology*, 1972, *222*, 1–15.

Lacey, B. C., & Lacey, J. I. Two-way communication between the heart and the brain: Significance of time within the cardiac cycle. *American Psychologist*, 1978, *33*, 99–113.

Lacey, J. I. Somatic response patterning and stress: Some revisions of activation theory. In M. H. Appley & R. Trumbull (Eds.), *Psychological stress: Issues in research*. New York: Appleton-Century-Crofts, 1967.

Lamb, L. E., Dermksian, G., & Sarnoff, C. A. Significant cardiac arrhythmias induced by common respiratory maneuvers. *American Journal of Cardiology*, 1958, *2*, 563–571.

Larson, S., & Porges, S. W. *The ontogeny of heart rate patterning in the rat*. Paper presented at the annual meeting of the International Society for Developmental Psychobiology, Cincinnati, 1980.

Levy, M. N. Sympathetic–parasympathetic interactions in the heart. *Circulation Research*, 1971, *29*, 437–445.

Levy, M. N., DeGeest, H., & Zieske, H. Effects of respiratory center activity on the heart. *Circulation Research*, 1966, *18*, 67–78.

Levy, M. N., Ng, M. L., & Zieske, H. Cardiac response to cephalic ischemia. *American Journal of Physiology*, 1968, *215*, 159–175.

Lopes, O. V., & Palmer, J. F. Proposed respiratory gating mechanism for cardiac slowing. *Nature*, 1976, *264*, 454–456.

Lowensohn, R. I., Weiss, M., & Hon, E. D. Heart-rate variability in brain-damaged adults. *Lancet*, 1977 (March 19), 626–628.

Lown, B., Verrier, R. L., & Rabinowitz, S. Neural and psychological mechanisms and the problem of sudden cardiac death. *American Journal of Cardiology*, 1977, *39*, 890–902.

Mannard, A., & Polosa, C. Analysis of background firing of single sympathetic preganglionic neurons of cat cervical nerve. *Journal of Neurophysiology*, 1973, *36*, 398–408.

Manzotti, M. The effect of some respiratory maneuvers on the heart rate. *Journal of Physiology*, 1958, *144*, 541–557.

Matta, R. J., Lawler, J. E., & Lown, B. Ventricular electrical instability in the conscious dog: Effects of psychologic stress and beta adrenergic blockade. *American Journal of Cardiology*, 1976, *38*, 594–598.

McCabe, P. M., Porges, S. .W., & Yongue, B. G. Spectral analysis of heart rate during depressor nerve stimulation: The validation of a non-invasive estimate of vagal tone. *Society for Neuroscience Abstracts*, 1979, *5*, 156.

McCrady, J. D., Vallbona, C., & Hoff, H. E. Neural origin of the respiratory–heart rate response. *American Journal of Physiology*, 1966, *211*, 323–328.

Melcher, A. Respiratory sinus arrhythmia in man: A study in heart rate regulating mechanisms. *Acta Physiologica Scandanavia*, 1976, Suppl 435.

Mills, E. Time course for development of vagal inhibition of the heart in neonatal rats. *Life Sciences*, 1978, *23*, 2717–2720.

Neil, E., & Palmer, J. F. Effects of spontaneous respiration on the latency of reflex cardiac chronotropic responses to baroreceptor stimulation. *Proceedings of the Physiological Society*, 1975, *247*, 16P.

Nelson, N. M. Respiration and circulation before birth. In C. A. Smith & N. M. Nelson (Eds.), *The physiology of the newborn infant*. Springfield, Ill.: Charles C Thomas, 1976.

Obrist, P. A., Webb, R. A., Sutterer, J. R., & Howard, J. L. Cardiac deceleration and reaction time: An evaluation of two hypotheses. *Psychophysiology*, 1970, *6*, 695–706.

Polosa, C., Mannard, A., & Laskey, W. Tonic activity of the autonomic nervous system: Functions, properties, and origins. In C. McC. Brooks, K. Koizumi, & A. Sato (Eds.), *Integrative functions of the autonomic nervous system*. Amsterdam: Elsevier, 1979.

Porges, S. W. Heart rate indices of newborn attentional responsivity. *Merrill–Palmer Quarterly*, 1974, *20*, 231–254.

Porges, S. W. The application of spectral analysis for the detection of fetal distress. In T. M. Fields, A. M. Sostek, S. Goldberg, & H. H. Shuman (Eds.), *Infants born at risk*. New York: Spectrum, 1979.

Porges, S. W., Arnold, W. R., & Forbes, E. V. Heart rate variability: An index of attentional responsivity in human newborns. *Developmental Psychology*, 1973, *3*, 85–92.

Porges, S. W., Bohrer, R., Cheung, M. N., Drasgow, F., McCabe, P. M., & Keren, G. A new time-series statistic for detecting rhythmic co-occurrence in the frequency domain: The weighted coherence and its application to psychophysiological research. *Psychological Bulletin*, 1980, *88*, 580–587.

Porges, S. W., & Raskin, D. C. Respiratory and heart rate components of attention. *Journal of Experimental Psychology*, 1969, *81*, 497–503.

Porges, S. W., & Smith, K. M. Defining hyperactivity: Psychophysiological and behavioral strategies. In C. K. Whalen & B. Henker (Eds.), *Hyperactive children: The social ecology of identification and treatment*. New York: Academic Press, 1980.

Porges, S. W., Srinivasan, G., Cheung, M. N., Shanker, H., Pildes, R., & Bohrer, R. *Spectral analysis of neonatal heart rate and respiratory patterns: Preliminary support for a new assessment technique*. Paper presented at the annual meeting of the International Society for Developmental Psychobiology, Atlanta, 1979.

Porges, S. W., Stamps, L. E., & Walter, G. F. Heart rate variability and newborn heart rate responses to illumination changes. *Developmental Psychology*, 1974, *10*, 507–513.

Priess, G., Kirchner, F., & Polosa, C. Patterning of sympathetic preganglionic neuron firing by the central respiratory drive. *Brain Research*, 1975, *87*, 363–374.

Reeve, R., & De Boer, K. Sinus arrhythmia: Data and patterns from groups of individuals followed from 1 month to 23 years of age. *Pediatrics*, 1960, *26*, 402–414.

Riege, W. H., & Peacock, L. V. Conditioned heart rate deceleration under different dimensions of respiratory control. *Psychophysiology*, 1968, *5*, 269–279.

Sayers, B. M. Analysis of heart rate variability. *Ergonomics*, 1973, *16*, 17–32.

Schifferli, P.-Y., & Caldeyro-Barcia, R. Effects of atropine and beta-adrenergic drugs on the heart rate of the human fetus. In L. Boreus (Ed.), *Fetal pharmacology*. New York: Raven Press, 1973.

Siddle, D. A. T., & Turpin, G. Measurement, quantification, and analysis of cardiac activity. In I. Martin & P. H. Venables (Eds.), *Techniques in psychophysiology*. Chichester, England: John Wiley & Sons, 1980.

Spyer, K. M. Baroreceptor control of vagal preganglionic activity. In C. McC. Brooks, K. Koizumi, & A. Sato (Eds.), *Integrative functions of the autonomic nervous system*. Amsterdam: Elsevier, 1979.

Sroufe, L. A. Effects of depth and rate of breathing on heart rate and heart rate variability. *Psychophysiology*, 1971, *8*, 648–655.

Stamps, L. E., & Porges, S. W. Heart rate conditioning in newborn infants: Relationships among conditionability, heart rate variability, and sex. *Developmental Psychology*, 1975, *11*, 424–431.

Tang, P. C., Maire, F. W., & Amassian, V. E. Respiratory influence on the vasomotor center. *American Journal of Physiology*, 1957, *191*, 218–224.

Vallbona, C., Cardus, D., Spencer, W. A., & Hoff, H. E. Neuropharmacological factors influencing the central regulation of the respiratory-heart rate response (RHR). *Archives of Internal Pharmacodynamics*, 1965, *153*, 256–266.

Yongue, B. G., McCabe, P. M., Kelley, S., Rivera, P., & Porges, S. W. *Changes in a respiratorily modulated component of heart period variability as a result of pharmacological manipulations of vagal tone in rats.* Paper presented at the meeting of the Society for Psychophysiological Research, Vancouver, B.C., 1980.

Yongue, B. G., Porges, S. W., & McCabe, P. M. *Changes in vagal control of the heart following signaled and unsignaled shock.* Paper presented at the meeting of the Society for Psychophysiological Research, Cincinnati, 1979.

# 8

## *Cardiac–Behavioral Interactions: A Critical Appraisal*

PAUL A. OBRIST

## INTRODUCTION

I have raised previously (Obrist, 1976, 1981) my growing doubts that the cardiovascular system will provide us with very much information when used as an index of behavioral processes such as emotion, motivation, learning, or attention. Rather, I believe that a psychophysiological strategy will contribute more to the human condition when its goal is to decipher the role of the organism's interactions with its environment in the etiology of cardiovascular disease. This chapter's purpose is to update this position, primarily commenting on the use of heart rate (HR) and blood pressure (BP)[1] as indices of behavioral states while only briefly alluding to the use of a psychophysiological strategy in research involving disease (e.g., hypertension), since this topic has been recently discussed elsewhere

---

1. While BP has not been a very commonly used measure to index behavioral states, in contrast to HR, some BP data are presented because they tend to reinforce the conclusions derived from the HR data.

Paul A. Obrist. Department of Psychiatry, University of North Carolina, Chapel Hill, North Carolina.

(Obrist, 1981; Obrist, Grignolo, Hastrup, Koepke, Langer, Light, McCubbin, & Pollak, in press). I rely mainly on our own research over the past 15 years to document my case, particularly those efforts that have attempted to delineate neurohumoral control mechanisms. The thrust of my argument is not to deny the importance of a psychophysiological strategy to index behavioral processes but to argue that the cardiovascular system is not particularly appropriate for this purpose. Rather, there are more direct ways to evaluate the neural substrate of behavior—namely, the activity of the central nervous system. The point is that we don't think, or learn, or emote, or attend with our hearts but with our brains. Our hearts, as is the entirety of the cardiovascular system, are much more involved in sustaining critical life processes.

This chapter looks at the use of indexing in two manners. First, I briefly consider what I believe to be a fundamental inadequacy in our research strategy; namely, the failure to view the cardiovascular system within the more global context for which it serves and, in turn, an indifference to evaluating neurogenic mechanisms of cardiovascular control. While such considerations do not in themselves present a prima facie case against indexing, they warn us that the problem is not a simple one that is apt to be resolved by the demonstration of a simple concomitance between some experimental manipulation and cardiovascular change.

Next, evidence is presented in which HR and BP were evaluated in different behavioral paradigms where the results are inconsistent with any simple indexing approach. First, only HR data are considered, without regard to neural mechanisms (the behavioral approach). Then both HR and BP data are considered under conditions where neurogenic influences were also evaluated. In this latter context, there is also a discussion of individual differences as well as the concept of "coping" since both present additional interpretive problems. In closing, there is a survey of the conceptual orientation guiding our current research on behavioral-cardiovascular interactions and hypertension since it stands in contrast in significant ways to an indexing approach.

## CARDIOVASCULAR FUNCTIONS AND METABOLIC ACTIVITY

There has never been a high priority in psychophysiological research of the necessity to view cardiovascular activity with regard to metabolic requirements and to delineate the neural mechanisms of cardiovascular control. There has even been an implicit argument against such efforts when the early visceral learning research thought it necessary to demonstrate nonmediated control of cardiovascular changes. There have been exceptions such as Schneiderman's (1974) and Cohen's (1974) work concerning mechanisms of HR control during classical conditioning. Also, there has been the Lacey mechanistic afferent feedback hypothesis where cardiovascular events were viewed to modify central nervous system activity via the baroreceptors, which in turn were held to influence both sensorimotor and cognitive processes (B. C. Lacey & Lacey, 1974; J. I. Lacey, 1959; J. I. Lacey, Kagan, Lacey, & Moss, 1963). This perhaps is the best example of a behaviorally relevant mechanistic model since it ties cardiovascular activity to specific behavioral events. Unfortunately, the vitality of this model is hardly agreed on (Carroll & Anastasiades, 1978; Elliott, 1972; Hahn, 1973; Iacono & Lykken, 1978), and one might view it as premature.

The requisite of delineating mechanisms should become even more apparent in the ensuing discussion. For now, it is sufficient to emphasize that when we deal with the cardiovascular system, we are dealing with a major life support system which is regulated by intricate neural and nonneural control mechanisms. In the healthy organism, it can efficiently carry out metabolic functions which include supplying the tissues with oxygen, removing metabolic waste produce, maintaining electrolyte and fluid balance, and controlling body temperature. Thus, anyone using the cardiovascular phenomena to serve additional functions such as indexing behavioral states must continually bear in mind the basic metabolic functions which the cardiovascular system continuously performs. Furthermore, any changes in cardiovascular function which are unique to our experimental manipulations must be superimposed on this background of metabolically relevant cardiovascular activity. Otherwise, cardiovascular changes would seem to have little direct relevance to our interests. However, there has been no great effort to ascertain the behavioral uniqueness of these cardiovascular changes, that is, their independence from metabolic function. This is likely because it was assumed that under the experimental conditions these metabolic functions were more or less a constant. Our faith in this possibility was shaken by the work evaluating cardiac somatic effects. Here we were able to demonstrate under certain circumstances a close concomitance between phasic HR and somatic activities (Obrist, 1981; Obrist, Howard, Lawler, Galosy, Meyers, & Gaebelein, 1974; Obrist, Webb, Sutterer, & Howard, 1970a). The relationship can be quite robust (Clifton, 1978; Obrist, 1981). It is evidenced when HR is under vagal control and with both increases and decreases in vagal excitation. From a quantitative point of view, the types of somatic activities as well as HR changes are not extensive, as in exercise, but do suggest that even at this level of activity they are a reflection of the means by which the central nervous system integrates cardiovascular and metabolic activities. To the extent that these HR changes are a reflection of such a central integrating mechanism, then, they have no particularly unique sensitivity to behavioral processes, or as Elliott (1974) stated it: "The cardiac somatic hypothesis, to the degree that it is sound and comprehensive, makes HR changes relatively uninteresting to the psychologist" (p. 537).

In more recent research, evidence has been found which is clearly suggestive of a disruption by the behavioral paradigm of the relationship between cardiac and somatic activities. In humans, this has taken the form of an independence between concomitant myocardial (sympathetically mediated) and somatic activities (Obrist, Gaebelein, Teller, Langer, Grignolo, Light, & McCubbin, 1978; Obrist, Lawler, Howard, Smithson, Martin, & Manning, 1974b). In dogs, it has been evidenced by an increase in both HR and cardiac output which is in excess of any increase in oxygen consumption (Langer, Obrist, & McCubbin, 1979). One might be tempted to conclude that under these conditions, the myocardial events are a reflection (index) of some behavioral state since they do not parallel metabolic events. However, aspects of these data which are presented next, specifically those from human studies, do not conform to a simple index approach. In any case, as we begin to obtain insight into the manner the cardiovascular system interacts with other aspects of organismic activity in the behaving organism, then we can better formulate our research strategies and goals.

HEART RATE AND BEHAVIORAL STATES:
THE BEHAVIORAL APPROACH

The Laceys (J. I. Lacey, 1959; J. I. Lacey & Lacey, 1970; Lacey et al., 1963) were among the first investigators to point out the difficulties in using cardiovascular events as "affect or arousal meters" (see J. I. Lacey, 1959, p. 161, for the use of this specific terminology). They called attention to two types of observations. One has been labeled "autonomic response specificity" or "interstressor stereotypy." It refers to the demonstration that different aspects of cardiovascular activity, as well as galvanic activity, show little consistency when used to rank subjects with respect to the "arousal" value of stimuli. A subject considered highly aroused by a stimulus according to one measure of autonomic activity may not be considered particularly aroused by another measure. The second observation has been referred to as "directional fractionation." It is illustrated by reports that some autonomic events, like galvanic activity, evidence sympathetic-like changes to motivationally or emotionally significant events, while other measures, like HR, evidence parasympathetic-like changes (i.e., decreases in HR). The Laceys also pointed out that fractionation can occur even with a single measure like HR. They noted that tasks which focus attention on external events (e.g., listening to a dramatic passage recited by a professional actor) commonly resulted in HR deceleration, while tasks which focus attention on internal events (e.g., solving mental arithmetic problems) resulted in HR acceleration.

The demonstration of stereotypy influenced the experimental design of one of my first psychophysiological efforts (Obrist, 1962). This study evaluated the relationship between "arousal" (Malmo, 1959) as indexed by HR and galvanic activity, and performance on a serial learning task using a within-subject design. The relationship was evaluated in each subject over a number of days (i.e., between 24 and 31), in the expectation that in any one subject, motivational levels would vary from day to day while other factors influencing HR, such as stereotypy essentially, would be constant. In all five subjects, a relationship was observed between autonomic activity and performance of one sort or another. However, the direction and linearity of the relationship varied among and even within subjects. For example, two subjects demonstrated a significant positive direct relationship between HR and performance but a significant inverse one between skin resistance and performance. In all, the results were not supportive of the notion that HR consistently indexed motivational states.

The data described so far have dealt with tonic levels of HR, in that the experimental procedures and tasks involved the measurement of HR over time periods of one minute or longer. There also began to appear at about the same time reports where phasic HR changes were evaluated, like anticipatory HR changes during classical aversive conditioning, which were not consistent with indexing affect or arousal with HR. Specifically, HR in humans was observed to decelerate at the point in time when the unconditioned stimulus (UCS) was expected (Notterman, Schoenfeld, & Bersh, 1952; Zeaman & Smith, 1965). This observation presented several complications and even paradoxes. First, it violated our Cannonean viewpoint that such conditions should evoke a diffuse sympathetic discharge which would manifest itself, among other ways, in the form of an accelerated HR. In fact, increased sympathetic activity was observed with galvanic and vasomotor activity (Obrist, Wood, & Perez-Reyes, 1965). Second, while the anticipatory response was a decrease in HR, the unconditioned response was an increase: an effect quite unprecedented in the classical conditioning literature. Third, in dogs the anticipatory response was observed to be an acceleration of HR (Dykman, Gantt, & Whitehorn, 1956). Finally, decreases in HR were observed to anticipate several types of nonaversive but motivationally significant events (Wood & Obrist, 1968), such as executing the motor response in a signaled reaction time (RT) task (J. I. Lacey, 1967).

For an indexing approach, several problems are created by this variety of observations. First, consider the fractionation observed with tonic HR. If we accept the assumption (Malmo, 1959) that increased HR reflects increased arousal, then those tasks and conditions resulting in a decrease in HR must reflect a decrease in arousal. Knowing the nature of the task, this hardly appears to be the case. Next, consider the species difference in the anticipatory HR change during aversive conditioning. This comparison would suggest that man and dog have different arousal or affective states as they ready themselves for the shock. This is conceivable—but, with respect to direction of change, why do cats (Hein, 1969) and rabbits (Schneiderman, 1974) decelerate their HR, while monkeys accelerate theirs (Smith & Stebbins, 1965)? And why is it that rats (Roberts, 1974) and several species of desert rodents (Hofer, 1970) can evidence both anticipatory increases and decreases of HR? It becomes very confusing and is hardly a very parsimonious situation. Finally, take the observation that in humans anticipatory decreases in HR occur in a variety of circumstances which reflect very different affective states. Obviously, we can't specify that these HR changes index some particular affect. Although some view these HR changes as indexing attention (Jennings, Averill, Opton, & Lazarus, 1971), the anticipatory deceleration seen with aversive stimulation makes me uncomfortable because it is not apparent what the individual is attending to when its HR decelerates as it expects a more or less painful aversive event. It might also be noted that HR decreases tonically in conjunction with alternating blasts of white noise (J. I. Lacey et al., 1963; Obrist, 1963) which at its peak exceeds 100 db, hardly sweet music to the ears (see also Zeaman & Smith, 1965).

To this point, then, even without considering the data provided by the exploration of neural control and the further complexities which they introduce, there are sufficient inconsistencies in the data to question the particular validity of HR to index behavioral processes. Such critical sentiments are shared by others. For example, when Rescorla and Solomon (1967) reviewed the literature concerning the use of HR to index the conditional emotional response in the context of two-factor learning theory, they found too little consistency in the evidence to conclude that HR can be used for this purpose. At one point, they concluded: "To expect simple heart rate changes, which are only a small portion of this system to mirror adequately a state such as fear is to oversimplify hopelessly the operation of the cardiovascular system" (p. 168). Elliott (1974), reviewing a literature concerning tonic HR, reached a similar conclusion when he stated: "There are in these data, in short, grounds for skepticism about any view of the motivational significance of HR" (p. 536), and "There is no obvious mandate in evidence for using HR to measure complex variables in social psychology and personality" (p. 527).

## HEART RATE, BLOOD PRESSURE, AND BEHAVIORAL STATES: NEUROGENIC MECHANISMS

### HEART RATE

We have evaluated the influence of the cardiac innervations in several paradigms and with respect to both phasic and tonic effects. Not surprisingly, during classical aversive conditioning, the anticipatory deceleration of HR was attributable to a phasic increase in vagal excitation as revealed by pharmacological blockade of the parasympathetic innervation (Obrist *et al.*, 1965). The situation is more complicated, however, as indicated in Figure 8-1, which depicts second-by-second changes on test trials (the UCS is omitted) under both conditions. With both innervations intact, the anticipatory response is actually a biphasic increase in HR followed by a decrease. With blockade, there is a uniphasic acceleration of HR concurrent to the deceleration of HR seen with the innervations intact. Thus, we see not only an increase in vagal excitation but, preceding

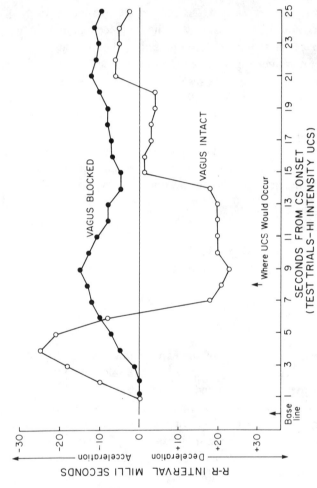

FIG. 8-1. Second-by-second changes in HR on test trials (UCS omitted) during classical aversive conditioning in humans with intact (open circles) and blocked (closed circles) vagal innervations. From "Heart Rate during Conditioning in Humans," by P. A. Obrist, D. M. Wood, and M. Perez-Reyes, *Journal of Experimental Psychology*, 1965, *70*, 32–42. Copyright 1965 by the American Psychological Association. Reprinted by permission.

it, a momentary loss of vagal restraint. Even this initial acceleration of HR cannot be considered as mediated by sympathetic activity. Furthermore, an increase in vagal excitation masks a sympathetic influence. Schneiderman (1974) observed this effect in rabbits with regard to the unconditioned HR response using brain stimulation as the unconditioned stimulus (see also Obrist, Webb, Sutterer, & Howard, 1970*b*).

The situation was complicated further when we changed the experimental paradigm from classical aversive conditioning to a shock-avoidance task (Obrist, Lawler, Howard, Smithson, Martin, & Manning, 1974). This study used a signaled RT task where avoidance was made contingent on performance and neural influences evaluated by sympathetic, rather than vagal, blockade. Figure 8-2 depicts the second-by-second HR changes over a 30-sec measurement period commencing with the ready signal on trials where shock was avoided (most of them). During the 8-sec preparatory interval and for several seconds after response execution, HR was under vagal control since a similar triphasic HR change is seen with both an intact and a blocked sympathetic innervation. The response in the signaled shock-avoidance RT task is characterized first by a decrease in vagal tone, then by an increase, and then by another decrease. It is only about the time that the aversive stimulus is expected that a sympathetic excitatory effect is seen. This effect continues throughout the measurement period.

More recently, we (Obrist *et al.*, 1978) evaluated sympathetic influences on tonic levels of HR under three conditions: the cold pressor, an erotic movie, and a shock-avoidance task using an unsignaled RT procedure. While all three procedures evoke increases in tonic levels of HR, the shock-avoidance task evokes the largest increase due to sympathetic excitation (see Figure 8-3). This is revealed again through the use of sympathetic pharmacological blockade ($\beta$-adrenergic),[2] which resulted in a significantly greater attenuation of HR during shock avoidance than during either the cold pressor or film. Thus, shock avoidance evokes both phasic and tonic sympathetic activity.

---

2. $\beta$-Adrenergic refers to receptor sites found in the myocardium and certain arterial beds (e.g., striate musculature). When stimulated, they result in myocardial excitation and vascular dilation. This is in contrast to adrenergic receptor sites found in the vasculature which upon stimulation result in vasoconstriction; these are referred to as $\alpha$-adrenergic.

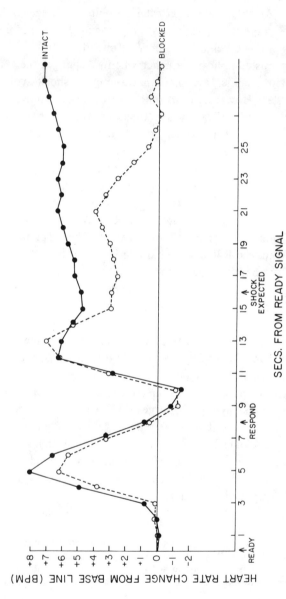

FIG. 8-2. Second-by-second changes in HR with an intact and blocked sympathetic innervation during a signaled shock-avoidance reaction time task. Based on trials when shock was not delivered. From "Sympathetic Influences on Cardiac Rate and Contractility during Acute Stress in Humans," by P. A. Obrist, J. E. Lawler, J. L. Howard, K. W. Smithson, P. L. Martin, and J. Manning, *Psychophysiology*, 1974, *11*, 405–427. Copyright 1974 by the Society for Psychophysiological Research. Reprinted by permission.

274

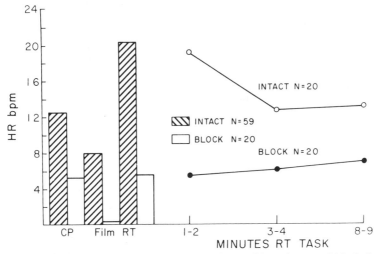

FIG. 8-3. Change from baseline in tonic levels of HR with an intact and blocked sympathetic innervation. Left: changes averaged over 90 sec of cold pressor and first 2 min of film and shock-avoidance task. Right: changes in first 9 min of shock-avoidance task. From "The Relationship among Heart Rate, Carotid dP/dt and Blood Pressure in Humans as a Function of the Type of Stress," by P. A. Obrist, C. J. Gaebelein, E. S. Teller, A. W. Langer, A. Grignolo, K. C. Light, and J. A. McCubbin, *Psychophysiology*, 1978, *15*, 102–115. Copyright 1978 by the Society for Psychophysiological Research. Reprinted by permission.

BLOOD PRESSURE

The primary focus of psychophysiological research in blood pressure has concerned visceral learning or biofeedback, and the question of hypertension. There has been less interest in using the BP to index behavioral states per se, probably because of the measurement problem. As will become apparent, it is important to discuss BP control because it is complex and, as with HR, not subject to simple generalizations about its significance to psychophysiological issues.

Blood pressure is a derived value resulting from the interaction of the cardiac output (CO) and vascular resistance. In studies using human subjects, the specific influence of each determinant has been difficult to ascertain with certainty because of the difficulty in measuring the cardiac output. This has not been the case in some animal preparations where the direct assessment of the CO has been obtained (Anderson & Tosheff, 1973; Anderson, Yingling, & Sagawa, 1979; Forsyth, 1971, 1976; Langer *et al.*, 1979; Lawler, Obrist, & Lawler, 1975). In these studies, the relative contributions of the output and vascular resistance have been observed to vary as a function of whether the animal is resting, where vascular influences are more dominant; or challenged by a behavioral task (e.g., shock avoidance), where myocardial influences become more pronounced. Over the course of a continuous 72-hour avoidance procedure, a shift from a more pronounced myocardial influence to a more pronounced vascular influence has been observed (Forsyth, 1971). Among other things, such data tell us that the influence of the two interacting determinants can vary as a function of conditions, and even within conditions. Thus, the BP is not a static event to be interpreted as a result of either vascular or myocardial events.

In humans, we cannot speak with as much authority about the respective influence of each determinant until we measure the cardiac output. However, through the use of pharmacological blocking agents, we have evidence which allows us to make some good guesses as to what controls the BP in the behaving organism. Also, the cardiac output has been observed to increase in conjunction with an accelerated HR during a behavioral challenge (Gliner, Bedi, & Horvath, 1979). Finally, it should be noted that the cardiac output has been assessed in clinical populations and found to make a significant contribution to the BP, particularly in some young adults evidencing marginally elevated levels of BP in the resting state (e.g., Lund-Johansen, 1967; Safar, Weiss, Levenson, London, & Milliez, 1973). But this latter work is not particularly germane to the current discussion since the significance of the behavioral–cardiac interaction remains uncertain under these conditions.

I would like to restrict my comments primarily to our own work since 1975, where we have measured the BP in most studies, usually noninvasively but on occasion, invasively. As with HR, the results present some perplexing interpretative difficulties concerning their behavioral significance.

Our first effort actually was reported in 1965 (Obrist *et al.*, 1965), where we measured the BP in five subjects invasively from the radial artery during classical aversive conditioning, first with and then without an intact $\alpha$-adrenergic vascular innervation. (See Footnote 2 for the distinction between $\alpha$- and $\beta$-adrenergic reactions.) Here, along with vagal excitatory influences on HR (i.e., HR deceleration), we observed a small anticipatory pressor response with increases in both systolic (SBP) and diastolic (DBP) pressure, peaking at around 3–4 mm Hg. These increases were blocked by the pharmacological agent. Thus, in the presence of a momentary increase in vagal excitation on HR, we observed a momentary increase in adrenergic excitation on the vasculature. A similar relationship has since been seen (Obrist, Lawler, Howard, Smithson, Martin, & Manning, 1974) during the foreperiod of a signaled RT task— that is, vagal-dominated phasic HR effects in the presence of small anticipatory BP responses. These two studies demonstrate simultaneous vagal influences on the myocardium along with sympathetic ($\alpha$-adrenergic) influences on the vasculature. This is not too profound an observation, other than to reinforce the point that the sympathetics do not necessarily act en masse.

More perplexing BP effects emerged in the studies which followed. When we evaluated sympathetic ($\beta$-adrenergic) influences on the myocardium during the cold pressor, erotic movie, and signaled shock-avoidance RT task, we also measured the SBP and DBP. Consistent with the HR effects, SBP was observed to be more appreciably elevated at the onset of the shock-avoidance task than with either the cold pressor or the film (see Figure 8-4). Moreoever, as with HR, pharmacological blockade attenuated SBP most at the onset of the shock-avoidance task.

FIG. 8-4. Change from baseline in tonic levels of systolic blood pressure with an intact and blocked sympathetic innervation, as in Figure 8-3. From "The Relationship among Heart Rate, Carotid dP/dt and Blood Pressure in Humans as a Function of the Type of Stress," by P. A. Obrist, C. J. Gaebelein, E. S. Teller, A. W. Langer, A. Grignolo, K. C. Light, and J. A. McCubbin, *Psychophysiology*, 1978, *15*, 102–115. Copyright 1978 by the Society for Psychophysiological Research. Reprinted by permission.

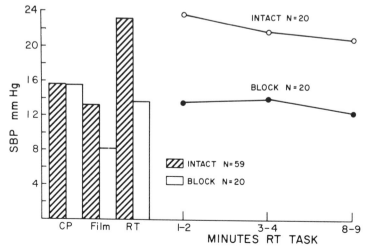

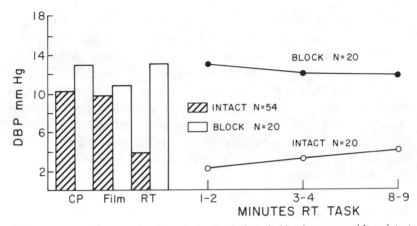

FIG. 8-5. Change from baseline in tonic levels of diastolic blood pressure with an intact and blocked sympathetic innervation, as in Figure 8-3. From "The Relationship among Heart Rate, Carotid dP/dt and Blood Pressure in Humans as a Function of the Type of Stress," by P. A. Obrist, C. J. Gaebelein, E. S. Teller, A. W. Langer, A. Grignolo, K. C. Light, and J. A. McCubbin, *Psychophysiology*, 1978, *15*, 102–115. Copyright 1978 by the Society for Psychophysiological Research. Reprinted by permission.

Diastolic blood pressure, on the other hand, presented a different and more complicated picture (Figure 8-5). In contrast to both HR and SBP, it increased less at the onset of the shock-avoidance task than with either the cold pressor or the film. In fact, at the onset of shock avoidance, the magnitude of the increase was significantly but marginally negatively correlated ($r = -.27, p < .05$) with the magnitude of the increase in SBP, indicating that the subjects with the largest SBP increase tended to have the smallest change in DBP. This was not the case with the cold pressor and the film. Here, not only was the DBP increase larger than with the shock-avoidance task, but the magnitude of the increase was directly correlated with the magnitude of the SBP increase (e.g., $r = +.42, p < .01$). Now, those subjects with the largest DBP increase tended to have the largest SBP increase. I have some confidence in these observations demonstrating the differential BP effects among conditions since they have now been replicated in an additional study (Obrist, Light, McCubbin, Hutcheson, & Hoffer, 1979). Also, a similar differential influence on SBP and DBP—that is, a large increase in SBP and little or no change in DBP—was seen in still another study involving shock avoidance (Light & Obrist, 1980a).

The effect on DBP of pharmacologically blocking the myocardial innervation further complicated the picture. During shock avoidance, DBP increased significantly more following blockade than with an intact innervation (see Figure 8-5), an effect just opposite to that seen with SBP. Pharmacological blockade, on the other hand, had no significant influence on the DBP increases evoked by the cold pressor and the film. Also, with blockade, SBP and DBP became positively correlated during shock avoidance, as they were with the cold pressor and film with either an intact or blocked myocardial innervation.

These observations warrant two comments: (1) At the onset of the shock avoidance, there is likely little change in vascular resistance; if anything, a decrease. How else could DBP essentially not change in the presence of an accelerated HR and an increased SBP? This is likely attributable to a $\beta$-adrenergic-mediated vascular dilation such as Forsyth (1976) observed in rhesus monkeys at the onset of a shock-avoidance task where direct measures of blood flow were made. He observed a decreased vascular resistance with an intact innervation but an increased vascular resistance with a blocked innervation, deriving vascular resistance from the CO and BP and measuring blood flow with a radioactive microsphere technique. (2) These data suggest that the relative contributions of the myocardium and vasculature in the control of the BP vary as a function of conditions. With the cold pressor and film, where $\beta$-adrenergic influences on the myocardium are minimal, both aspects of the BP change are primarily under vascular control (i.e., increased resistance). But with shock avoidance, myocardial influences are more evident, particularly as seen with SBP; whereas vascular influences are minimal, as indicated by the small changes in DBP. In summary, the control of the BP under these rather simple yet differing behavioral challenges appears to reflect different BP control mechanisms.

INTERPRETATIVE PROBLEMS

The various lines of evidence concerning both myocardial and BP control raise significant issues concerning our view of these cardiovascular events with regard to behavioral processes. First, it is obvious that we can no longer consider increased parasympathetic excitation on the heart as reflecting only vegetative influences (Hassett, 1978; Sternbach, 1966) since we see, in anticipation of aversive events, vagal influences dominating HR in some paradigms (e.g., classical conditioning; Obrist *et al.*, 1965). There is also the observation that vagally mediated HR decreases occur in conjunction with sympathetic (α-adrenergic) mediated anticipatory increases in BP.[3] Such observations warn us that the myocardium is not invariantly dominated by sympathetic influences as the individual interacts with significant life events, and that even within the cardiovascular system, directional fractionation can occur. Second, the observation that the dominant innervation of the heart varies among paradigms, and even at different points in time within the same paradigm, presents additional interpretational problems for any unidimensional index interpretation. For example, are we to understand that the two innervations whose excitatory effects are antagonistic (i.e., one decelerating the heart— the other accelerating it) provide comparable meaning when similar behavioral states are evoked? Furthermore, even when we observe only vagal excitatory effects (i.e., HR deceleration) in paradigms with quite different demand characteristics such as are reported with reaction time and aversive conditioning procedures, what basis do we have for attributing different meanings to similarly mediated HR changes? That is, the anticipatory HR change is thought to reflect attentional states in one circumstance and affective states in another. The most parsimonious explanation in both cases is that the anticipatory decreases in HR reflect similar central nervous system mechanisms, which involve not only vagal excitation but still other processes such as we have proposed with regard to somatomotor activity. As such, HR has no direct behavioral significance since it does not bear any one-to-one relationship with behavioral states.

The tonic BP data present some additional interpretational difficulties. Suppose that in the study using the cold pressor and the shock-avoidance task, we had asked which of these two challenges was the most arousing and had sought the answer by measuring BP. If we had resorted to measuring only the SBP, the avoidance task would get the nod. Had we measured only the DBP, then the cold pressor would be favored. If we had measured both, there would not be a definitive answer.

Next, consider the effects of pharmacological blockade during shock avoidance. Since the SBP changes are attenuated, we could conclude that

---

3. The vagal influence on HR is not secondary to the BP increase via baroreceptor mechanisms since the vagal effects are still seen after pharmacological blockade of the BP increase (Obrist *et al.*, 1965).

the task has become less arousing. However, since the DBP increased more, the task could be judged more arousing. The point is that the BP, like HR, is too complexly controlled in regard to situational determinants and their influence on control mechanisms to make any blanket generalizations about underlying behavioral states.

## INDIVIDUAL DIFFERENCES

The situation is complicated further by the recent observations with our various experimental procedures (Obrist, 1981; Obrist *et al.*, in press) of appreciable individual differences in myocardial and SBP reactivity. The data are derived from two experiments (Obrist *et al.*, 1978; Obrist, Light, McCubbin, Hutcheson, & Hoffer, 1979) and are illustrated in Table 8-1 for tonic levels of HR and in Table 8-2 for tonic levels of SBP. These data are derived from 56 young adult male undergraduates who were exposed to the battery of challenges consisting of the cold pressor, the film, and the shock-avoidance task, as well as two resting, or baseline, conditions. One baseline occurred just prior to exposure to the challenges and is referred to as the "pretask baseline." The other occurred anywhere from 1–2 weeks or a year or more later, when the subjects returned to the lab on two occasions. This latter condition is referred to as the "relaxation baseline." With both baselines, the subjects were instructed to rest and relax. With the pretask baseline, the subjects knew they were about to be exposed to the three experimental challenges. With the relaxation base-

TABLE 8-1. Mean HR during Two Types of Baselines and Experimental Tasks (Cardiac Innervations Intact)

| Heart rate reactivity | Relaxation baseline | Pretask baseline | Cold pressor | Film | Shock avoidance |
|---|---|---|---|---|---|
| Most | 63 | 80 ( 26) | 96 (51) | 86 (35) | 120 (90) |
| ↓ | 65 | 78 ( 20) | 92 (40) | 80 (23) | 103 (57) |
| | 68 | 75 ( 11) | 88 (29) | 80 (18) | 93 (37) |
| Least | 67 | 66 (−2) | 80 (19) | 72 ( 7) | 76 (13) |
| $\bar{x}$ | 66 | 75 | 89 | 79 | 98 |

*Note.* Data quartiled on the basis of HR reactivity during shock avoidance. $n = 56$ (see text for details). Percent change data are given in parentheses.

TABLE 8-2. Mean SBP during Two Types of Baselines and Experimental Tasks (Cardiac Innervations Intact)

| Heart rate reactivity | Relaxation baseline | Pretask baseline | Cold pressor | Film | Shock avoidance |
|---|---|---|---|---|---|
| Most | 124 | 137 (10) | 157 (26) | 149 (20) | 170 (37) |
| ↓ | 121 | 139 (7) | 142 (17) | 137 (13) | 154 (27) |
| | 124 | 126 (2) | 137 (11) | 137 (11) | 150 (22) |
| Least | 121 | 124 (2) | 141 (17) | 133 (9) | 137 (13) |
| $\bar{x}$ | 125 | 129 | 144 | 139 | 153 |

Note. Data quartiled on the basis of HR reactivity during shock avoidance (see Table 8-1). $n = 56$. Percent change data are given in parentheses.

line, they were instructed that they would not be involved in any other procedures.[4]

Based on the difference in average HR values between the relaxation baseline and the first 2 min of the shock-avoidance task, the 56 subjects were divided into quartiles of reactivity. The 14 subjects in the first row of Table 8-1 were the most reactive, while the 14 in the last row were the least reactive. Subjectives in Rows 2 and 3 were intermediate in reactivity. Several details should be noted. (1) The four subgroups demonstrated very similar average HR values during the follow-up or relaxation baseline. These values are comparable to those obtained when sympathetic myocardial influences were blocked in the resting state (i.e., $\bar{x}$ HR, 66 vs. 67 bpm; Obrist et al., 1978), suggesting that sympathetic influences are minimal under this baseline condition. (2) The difference in HR reactivity between the relaxation baseline and shock-avoidance task is appreciable among the most and least reactive quartiles, averaging 57 and 9 bpm, respectively. (3) These individual differences in reactivity extend to the other conditions including the pretask baseline, although they are not as pronounced. (4) If we had used the pretask baseline as the reference point, the individual differences in reactivity would be considerably less since it

4. Although 154 subjects participated in these two studies, complete data were available only on 56, primarily because of the unavailability of data from the follow-up relaxation baseline. Even though the time between the two baselines varied among subjects, this does not appear to influence baseline differences since in a more recent study involving 72 subjects (Light & Obrist, 1980b) as well as an additional 18 pilot subjects, the two baselines were obtained within 1–2 weeks of each other. Identical baseline effects were seen in these 90 subjects as in the 56 subjects of the earlier studies (Obrist, 1981).

was already elevated in the most reactive subjects. Also, we would have been forced to conclude that individual differences in reactivity were unique to shock avoidance, as was erroneously reported in an earlier publication (Obrist, Langer, Grignolo, Sutterer, Light, & McCubbin, 1979). For example, the HR differences between the pretask baseline and shock avoidance were 40, 25, 18, and 10 bpm for the four reactivity groups going from most to least reactive. During the cold pressor, these differences would have been 16, 14, 13, and 14 bpm for those respective quartiles.

The important conclusions to be drawn from these data are as follows. There are appreciable individual differences in sympathetic reactivity.[5] These individual differences are most pronounced when a follow-up relaxation baseline is used. Most importantly, hyperreactivity generalizes to a variety of conditions with distinct qualitative differences, including a pretask resting baseline. It appears that the more reactive individuals evidence hyperreactivity to any novel, challenging event. Finally, it should be noted that we have observed individual differences in HR reactivity in a variety of other experimental challenges, for example, preparing and then making a public speech (Hastrup, Swaney, Obrist, Beeler, & Chaska, 1981), difficult mental arithmetic tasks, and reaction time tasks where the subjects perform for financial bonuses, competing either against some instructed criterion or against another subject. Also, we find HR reactivity to be a fairly stable characteristic of an individual in that it can be reproduced within the same task, for up to one year, as well as between tasks (Light, 1981, unpublished observations). Thus, reactivity is not unique to some contrived laboratory task like shock avoidance and appears to be a stable characteristic of an individual (see also Manuck & Garland, 1980; Manuck & Schaefer, 1978).

With respect to SBP, we find a comparable situation in regard to individual differences and the generalizability of SBP reactivity over conditions. Furthermore, SBP reactivity is related to HR reactivity in that the HR reactors are the SBP reactors, etc. Table 8-2 presents the

5. We cannot with absolute certainty claim that we are dealing only with individual differences in sympathetic excitation. But most available evidence indicates that $\beta$-adrenergic influences are quite significant in the more reactive subjects. For example, in an earlier study (Obrist *et al.*, 1978), the average HRs with the sympathetics blocked for the cold pressor, the film, and the shock-avoidance task were 72, 68, and 72 bpm, respectively. This is in contrast to 89, 79, and 98 bpm, respectively, with an intact innervation (Table 8-1).

average SBP values for the five conditions depicted in Table 8-1, using the same 56 subjects. The data are quartiled on the basis of HR reactivity. Thus, in both tables, the same subjects appear in the same rows (quartiles). Again, we see the similarity among subgroups during the relaxation baseline, but the similarity ends there, as with HR. The most reactive HR subjects demonstrated greater SBP reactivity across all other conditions, with the most pronounced effect seen in the shock-avoidance task. Again, the least reactive HR subjects remained minimally reactive with SBP under all conditions.

We have little insight into the basis of these individual differences. One possibility to consider is that the more reactive subjects are more emotional. The reactive subjects may be more apprehensive during the pretask baseline, experience the cold pressor as more painful, be more aroused sexually by the erotic movie, and be more challenged and/or frightened by the shock-avoidance task. However, this conjecture seems unlikely because of the lack of evidence indicating the existence of such a generalized state of emotionality (at least to our knowledge). We also cannot attribute the individual differences to certain differences in the nature of our subject population such as age, sex, educational background, etc., because they are all very homogeneous in this regard. We have assessed these subjects on a number of personality scales such as the Jenkins (1976) Activity Questionnaire, with no success. In one study, we did find that the more reactive subjects were slightly but significantly faster in performance time during the RT shock-avoidance task (Light & Obrist, 1980b). Also, in two other studies, more reactive subjects claimed to be more challenged and stressed by the task (McCubbin, 1980; Obrist et al.; 1978). But these effects are not substantive and do not account for the individual differences during the pretask baseline, the cold pressor, or the film. In short, we do not have a compelling basis for attributing meaning to these individual differences, and until we develop such a basis, these data warn us that these two aspects of cardiovascular activity, as used in these paradigms, offer us little help in understanding behavioral processes.

## THE COPING CONCEPT

We originally attributed the differential influences of classical conditioning and shock avoidance on the cardiac innervations (i.e., vagal dominance during classical conditioning and sympathetic dominance during shock avoidance) to the stimulus parameter of coping (Obrist, 1976; Obrist *et al.*, 1978). It was hypothesized that passive coping evokes parasympathetic effects, while active coping evokes sympathetic effects. We have even manipulated in still another manner the ability for subjects to control (i.e., cope with) aversive events and again found that tonic HR among other cardiovascular events is significantly more accelerated in subjects given some control (active coping) of aversive stressors than a yoked control (passive coping) (Light & Obrist, 1980*a*). Thus, it can be concluded that HR can be used to index coping strategies.

However, this conclusion must be viewed in another perspective. Recalling the large individual differences we see in HR reactivity during shock avoidance (active coping), can we conclude that the *hyper*reactor is coping with greater effort than the *hypo*reactor? Some of the latter never increase their HR from baseline; are they not coping at all? They do perform well on the shock-avoidance task, although in one study (Light & Obrist, 1980*b*), with marginally less rapidity.

One might question why the manipulation of active coping works if HR is such a poor index of behavioral processes. Previously, I (Obrist, 1976, 1981) have answered this question with recourse to the notion that coping, whether passive or active, involves an element of action or inaction, and that it is action that the cardiovascular system is significantly concerned with. Since the cardiovascular system has evolved to facilitate the metabolic requirements of the working muscles, it is not too surprising in situations requiring action or the anticipation of action such as flight or fight (active coping), that the cardiovascular system mobilizes accordingly (e.g., an accelerated HR). On the other hand, in situations where action is to no avail to start with (classical aversive conditioning), is found to be futile (impossible condition, shock avoidance), or is found to require little effort (easy condition, shock avoidance), it is not surprising that we see a dampening of cardiovascular activity (i.e., vagal dominance or a lessening of sympathetic influences). Because of the association of active coping with action, I find it easier conceptually to link cardiovascular activity with it than with behavioral processes such as motivation or emotion or attention, unless the latter can be viewed along an activity continuum. But have caution with this conceptualization. It still does not explain the individual differences; nor does it explain cardiac–somatic coupling and uncoupling (see Obrist, 1981).

## A PSYCHOPHYSIOLOGICAL STRATEGY
## IN HYPERTENSION RESEARCH

This section presents an overview of our current research strategy concerning the role of the behavioral–cardiac interaction in the etiology of hypertension (see Obrist, 1981; Obrist et al., 1981).

Concern with neurogenic mechanisms of cardiac and vascular control, as well as myocardial and vascular influences on BP, is but one necessary phase of our strategy. Another aspect of it is an evaluation of a conceptual model which has several components. But before outlining these, it should be emphasized that this model is basically a series of working hypotheses which act as guidelines for our experimental efforts, and it is subject to modification or elaboration contingent on the data. It is not meant to be a hard-and-fast theory but rather a series of speculative sojourns.

One aspect of the model focuses on the hemodynamics in the development of hypertension. This proposes that in the early stages of hypertension, where the BP is only marginally elevated, the cardiac output is significantly increased, while the vascular resistance has not changed. As such, the BP is more under myocardial than vascular control. As the hypertension progresses, hemodynamic control shifts from myocardial to vascular control. Thus, in established hypertension, the elevated BP is almost exclusively due to an elevated vascular resistance (Lund-Johansen, 1967, 1979). This hypothesis was derived from research that did not evaluate behavioral influences. However, evidence was presented that the elevated resting cardiac output observed with a marginally elevated BP was due to increased sympathetic drive on the myocardium (Julius & Esler, 1975), suggesting a behavioral influence. Although we have not as yet measured the cardiac output in humans, our evidence that increased sympathetic drive on the myocardium is in association with certain behavioral challenges points to the potential role of behavioral influences.

A second facet of the model hypothesizes that hypertension is a consequence of a breakdown in the efficiency of at least two metabolic processes associated with cardiovascular functions, the cardiac output and renal mechanisms associated with electrolyte (sodium) balance. The elevated output observed in borderline hypertension is proposed to be excessive (exaggerated) relative to tissue requirements. This triggers non-neurogenic vascular mechanisms to return the output to normal, but in the process, the peripheral resistance is elevated (Birkenhager & Schale-kamp, 1976; Folkow, Hallback, Lundgren, Sivertsson, & Weiss, 1973; Guyton, 1977, 1980). While this possibility has not been systematically evaluated in clinical populations evidencing marginally elevated pressures, there is evidence that behavioral challenges in still other populations can evoke such an effect. For example, an exaggerated increase in the output has been observed in a shock-avoidance task with a chronic dog preparation (Langer, 1978; Langer et al., 1979).

In regard to kidney involvement, it has been proposed (Guyton, 1977, 1980) that established hypertension is necessary to maintain sodium balance, because over time, the kidney has developed an abnormality (or inefficiency) whereby it can no longer maintain balance at normotensive levels of the BP. The basis of this breakdown in metabolic efficiency is obscure, but we have recently demonstrated again in a chronic dog preparation that a behavioral challenge (i.e., shock avoidance) facilitated sodium and water retention under conditions where excretion rates of both are normally increased (Grignolo, 1980; Grignolo, Koepke, & Obrist, 1982). This effect appears to be influenced by increased $\beta$-adrenergic drive (Koepke, Grignolo, & Obrist, 1981). It remains unknown how these behaviorally evoked renal phenomena result in the inefficient development of kidney functioning, and how they may interact with a metabolically exaggerated elevated cardiac output in relation to the organism's interaction with its environment. But such observations clearly emphasize the importance of behavioral factors and point to future directions for research.

These are the two major aspects of the model. There are also two corollaries to it. One proposes that since hypertension is a progressive disorder, it is more appropriate in the study of its etiology to begin our evaluation of the behavioral–cardiac interaction as early in the inception of the disease process as possible. If we focus on older individuals with an already established hypertension, we may miss critical events and transition in the etiological process. Those mechanisms which are involved in BP control early in the process may differ appreciably from those that sustain the BP once hypertension is more established (Brown, Fraser, Lever, Morton, Robertson, & Schalekamp, 1977). Furthermore, the significance of behavioral factors may differ in the course of the progression, being greater early than later in the process, since neurogenic influences may lessen in time. Because of this consideration, the role of the behavioral–cardiac interaction needs to be evaluated as early in the disease process as possible. This creates the problem of how one identifies the prehypertensive. An encouraging lead that we are pursuing is working with our young adult population, concentrating on the individual differences in myocardial and SBP reactivity which were previously described, and evaluating whether the hyperresponders are prehypertensive.

A second corollary concerns the significance we can attribute to acute elevations of the BP in young adults with regard to an eventual established hypertension. There is abundant evidence that the BP is very labile, even in individuals considered normotensive (Pickering, 1977), and it is likely that acute elevations of the BP in some individuals may have no ominous consequences. We propose that they are predictors of sustained hypertension only when they reflect the influence of an inappropriate adjustment in basic metabolic function on BP control mechanisms, such as an inappropriately elevated cardiac output or excessive sodium retention. If an acute BP rise does not reflect some disruption of one or more metabolic processes, then its ultimate significance to pathophysiology is questionable. An example of the latter is an acute elevation of the BP due to an increase in vascular resistance in reaction to some stimulus without any metabolically justified change (disruption) of cardiac output, tissue perfusion, or sodium retention.

Finally, the problem with hypertension can be seen in another perspective. An elevated BP is a symptom like an elevated body temperature. A fever does not inform you of the type of infecting organism, where in the body the infection may have localized or originated from, the conditions under which the infection was incurred, nor how to prevent future infections. Without further understanding, an elevated BP is similarly uninformative. This is the reason for the importance of delineating BP control mechanisms and the internal events that influence these mechanisms. As we unravel the complexities, we can evaluate the influence of behavioral factors and the means by which they interact, not with the symptom per se but with those processes that modify the control mechanisms.

In summary, I have attempted to outline some of the events that may be involved in the etiology of hypertension which can serve as a means of directing the efforts of those of us coming out of behavioral science in evaluating the etiological process. I wish to emphasize, however, as Page (1977) has done, that the "causes" of hypertension are probably numerous. The etiological scheme presented here, even if eventually shown to have some validity, may only apply to a certain percentage of individuals who eventually evidence established hypertension. In others, there may be differing etiological processes. The significance of behavioral factors may vary similarly and be of primary importance in some individuals and of lesser significance in others.

## SUMMARY AND DISCUSSION

The intention of this chapter is to question whether cardiovascular activity as used in psychophysiological research, particularly HR, provides sensitive and useful quantitative information about behavioral states.[6] On the basis of the data cited, one can raise serious doubts that the cardiovascular system will serve this purpose. There are several types of evidence on which this conclusion is based. (1) There are data indicating that certain experimental manipulations produce inconsistent effects such as fractionation of autonomic responding or the interspecies difference in anticipatory HR changes seen during classical aversive conditioning. (2) There are data obtained from the evaluation of neurogenic mechanisms where there is demonstrated a complex interplay between the two innervations. (3) There are the observations of appreciable individual differences in HR reactivity across a variety of circumstances, which cannot be argued in any convincing manner to reflect quantitative differences in some behavioral state. Finally, some BP data are introduced, not because BP has been used that extensively to index, but because it demonstrates in still another way the complexities of cardiovascular control.

The position taken can be accused of ignoring a considerable amount of research that has quite consistently shown an influence of behavioral events and manipulation on cardiovascular activity. The phasic anticipatory deceleration of HR in anticipation of response execution during a signaled RT task is an example of such an effort, and as a result, HR has been viewed to index attention. But has it told us much about the

6. By "sensitive," is meant providing quantitative values that reliably and validly depict either between- or within-individual differences in some behavioral state such as how attentive an organism is to a given event. By "useful," is meant that the information obtained provides insight into existing issues not readily obtained by other procedures (e.g., behavioral observations).

attention process, such as the degree the individual is attending, the sensitivity of HR to individual differences in attention, or within-subject differences in attentional states? The demonstration that HR provides such information is important; otherwise, how useful is HR in our efforts to understand this or any other behavioral process? However, there are few available data demonstrating a particular sensitivity of HR to manipulations of behavioral states. If anything, the available data are either negative, inconsistent, or, at best, demonstrate a very modest degree of covariation between HR and some behavioral manipulation.

A recent study by Iacono and Lykken (1978) illustrates the point; here they directed their efforts at just such questions and came up with essentially negative results. Phasic anticipatory HR changes were not sensitive to differing attentional demands placed on the individual and appeared to be insensitive to trial-to-trial alterations in attentional states as indexed by performance (see also Obrist, 1981). Of course, a single study does not decide significant issues, but it is more studies of this kind that are needed to determine how sensitive and useful HR is to these central nervous system processes which are directly involved in the control of behavioral processes and events.

One could even question whether efforts aimed at evaluating the sensitivity of HR to index any behavioral state is not premature, at least until we first elaborate neurogenic mechanisms and resolve the inconsistencies in the data discussed earlier in this chapter. For example, how do we handle the individual differences? What can we say about the hyporesponder, particularly the individual who demonstrates no change in HR during our various challenges? Can we conclude that he/she failed to attend or emote or be aroused? This is an unlikely conclusion in the light of available evidence.

To repeat a point made earlier, our first serious apprehensions about using HR as a behavioral index developed when we formulated the cardiac–somatic relationship (Obrist et al., 1970a), since it makes behaviorally evoked HR changes more or less coincidental to the modification of somatic activity. The evidence presented earlier in this chapter concerning neurogenic control and individual differences is equally disconcerting to an index approach and acts to complement that raised by the cardiac–somatic formulation.

In closing, it should be reemphasized that our belief in the value of a cardiovascular psychophysiological strategy in the study of pathophysiology is based on the fact that the cardiovascular system is foremost concerned in sustaining critical life processes. Furthermore, a case can be made that when the efficiency with which these processes are sustained is compromised, then disease evolves. Our role as cardiovascular psychophysiologists should be to shed insight as to how behavioral events might influence this breakdown in metabolic efficiency. In this context, the cardiovascular system is not secondary or peripheral to the disease process, as it is when we attempt to index central nervous system processes. As was stated in the introduction, we do not think, emote, etc., with our hearts but with our brains. Thus, if our concern is with these processes, let us focus on the brain.

## ACKNOWLEDGMENT

The research performed by the author was supported by research grants MH 07995, National Institute of Mental Health; and HL 18976, National Heart, Lung, and Blood Institute.

## REFERENCES

Anderson, D. E., & Tosheff, J. G. Cardiac output and total peripheral resistance changes during pre-avoidance periods in the dog. *Journal of Applied Physiology*, 1973, *34*, 650–654.

Anderson, D. E., Yingling, J. E., & Sagawa, K. Minute to minute covariations in cardiovascular activity of conscious dogs. *American Journal of Physiology: Heart and Circulatory Physiology*, 1979, *5*, H434–H439.

Birkenhager, W. H., & Schalekamp, M. A. D. H. *Control mechanisms in essential hypertension*. New York: American Elsevier, 1976.

Brown, J. J., Fraser, R., Lever, A. F., Morton, J. J., Robertson, J. I. S., & Schalekamp, M. A. D. H. Mechanisms in hypertension: A personal view. In J. Genest, E. Koiw, & O. Kutchel (Eds.), *Hypertension: Physiopathology and treatment*. New York: McGraw-Hill, 1977.

Carroll, D., & Anastasiades, P. Behavioral significance of heart rate: Lacey's hypothesis. *Journal of Biological Psychology*, 1978, *7*, 249–275.

Clifton, R. K. The relation of infant cardiac responding to behavioral state and motor activity. *Minnesota Symposia on Child Psychology*, 1978, *11*, 64–97.

Cohen, D. H. Analysis of the final common path for heart rate conditioning. In P. A. Obrist, A. H. Black, J. Brener, & L. V. DiCara (Eds.), *Cardiovascular psychophysiology: Current issues in response mechanisms, biofeedback and methodology*. Chicago: Aldine, 1974.

Dykman, R. A., Gantt, W. H., & Whitehorn, J. C. Conditioning as emotional sensitization and differentiation. *Psychological Monographs*, 1956, *70*(Whole No. 15), 1–17.

Elliott, R. The significance of heart rate for behavior: A critique of Lacey's hypothesis. *Journal of Personality and Social Psychology*, 1972, *22*, 398–409.

Elliott, R. The motivational significance of heart rate. In P. A. Obrist, A. H. Black, J. Brener, & L. V. DiCara (Eds.), *Cardiovascular psychophysiology: Current issues in response mechanisms, biofeedback and methodology.* Chicago: Aldine, 1974.

Folkow, B. U. G., Hallback, M. I. L., Lundgren, Y., Sivertsson, R., & Weiss, L. Importance of adaptive changes in vascular design for establishment of primary hypertension, studies in man and in spontaneously hypertensive rat. *Circulation Research,* 1973, *32–33* (Suppl. 1), I-2–I-16.

Forsyth, R. P. Regional blood flow changes during 72 hour avoidance schedules in monkeys. *Science,* 1971, *173,* 546–548.

Forsyth, R. P. Effect of propranolol on stress-induced hemodynamic changes in monkeys. In P. R. Saxena & R. P. Forsyth (Eds.), *Beta-adrenoceptor blocking agents.* Amsterdam: North-Holland, 1976.

Gliner, J. A., Bedi, J. F., & Horvath, S. M. Somatic and non-somatic influences on the heart: Hemodynamic changes. *Psychophysiology,* 1979, *16,* 358–362.

Grignolo, A. *Renal function and cardiovascular dynamics during treadmill exercise and shock-avoidance in dogs.* Unpublished doctoral dissertation, University of North Carolina at Chapel Hill, 1980.

Grignolo, A., Koepke, J. P., & Obrist, P. A. Renal function and cardiovascular dynamics during treadmill exercise and shock avoidance in dogs. *American Journal of Physiology,* 1982, in press.

Guyton, A. C. Personal views on mechanisms of hypertension. In J. Genest, E. Koiw, & O. Kuchel (Eds.), *Hypertension: Physiopathology and treatment.* New York: McGraw-Hill, 1977.

Guyton, A. C. *Circulatory physiology III: Arterial pressure and hypertension.* Philadelphia: W. B. Saunders, 1980.

Hahn, W. W. Attention and heart rate: A critical appraisal of the hypothesis of Lacey and Lacey. *Psychological Bulletin,* 1973, *79,* 59–70.

Hassett, J. *A primer of psychophysiology.* San Francisco: Freeman, 1978.

Hastrup, J. L., Swaney, K., Obrist, P. A., Beeler, C., & Chaska, L. Relationship of parental history of hypertension to cardiovascular reactivity: Public speaking and reaction time task. *Psychophysiology,* 1981, *18,* 186.

Hein, P. L. Heart rate conditioning in the cat and its relationship to physiological responses. *Psychophysiology,* 1969, *5,* 455–464.

Hofer, M. A. Cardiac and respiratory function during sudden prolonged immobility in wild rodents. *Psychosomatic Medicine,* 1970, *32,* 633–647.

Iacono, W. G., & Lykken, D. T. Within subject covariation of reaction time and fore-period cardiac deceleration: Effects of respiration and imperative stimulus intensity. *Journal of Biological Psychology,* 1978, *7,* 287–302.

Jenkins, C. D. Recent evidence supporting psychologic and social risk factors for coronary disease. *New England Journal of Medicine,* 1976, *292,* 987–994; 1033–1038.

Jennings, J. R., Averill, J. R., Opton, E. M., & Lazarus, R. S. Some parameters of heart rate change: Perceptual versus motor task requirements, noxiousness, and uncertainty. *Psychophysiology,* 1971, *7,* 194–212.

Julius, S., & Esler, M. D. Autonomic nervous cardiovascular regulation in borderline hypertension. *American Journal of Cardiology,* 1975, *36,* 685–696.

Koepke, J. P., Grignolo, A., & Obrist, P. A. Decreased urine and sodium excretion rates during unsignaled shock avoidance in dogs: Role of beta-adrenergic receptors. *Federation Proceedings,* 1981, *40,* 553.

Lacey, B. C., & Lacey, J. I. Studies of heart rate and other bodily processes in sensorimotor behavior. In P. A. Obrist, A. H. Black, J. Brener, & L. V. DiCara (Eds.), *Cardio-*

vascular psychophysiology: Current issues in response mechanisms, biofeedback and methodology. Chicago: Aldine, 1974.

Lacey, J. I. Psychophysiological approaches to the evaluation of psychotherapeutic process and outcome. In E. A. Rubenstein & M. B. Parloff (Eds.), Research in psychotherapy. Washington, D.C.: American Psychological Association, 1959.

Lacey, J. I. Somatic response patterning and stress: Some revisions of activation theory. In M. H. Appley & R. Trumbull (Eds.), Psychological stress: Issues in research. New York: Appleton-Century-Crofts, 1967.

Lacey, J. I., Kagan, J., Lacey, B. C., & Moss, M. A. H. The visceral level: Situational determinants and behavioral correlates of autonomic response patterns. In P. N. Knapp (Ed.), Expression of the emotions in man. New York: International Universities Press, 1963.

Lacey, J. I., & Lacey, B. C. Some autonomic–central nervous system interrelationships. In P. Black (Ed.), Physiological correlates of emotion. New York: Academic Press, 1970.

Langer, A. W. A comparison of the effects of treadmill exercise and signaled shock avoidance training on hemodynamic processes and the arterial–mixed venous oxygen content difference in conscious dogs. Unpublished doctoral dissertation, University of North Carolina, Chapel Hill, 1978.

Langer, A. W., Obrist, P. A., & McCubbin, J. A. Hemodynamic and metabolic adjustments during exercise and shock avoidance in dogs. American Journal of Physiology: Heart and Circulatory Physiology, 1979, 5, H225–230.

Lawler, J. E., Obrist, P. A., & Lawler, K. A. Cardiovascular function during pre-avoidance, avoidance and post-avoidance in dogs. Psychophysiology, 1975, 12, 4–11.

Light, K. C. Cardiovascular responses to effortful active coping: Implications for the role of stress in hypertension development. Psychophysiology, 1981, 18, 216–225.

Light, K. C., & Obrist, P. A. Cardiovascular response to stress: Effects of opportunity to avoid shock experience and performance feedback. Psychophysiology, 1980, 17, 243–252. (a)

Light, K. C., & Obrist, P. A. Cardiovascular reactivity to behavioral stress in young males with and without marginally elevated systolic pressures: A comparison of clinic, home and laboratory measures. Hypertension, 1980, 2, 802–808. (b)

Lund-Johansen, P. Hemodynamics in early essential hypertension. Acta Medica Scandinavica, 1967 (Suppl. 182), 1–101.

Lund-Johansen, P. Spontaneous changes in central hemodynamics in essential hypertension—A 10-year follow-up study. In G. Onesti & C. R. Klimt (Eds.), Hypertension—Determinants, complications and intervention. New York: Grune & Stratton, 1979.

Malmo, R. B. Activation: A neuropsychological dimension. Psychological Review, 1959, 66, 367–386.

Manuck, S. B., & Garland, F. M. Stability of individual differences in cardiovascular reactivity: A thirteen-month follow-up. Physiology and Behavior, 1980, 24, 621–624.

Manuck, S. B., & Schaefer, D. C. Stability of individual differences in cardiovascular reactivity. Physiology and Behavior, 1978, 21, 675–678.

McCubbin, J. A. Hemodynamic and neurohumoral correlates of behavioral stress in young adult males. Unpublished doctoral dissertation, University of North Carolina at Chapel Hill, 1980.

Notterman, J. M., Schoenfeld, W. N., & Bersh, P. J. Conditioned heart rate responses in human beings during experimental anxiety. Journal of Comparative and Physiological Psychology, 1952, 45, 1–8.

Obrist, P. A. Some autonomic correlates of serial learning. *Journal of Verbal Learning and Verbal Behavior*, 1962, *1*, 100–104.

Obrist, P. A. Cardiovascular differentiation of sensory stimuli. *Psychosomatic Medicine*, 1963, *25*, 450–458.

Obrist, P. A. The cardiovascular behavioral interaction—As it appears today. *Psychophysiology*, 1976, *13*, 95–107.

Obrist, P. A. *Cardiovascular psychophysiology—A perspective*. New York: Plenum, 1981.

Obrist, P. A., Gaebelein, C. J., Teller, E. S., Langer, A. W., Grignolo, A., Light, K. C., & McCubbin, J. A. The relationship among heart rate, carotid dP/dt and blood pressure in humans as a function of the type of stress. *Psychophysiology*, 1978, *15*, 102–115.

Obrist, P. A., Grignolo, A., Hastrup, J. L., Koepke, J. P., Langer, A. W., Light, K. C., McCubbin, J. A., & Pollak, M. H. Behavioral–cardiac interactions in hypertension. In D. S. Krantz, A. Baum, & J. E. Singer (Eds.), *Handbook of psychology and health* (Vol. 1: *Cardiovascular disorders*). Hillsdale, N.J.: Erlbaum, in press.

Obrist, P. A., Howard, J. L., Lawler, J. E., Galosy, R. A., Meyers, K. A., & Gaebelein, C. J. The cardiac somatic interaction. In P. A. Obrist, A. H. Black, J. Brener, & L. V. DiCara (Eds.), *Cardiovascular psychophysiology: Current issues in response mechanisms, biofeedback and methodology*. Chicago: Aldine, 1974.

Obrist, P. A., Langer, A. W., Grignolo, A., Sutterer, J. R., Light, K. C., & McCubbin, J. A. Blood pressure control mechanisms and stress: Implications for the etiology of hypertension. In G. Onesti & L. R. Klimt (Eds.), *Hypertension: Determinants, complications and intervention*. New York: Grune & Stratton, 1979.

Obrist, P. A., Lawler, J. E., Howard, J. L., Smithson, K. W., Martin, P. L., & Manning, J. Sympathetic influences on cardiac rate and contractility during acute stress in humans. *Psychophysiology*, 1974, *11*, 405–427.

Obrist, P. A., Light, K. C., McCubbin, J. A., Hutcheson, J. S., & Hoffer, J. L. Pulse transit time: Relationship to blood pressure and myocardial performance. *Psychophysiology*, 1979, *16*, 292–301.

Obrist, P. A., Webb, R, A., Sutterer, J. R., & Howard, J. L. The cardiac–somatic relationship: Some reformulations. *Psychophysiology*, 1970, *6*, 569–587. (a)

Obrist, P. A., Webb, R. A., Sutterer, J. R., & Howard, J. L. Cardiac deceleration and reaction time: An evaluation of two hypotheses. *Psychophysiology*, 1970, *6*, 695–706. (b)

Obrist, P. A., Wood, D. M., & Perez-Reyes, M. Heart rate during conditioning in humans: Effects of UCS intensity, vagal blockade and adrenergic block of vasomotor activity. *Journal of Experimental Psychology*, 1965, *70*, 32–42.

Page, I. H. Some regulatory mechanisms of renovascular and essential arterial hypertension. In J. Genest, E. Koiw, & O. Kuchel (Eds.), *Hypertension: Physiopathology and treatment*. New York: McGraw-Hill, 1977.

Pickering, T. G. Personal views on mechanisms of hypertension. In J. Genest, E. Koiw, & O. Kuchel (Eds.), *Hypertension: Physiopathology and treatment*. New York: McGraw-Hill, 1977.

Rescorla, R. A., & Solomon, R. L. Two process learning theory: Relationships between Pavlovian conditioning and instrumental learning. *Psychological Review*, 1967, *74*, 151–182.

Roberts, L. E. Comparative psychophysiology of the electrodermal and cardiac control systems. In P. A. Obrist, A. H. Black, J. Brener, & L. V. DiCara (Eds.), *Cardiovascular psychophysiology: Current issues in response mechanisms, biofeedback and methodology*. Chicago: Aldine, 1974.

Safar, M. E., Weiss, Y. A., Levenson, J. A., London, G. M., & Milliez, P. L. Hemodynamic study of 85 patients with borderline hypertension. *American Journal of Cardiology*, 1973, *31*, 315–319.

Schneiderman, N. The relationship between learned and unlearned cardiovascular responses. In P. A. Obrist, A. H. Black, J. Brener, & L. V. DiCara (Eds.), *Cardiovascular psychophysiology: Current issues in response mechanisms, biofeedback and methodology*. Chicago: Aldine, 1974.

Smith, O. A., & Stebbins, W. C. Conditioned blood flow and heart rate in monkeys. *Journal of Comparative and Physiological Psychology*, 1965, *59*, 432–436.

Sternbach, R. A. *Principles of psychophysiology*. New York: Academic Press, 1966.

Wood, D. M., & Obrist, P. A. Minimal and maximal sensory intake and exercise as unconditioned stimuli in human heart rate conditioning. *Journal of Experimental Psychology*, 1968, *76*, 254–262.

Zeaman, D., & Smith, R. W. Review of some recent findings in human cardiac conditioning. In W. F. Prokasy (Ed.), *Classical conditioning: A symposium*. New York: Appleton-Century-Crofts, 1965.

# 9

## The Modification of Elicited Cardiovascular Responses by Operant Conditioning of Heart Rate

ALEKSANDER PERSKI
BERNARD T. ENGEL
JAMES H. MCCROSKERY

## INTRODUCTION

The cardiovascular (CV) system is capable of exquisite adjustments in response to alterations in environmental conditions. One application of operant cardiac conditioning is to reveal these adjustments and to elucidate the mechanisms that underlie them. In this chapter we describe experiments in which heart rate (HR) was brought under stimulus control while the subject was responding to different types of stimulation. The first section deals with modification of HR during aversive or taxing stimuli. An animal model is described, and some of the relevant studies with human subjects are reviewed briefly. The major portion of the chapter focuses on the modification of HR elicited by physical effort, with

Aleksander Perski and Bernard T. Engel. Laboratory of Behavioral Sciences, National Institute on Aging, Gerontology Research Center, Baltimore City Hospital, Baltimore, Maryland.

James H. McCroskery. Department of Psychology, State University of New York, Oswego, New York.

results from experiments using both animals and healthy human subjects. Finally, we consider some possible clinical applications of operant cardiac rate conditioning during exercise in patients with cardiac disorders.

## MODIFICATION OF CARDIOVASCULAR RESPONSES TO AVERSIVE STIMULI OR TAXING CONDITIONS

In 1974 Ainslie and Engel conducted a study in which they asked whether operant learning of HR could modify a monkey's cardiac response to impending electric shock. This response has generally been reported to be an increase in HR, often followed by a decrease which may reach or go below baseline level as shock approaches (Smith & Stebbins, 1965).

Six monkeys (*Macaca mulatta*) were presented with two types of auditory stimuli: 2/sec clicks and 20/sec clicks. After it was determined that there were no differences in HR in response to the two click frequencies, one click pattern was designated as a warning cue, indicating that an inescapable electric shock to the tail would be administered at the termination of the cue. The other click pattern became the neutral cue. Each 2048-sec training session was divided into 16 contiguous 128-sec segments. Warning clicks were presented during the 1st, 5th, 9th, and 13th segments, while neutral clicks occupied the 3rd, 7th, 11th, and 15th segments. Following this classical conditioning paradigm, the animals responded consistently to the presentation of warning clicks relative to neutral clicks with HR acceleration and a rise in systolic blood pressure (SBP). Subsequently, the animals were subjected to operant conditioning training in which a desired change in HR was required to avoid the shock to the tail. Four monkeys were trained to slow HR to avoid the shock, while the other two were trained to speed HR. The duration of each session was again 2048 sec. After the animals learned to produce reliable operant responses, the two procedures were put in effect concurrently. The monkeys received tail shocks when they failed to keep their HR within the operant criteria, and they received unavoidable shocks at the end of each warning cue presented throughout the session, as it had been during the classical conditioning procedure. As a result of this combination, the classically elicited tachycardia to clicks was now changed by the operant procedure to a bradycardia in the monkeys taught to slow HR. The HR increase evoked by clicks was maintained in the two animals taught to accelerate HR (Figure 9-1).

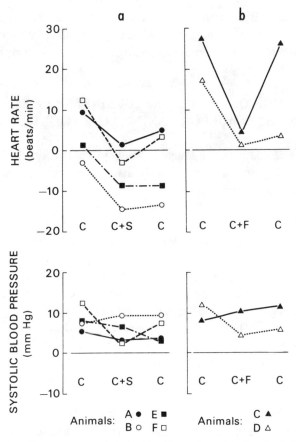

FIG. 9-1. HR and SBP responses (warning cues–neutral cues) during classical conditioning sessions of: (a) animals operantly trained to slow HR and (b) animals operantly trained to speed HR. Abbreviations: C = classical conditioning; C + S = combined classical conditioning and operant HR slowing; C+F = combined classical conditioning and operant HR speeding.

Following this part of the study the animals were again exposed to the classical paradigm alone. The effect of the operant training persisted: Bradycardia to warning clicks persisted in the monkeys taught to slow HR, and the HR increase was observed in the animals taught to speed HR. Furthermore, when the animals which had been taught to speed HR received additional sessions in HR-slowing training, their response to the warning clicks also was modified: They responded with bradycardia to warning clicks. Thus, it was shown that classically conditioned cardiac responses could be permanently modified by operant training. In addition, throughout all of these training procedures, all animals continued to emit a pressor response. Thus, the training effect was shown to be specific to the HR contingency *and* specific to the HR response.

This model demonstrates the power which operant conditioning might have in altering elicited responses. Similar models using operant conditioning to modify responses to aversive stimuli or taxing conditions such as psychomotor performance or mental arithmetic have been studied in man. For example, behavioral control of anticipatory HR reaction to mild electric shock has been demonstrated by Sirota, Schwartz, and Shapiro (1974). In their study 20 women were given a series of mild electric shocks, each of which was preceded by a warning signal. Ten of the subjects were instructed to slow HR on every second aversive trial, and 10 were instructed to speed HR. Feedback from their performance was given during HR control trials. Subjective ratings of shock intensity also were collected after each trial. The results showed that the HR responses during the warning signal (anticipation) and during the shock (aversive stimulation) were altered. Furthermore, the judgment of shock intensity changed depending on the feedback condition. Electrical shocks were labeled as more intense by the HR-speeding group and milder by the HR-slowing group. This experiment was successfully replicated on a second sample 2 years later in the same laboratory (Sirota, Schwartz, & Shapiro, 1976). DeGood and Adams (1976) also demonstrated that HR acceleration as a response to mild electric shock can be reversed by operantly conditioned HR slowing. Victor, Mainardi, and Shapiro (1978) showed that the tachycardia elicited by immersion of the hand in ice water (cold-pressor test) also could be modified by training in HR slowing. These investigators also replicated another finding of Sirota *et al.* (1974, 1976): Ratings of painfulness during the test were reduced during HR-slowing training. Several studies also have appeared in which this paradigm was used to alter physiological and subjective reactions to phobic or feared stimuli. For example, Gatchel and Proctor (1976) showed that HR control training was effective in reducing public-speaking phobia. Blanchard and Abel (1976), in a single case study, showed that operant training could reduce the tachycardia which was elicited by recall of a traumatic experience (rape). The use of operant conditioning to modify responses during taxing conditions has received relatively little attention. The ability to learn HR control while carrying out a visual tracking task was demonstrated by Perski and Dureman (1979). Steptoe (1978) has reported that pulse transit time (which is correlated with HR and SBP) can be operantly modified during reaction time and rapid mental arithmetic tasks.

The studies cited in this section have shown that animals and human subjects can be taught to control HR reliably while anticipating or while experiencing a variety of aversive stimuli or taxing conditions. These studies also suggest that the perception of those stimuli or conditions is altered by the operant conditioning procedure. These findings raise a number of interesting questions such as: What are the mechanisms by which the cardiovascular effects are mediated? What are the mechanisms by which the perceptual effects are mediated (e.g., the judgment of pain intensity during the cold-pressor test)? What are the limitations on the cardiovascular or perceptual effects? And what are the conditions which determine the transfer of such skills from the laboratory to the field? Discussion of some of these issues can be found in Chapter 7 of this volume.

## MODIFICATION OF CARDIOVASCULAR RESPONSE TO EXERCISE

Exercise is a ubiquitous stimulus which has elicited considerable interest among physiologists and cardiologists. At one time it was believed that the CV adjustments to exercise were determined by the metabolic changes in the exercising muscles. However, a number of systematic studies have shown that these muscular effects are neither necessary nor sufficient to mediate the CV adjustments to exercise. Rather, the adjustments are neurally mediated. Until recently, it was widely believed that the neural adjustments were reflexly elicited. However, a number of experiments now suggest that many of the responses may be conditioned, indicating that the central nervous system has a major role in regulating them. The demonstration that CV adjustments can be brought under operant control provides us with a powerful tool for exploring control mechanisms and a potentially significant means of producing clinically useful effects.

We begin this section with a description of an animal model in which operant conditioning of HR during dynamic exercise is being studied in this laboratory. (This work is being carried out collaboratively by B. T. Engel and his colleagues, James A. Joseph and Stephen P. Tzankoff.) This experiment is similar to the Ainslie and Engel (1974) study described earlier in that it combines two procedures in a single experiment. In this case the procedures are dynamic exercise and operant HR conditioning. In the first phase of the study, the monkey is trained to exercise by pulling a bar with weights attached (10–12 kg depending on the size of monkey). Food (banana pellets) is used as reinforcement. This phase is conceptually similar to the classical conditioning phase of the Ainslie and Engel study. During each 34-min exercise session, oxygen consumption, HR, and SBP are monitored. After reliable exercise performance is established, the animal is trained to slow its HR using shock avoidance as the reinforcement for HR slowing. In the third phase of the study, exercise and HR slowing are combined in a single experiment. The animal is required to pull the bar as well as to maintain its HR below a selected level. The performance of one monkey is considered here. That animal responded to exercise with about a 33% increase in both HR and SBP. HR-slowing training also resulted in reliable performance. When the exercise and HR slowing were combined, the animal was found to be able to perform considerably more work with the same increase in HR. Thus, the change in HR per unit work was attenuated significantly. Figure 9-2 presents these results. As can be seen, average HR in beats per minute (bpm) is similar during the exercise (199.4 bpm) and combined sessions (197.3 bpm).

FIG. 9-2. HR levels as a function of work during exercise and combined exercise and HR-slowing sessions. Circles are means (based on five sessions of each condition), and line segments show the linear relationship between HR and work. The data have been divided into first (early) and second (late) halves of the session to show the stability of the performance.

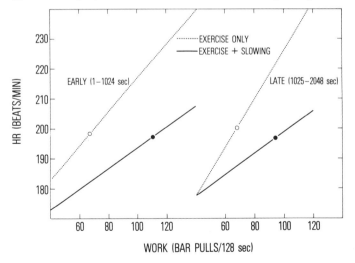

However, work (67.3 and 104.8 bar pulls, respectively) differs significantly. Thus, the rate of change of HR per unit work (i.e., the slope of the line of best fit relating HR to work) is significantly attenuated during the combined sessions (.68 and .26 bpm/bar pull, respectively). Since SBP change from baseline was similar between the conditions, cardiac work was reflected in the HR data. Cardiac work is indexed by the product of HR and SBP (Robinson, 1967). We refer to this index as "rate–pressure product" (RPP).

The role of operant cardiac conditioning in the physiological adjustments to exercise also has been studied in man. Goldstein, Ross, and Brady (1977) showed that operant HR training during exercise on a treadmill could modify the CV responses elicited by the exercise. Eighteen healthy subjects participated in 10 weekly sessions. In each session, after 2 min of rest, each subject was instructed to walk on a treadmill at a fixed rate of 2.5 mph and 6% grade for 10 min. This sequence was repeated four more times during each session. Subjects were randomly assigned to either group E-C (experimental–control) or group C-E (control–experimental). During the first five sessions of the program, subjects in the E-C group received HR visual feedback and were asked to slow HR while exercising; subjects in the C-E group exercised without feedback or instruction to slow. The resulting pattern of HR change was significantly different between groups during the five sessions. E-C subjects' average HR decreased from 105.2 bpm in Trial 1 to 99.3 in Trial 5. HR in the C-E group did not change across the trials but was maintained at a rate of 110 bpm. SBP responses paralleled changes in HR. Thus, these data are similar to our findings obtained in the monkey in that the feedback group attenuated HR response, whereas the control did not. Furthermore, the findings are similar in that RPP also was attenuated. However, the results differed in that we saw no differences in SBP across conditions, whereas Goldstein, Ross, and Brady (1977) did. During Sessions 6–10 of their experiment, the E-C group was instructed to slow HR but received no feedback. The results showed that the transfer to no-feedback conditions was readily obtained. The C-E group was trained with feedback and instruction to slow HR during Sessions 6–10. The results showed no evidence of learning.

We recently replicated this experiment in our laboratory using a similar experimental design, but instead of a treadmill exercise, our subjects exercised on an electrically braked stationary bicycle (Perski & Engel, 1980). Ten subjects (both men and women) were divided into an experimental (E) and a control (C) group. Subjects in the E group participated in seven daily sessions; subjects in the C group participated in 10 daily sessions. Each session consisted of a 10-min baseline and five 4-min exercise trials separated by 2-min rest periods. The first five sessions were similar to those of Goldstein, Ross, and Brady (1977). The E subjects received feedback and instruction to slow HR; the C subjects merely exercised. Sessions 6 and 7 were transfer sessions for E subjects; that is, they exercised without feedback but were instructed to continue to control HR. Sessions 6–10 were cross-over sessions for the C subjects; that is, they received the same feedback and instructions that the E subjects had received during Sessions 1–5. Thus, our experimental design permitted us to evaluate the effect of visual feedback and instructions to slow HR both between two groups of subjects and within one group of subjects. The average work load was set at 380 kg-m/min, which could be considered moderate. Figure 9-3 presents our main findings.

Subjects in the C group, exercising without feedback and instructions to slow, increased HR an average of 32.4 bpm, while E subjects increased only 17.2 bpm. This significant attenuation of HR response was repeated within the C group, in whom the increase of 32.4 bpm during nonfeedback sessions was reduced to 19.4 bpm during feedback sessions. Contrary to the Goldstein, Ross, and Brady (1977) findings, SBP did not systematically vary with HR; consequently, the statistically significant reduction in RPP was achieved through HR modulation only.

Our next experiment was designed to study the effect of level of exercise on ability to control HR. A group of young college athletes from

FIG. 9-3. HR changes from resting levels to exercise on stationary bicycle. Each session comprises five trials. Thus, Trial 6 is the first trial of Session 2, etc.

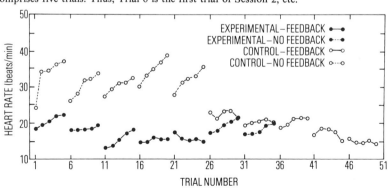

various athletic specialities were studied, since more demanding exercise conditions were introduced. The basic design of the study was similar to our first study (just described). In addition, maximal exercise–stress tests were included at the beginning and end of each phase of the training. The first session was identical for all subjects and consisted of exercising five times, 4 min at a time with a 2-min rest period following each exercise trial. The E subjects were instructed to slow HR and received visual feedback of performance during the subsequent five sessions. C subjects exercised without feedback, and in Sessions 6 to 11 they crossed over to the feedback and instruction condition. The exercise load was much higher in these experiments: The average work load was 750 kg-m/min, which elicited about 70% of maximal HR. The results are presented in the upper part of Figure 9-4.

In this figure we have included results from the appropriate sessions of the previous study for comparison. In the present experiment the C group increased HR during no-feedback sessions 54.6 bpm as compared to 42.6 bpm for E subjects ($F(1,8) = 3.87, p < .08$). HR increased through

FIG. 9-4. Changes in HR from resting levels to exercise. The high-exercise group results are presented in the upper panel. The low-exercise group results are taken from Figure 9-2 for comparison.

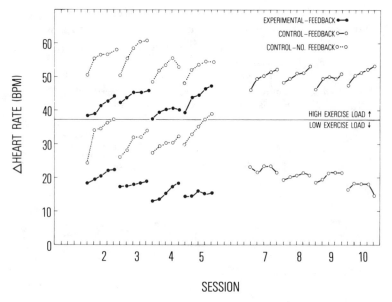

trials within each session (trial $F$ (4,32) = 11.40, $p < .001$), but there were no differences between groups in this respect. The control subjects decreased HR from 54.6 bpm (to 49.9 bpm in the feedback sessions ($F$ (1,4) = 13.71, $p < .02$). The trial ($F$ (4, 16) = 3.40, $p < .03$) and trial $\times$ feedback condition interactions were significant ($F$ (4,16) = 5.55, $p < .005$), indicating that control subjects not only had lower HR during feedback sessions but also that within each trial there was an attenuation of HR increase. Again, HR changes were not paralleled by changes in SBP. Thus, these findings not only replicated our original results but also showed that this behavioral conditioning effect could occur even at relatively high levels of exercise.

We have been dealing with the modification of cardiovascular response to dynamic exercise. There is some indication that HR response during static, muscular effort also can be modified. Magnusson (1976) showed that subjects performing a handgrip task were able to obtain larger HR increases while presented with feedback than subjects without feedback. Clemens and Shattock (1979) recently demonstrated that voluntary HR speeding or slowing during a handgrip task was possible at levels ranging from 0% to 50% of maximal voluntary contraction.

Taken together, the data from these experiments show that at least some aspects of what has been ascribed to the physical conditioning effects of exercise also can be explained on the basis of behavioral conditioning. There is still a great deal of work to be done before we will understand the psychophysiological mechanisms that mediate these effects, or the limits of behavioral conditioning in exercise performance. However, it is reasonable to ask whether individuals who are limited in their capacity to exercise can benefit from this technique. Such clinical studies not only should provide additional information about control mechanisms, but also they should show whether clinically meaningful changes can be effected with behavioral training procedures.

## CLINICAL APPLICATIONS

In this section we focus on the application of HR conditioning in the control of cardiac adjustments to exercise in patients with ischemic heart disease. Before considering those experiments, we would like to cite a relevant and interesting single case study by Pickering and Gorham (1975). They saw a 31-year-old woman with ventricular parasystolic arrhythmia. (This is a cardiac rhythm irregularity characterized by the interaction of two beats—one is the normally conducted impulse; and the other, an aberrantly conducted impulse whose site of origin is electrically isolated from the normal conduction system. The two impulses independently initiate ventricular beats at different rates.) She was taught to speed and to slow her HR using a biofeedback paradigm. Before training, the threshold at which her parasystolic rhythm appeared was 79.1 bpm. When the patient became successful at the HR acceleration and deceleration tasks, her threshold for aberrant rhythm shifted to a much higher HR of 94.1 bpm. This effect was present both during voluntary speeding and during exercise-induced HR acceleration. These findings suggest that at least some aspects of cardiac function which can be induced by exercise in patients can be modified by biofeedback training as well.

Pickering and Gorham's (1975) findings also illustrate an important clinical principle: In many patients aberrant function will be elicited only when the patient is being challenged. At rest, there may be no abnormal responses present. This is especially evident in the case of ischemic heart disease. In these patients any deficiency between cardiac oxygen supply and demand causes temporary ischemia in cardiac muscle, which manifests itself as a chest discomfort that is often described by the patients as pain, tightness, or heaviness. An ischemic episode typically occurs during some taxing condition in which demand for oxygen—driven by an increase in HR or SBP, or by elevated wall tension in the left ventricle—exceeds supply, which is impaired by atherosclerotic occlusion and/or coronary artery spasms (Oliva, Potts, & Pluss, 1973). Medical management of patients usually is aimed at the reduction of the oxygen demand through the use of long-acting nitrates or $\beta$-adrenergic blocking agents (propranolol). Physical conditioning programs are used frequently because it is believed that increased efficiency of performance of the skeletomuscular or cardiovascular system will result in reduced HR, and this might be beneficial for the patient (Clausen & Trap-Jensen, 1976).

For each patient there exists a threshold of RPP elicited during physical effort, where an imbalance between supply and demand for oxygen will occur. This threshold is relatively constant over an extended period of time. Therefore, any reduction of HR, SBP, or both during exercise would enable a patient to perform more work before ischemia and discomfort occurred. If operant cardiac conditioning can reduce RPP in patients as it seems to do in normal subjects, it could have some beneficial effects.

One attempt to apply this procedure to angina pectoris patients was conducted in this laboratory (McCroskery, Engel, Gottlieb, & Lakatta, 1978). Six patients with "stable" angina pectoris (see Table 9-1 for patient descriptions) were trained to slow HR at rest. Each patient participated in 18 training sessions, and each session consisted of two 1024-sec feedback-assisted training periods. At the final stage of training, patients were gradually weaned from the feedback displays. After every third session patients were asked to slow HR while walking a distance of 81 m along a fixed course. No feedback was available during this time. At the beginning and the end of the program, two treadmill stress tests were conducted. Each patient was asked to walk on the treadmill while the speed and elevation were gradually increased until he reported fatigue or cramps, or reached a level of anginal pain which would ordinarily force him to stop what he was doing and rest.

The patients also filled out self-report checklists daily during the month before and after training. On these forms they were asked to report the frequency and severity of anginal episodes.

TABLE 9-1. Patient Status

| Patient | Age | NYHA functional classification | Clinic stress test | Cardiac history | Medications |
|---------|-----|-------------------------------|--------------------|-----------------|-------------|
| 1 | 50 | I | +(4/75) | Angina since 1/75 | Inderal<br>TNG |
| 2 | 47 | II | +(3/75) | MI, 2/74<br>Angina since 2/74 | Inderal<br>Valium<br>Cardilate<br>TNG |
| 3 | 44 | I–II | +(8/76) | Angina since 6/74<br>(Angiography, 9/74) | Inderal<br>Benedryl<br>Tranxene |
| 4 | 48 | III | +(3/74)<br>+(3/75)<br>+(9/76) | Angina since 6/74<br>Bypass surgery, 9/75<br>Angina recurred, 9/76 | Lasix<br>KCI<br>TNG |
| 5 | 54 | III–IV | No test | MI, '64, '72, '72<br>Angina since '72 | Inderal<br>Digoxin<br>Cardilate<br>Hydrochlorathiazide<br>TNG |
| 6 | 59 | III | No test | MI, '69, '72<br>Angina since '69 | Inderal<br>Digoxin<br>Hydrochlorathiazide<br>TNG |

All patients were able to decrease HR at rest during the laboratory training sessions, and this ability was maintained during sessions in which feedback displays were withheld. There was no indication that this ability was transferred to the walking conditions. The comparison of performance during the stress tests before and after the training program is presented in Table 9-2. In four of the six patients there was a large increase in exercise capacity after training, as evidenced by increased time of exercise (54%) and increased work capacity (159%). Five of the eight posttraining stress tests were terminated due to leg cramps or fatigue rather than chest pain. However, only Patient 3 achieved this improvement due to significant attenuation of HR. In the other three successful patients this effect was achieved mainly by attenuating SBP. An average decrease of 23% in daily anginal episodes was noted in the self-report checklists.

An apparent difficulty in transfer of the slowing ability from the resting to the exercise condition was encountered in this study. Despite the obvious importance of this issue, only a few studies have been devoted to the question of transfer of learned HR control. The major emphasis in these studies (e.g., Colgan, 1977; Perski & Dureman, 1977) was on the deterioration of performance due to feedback withdrawal, or on techniques to deal with that phenomenon. The issue of improvement of transfer of learning from laboratory, resting conditions to field, taxing conditions has received no attention.

TABLE 9-2. Exercise Stress Test: Percent Change from Pretraining to Posttraining

| Patient | Exercise tolerance | | Cardiovascular function | | |
|---|---|---|---|---|---|
| | Time (min) | Work (kg-m/min) | HR (bpm) | SBP (mm Hg) | RPP ([HR×SBP]/100) |
| 1 | +30 | +42 | +1 | +13 | +14 |
| 2 | +113 | +461 | +9 | +48 | +66 |
| 3 | +37 | +69 | 0 | +1 | +1 |
| 4 | +36 | +63 | +17 | +19 | +39 |
| 5 | +5 | +16 | 0 | +10 | +11 |
| 6 | −1 | −3 | +6 | −5 | +1 |
| Mean percent change | +37 | +108 | +5.5 | +13.4 | +22 |
| Mean absolute change | +2.05 | +1442 | +7 | +27 | +48 |

One technique for enhancing transfer of learning would be to teach HR control during exercise itself. Encouraged by the results from the studies with healthy subjects described in the previous section, we have designed such a study with angina pectoris patients. Three questions are being asked in this study: (1) Is it possible to teach patients voluntary HR control during submaximal exercise? (2) If so, does this procedure result in significant clinical improvement, manifested by increased work tolerance and reduction in incidence of anginal episodes? (3) Is the combination of biofeedback and exercise superior to an exercise program alone? Although this study still is going on, a few patients have completed testing, and here we consider the data from two of them. One patient was in the experimental (E) group, and the other was in the control (C) group. In the first phase of the study, after completing a 21-day observation period in which self-report checklists were completed and two exercise stress tests were taken, both patients participated in a 2.5-month mild exercise program on a stationary bicycle. The experimental patient was instructed to slow his HR while exercising and was given visual feedback during exercise. Another two stress tests followed during which he was asked to attenuate his HR response while no feedback was presented. Another period of self-observation followed. The patient in the control group exercised only in phase one. Subsequently, he received additional training sessions with feedback and instructions to slow. Stress tests and a self-observation period followed, as in the case of the experimental patient.

The experimental patient was a 48-year-old man who had suffered an inferior wall myocardial infarction 2 years prior to the study. His chest pain was well controlled by medication (propranolol). He had excellent work tolerance, he was able to hunt, and he had only five anginal episodes during the 25 days of self-monitoring. His initial exercise stress test had to be terminated after 14 min when marked ST-segment depressions occurred in ECG lead $V_5$. The patient underwent 25 training sessions of mild exercise and biofeedback training. He also was asked to slow his HR at the final stress test, which was terminated after 15 min when marked ST-segment depressions were observed. His HR, SBP, and RPP levels during the stress tests are presented in Figure 9-5. Notice the remarkable ability of this patient to attenuate his cardiovascular responses even during strenuous exercise. His HR was 10–15 bpm below the pretraining values by the end of the test. There also was a marked reduction in SBP. Consequently, much lower RPP was achieved throughout the stress test. No pain episodes occurred during 20 days of self-observation.

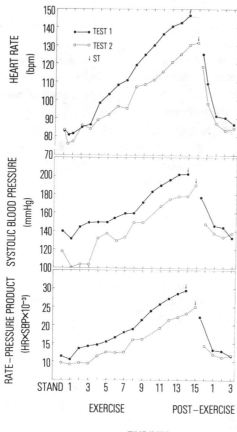

FIG. 9-5. HR, SBP, and RPP to treadmill exercise in experimental Patient 1. Exercise load increased every 2 min. ST indicates clinically significant depression of ST segment in the ECG.

The control patient was greatly impaired by his disease. He was a 60-year-old, self-employed plumber, hospitalized 2 years earlier with a diagnosis of anteroseptal myocardial infarction. Anginal pain—related to specific activities like driving his car, brisk walking, or pushing—was present a few months before admission. The pain was more frequent when ambient temperature was lower and after meals. An exercise stress test performed a few months after hospitalization confirmed the diagnosis of ischemic heart disease, since typical chest pain occurred at moderate exercise load and it was accompanied by 1–2 mm ST-segment depressions in leads $V_5$ and $V_6$. Occasional premature ventricular contractions were present for about 30 sec after termination of exercise. When first seen in our laboratory, the patient appeared to be very limited by his disease since he did not tolerate β-receptor blockers well, and his medication (nitroglycerin ointment) was not effective in controlling his symptoms. Self-reports revealed one or several episodes of chest pain in 13 out of 21 days, and he developed chest pains after 2.5 min of exercise on the treadmill. Exercise tolerance and clinical status did not change after 25 sessions of mild exercise training without feedback. Comparisons among his cardiovascular responses to the stress test can be seen in Figure 9-6. An additional 25 exercise sessions coupled with biofeedback training did result in some change of exercise tolerance (1 min). This effect occurred due to an attenuation of HR and SBP, but not because of a change in pain tolerance since his angina threshold did not change on three separate occasions. Self-reports did not indicate any clinical improvement, since he reported pain in 10 out of 18 consecutive days after biofeedback training.

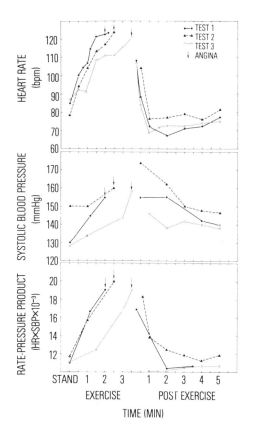

FIG. 9-6. HR, SBP, and RPP to treadmill exercise in control Patient 2. Exercise load increased every 2 min as in Figure 9-5.

## DISCUSSION

Much of the early research on operant training of HR was designed to demonstrate the phenomenon. Only a few experiments focused on mechanisms, and most of these studies either looked at procedural variables— for example, Lang (1974) and McCanne and Sandman (1975)—or at subject characteristics—for example, Stephens, Harris, Brady, and Shaffer (1975). Very few of these earlier studies utilized *both* psychological *and* physiological procedures to study regulatory mechanisms. In this chapter we have tried to show how one might proceed to carry out psychophysiological studies of cardiac control. Our model was exercise. However, one could explore other stimuli such as baroreceptor regulation (e.g., see Goldstein, Harris, & Brady, 1977) or reflexly induced HR deceleration (Furedy & Paulos, 1976). We believe that such studies are sorely needed because they will tell us a great deal about the psychophysiological mechanisms which mediate cardiovascular function under naturally occurring conditions.

Our analyses of the interaction between behavioral conditioning and physical conditioning have just begun. Our experiments with normal human subjects have shown that behavioral conditioning can occur not only at mild levels of exercise but also at heavy work loads. However, we still do not know what the upper limit of this training is. Nor do we know how the behavioral training operates. For example, we do not know how important attending to the display is. It is difficult to see how attention, per se, could produce effects of the magnitude we have reported. However, these experiments need to be done. Meanwhile, the results of these experiments already have revealed one important finding. At least some aspects of CV adjustments to exercise clearly are under behavioral control. This indicates that the central nervous system plays an important role in the process of organizing physiological adjustments to exercise, a fact seemingly overlooked by exercise physiologists who appear to be mainly interested in the peripheral adjustments to exercise. It is possible that behavioral techniques could be used to enhance a desired configuration of physiological adjustments in the course of physical training or even in athletic performance. Behavioral conditioning also provides an excellent tool to study the role of the nervous system in mobilizing and adjusting physiological performance during exercise or other demanding environmental conditions since it is possible to use such conditioning to observe the integrative effect of bringing specific responses under control—for example, what would be the effect of controlling HR on baroreceptor-mediated adjustments to blood pressure responses?

Our clinical findings are much too few to permit us to speculate about their importance. It seems likely from the data that we have reported here that at least some patients can be operantly conditioned to improve their CV adjustments to exercise. However, the self-report data warn us that many more stimuli besides exercise elicit the pain of angina pectoris. And the clinical literature warns us that physical conditioning in these patients improves peripheral function (i.e., oxygen demand) but does not change cardiac capacity (i.e., the oxygen supply system). It is unlikely that behavioral conditioning will succeed where physical training does not, since the peripheral effects of conditioning are likely to be the same irrespective of the mechanism by which they are induced. However, operant training of HR still could improve performance within the limits set by the structural determinants of ischemic heart disease. Operant training of HR might facilitate coping and thereby improve function over the range of response which is still available to the patient. It also might facilitate recovery from an ischemic episode.

## REFERENCES

Ainslie, G. W., & Engel, B. T. Alternation of classically conditioned heart rate by operant reinforcement in monkeys. *Journal of Comparative and Physiological Psychology*, 1974, *87*, 373–382.

Blanchard, E. B., & Abel, G. G. An experimental case study of the biofeedback treatment of a rape-induced psychophysiological disorder. *Behavior Therapy*, 1976, *7*, 113–119.

Clausen, J. P., & Trap-Jensen, J. Heart rate and arterial blood pressure during exercise in patients with angina pectoris. *Circulation*, 1976, *53*, 436–442.

Clemens, W. J., & Shattock, R. J. Voluntary heart rate control during static muscular effort. *Psychophysiology*, 1979, *16*, 327–332.

Colgan, M. Effect of binary and proportional feedback on bidirectional control of heart rate. *Psychophysiology*, 1977, *14*, 187–191.

DeGood, D. E., & Adams, A. S. Control of cardiac responses under aversive stimulation. *Biofeedback and Self-Regulation*, 1976, *1*, 373–385.

Furedy, J. J., & Paulos, C. X. Heart rate decelerative Pavlovian conditioning with tilt as UCS: Towards behavioral control of cardiac dysfunction. *Biological Psychology*, 1976, *4*, 93–105.

Gatchel, R. J., & Proctor, J. D. Effectiveness of voluntary heart rate control in reducing speech anxiety. *Journal of Consulting and Clinical Psychology*, 1976, *44*, 381–389.

Goldstein, D. S., Harris, A. H., & Brady, J. V. Baroreflex sensitivity during operant blood pressure conditioning. *Biofeedback and Self-Regulation*, 1977, *2*, 127–138.

Goldstein, D. S., Ross, R. S., & Brady, J. V. Biofeedback heart rate training during exercise. *Biofeedback and Self-Regulation*, 1977, *2*, 107–126.

Lang, P. J. Learned control of human heart rate in a computer directed environment. In P. A. Obrist, A. H. Black, J. Brener, & L. V. DiCara (Eds.), *Cardiovascular psychophysiology*. Chicago: Aldine, 1974.

Magnusson, E. The effect of controlled muscle tension on performance and learning of heart-rate control. *Biological Psychology*, 1976, *4*, 81–92.

McCanne, T. R., & Sandman, C. A. Determinants of human operant heart rate conditioning: A systematic investigation of several methodological issues. *Journal of Comparative and Physiological Psychology*, 1975, *88*, 609–618.

McCroskery, J. H., Engel, B. T., Gottlieb, S. M., & Lakatta, E. G. Operant conditioning of heart rate in patients with angina pectoris. *Psychosomatic Medicine*, 1978, *40*, 89–90.

Oliva, P. B., Potts, D. E., & Pluss, R. G. Coronary arterial spasm in Printzmetal angina. *New England Journal of Medicine*, 1973, *288*, 745–751.

Perski, A., & Dureman, I. Voluntary control of heart rate: The effect of type of feedback withdrawal on acquisition and transfer of learning. *Department of Psychology Report, University of Uppsala, Sweden*, 1977, *229*, 1–30.

Perski, A., & Dureman, I. Voluntary control of heart rate: An extended replication study. *Scandinavian Journal of Behavior Therapy*, 1979, *8*, 83–96.

Perski, A., & Engel, B. T. The role of behavioral conditioning in the cardiovascular adjustment to exercise. *Biofeedback and Self-Regulation*, 1980, *5*, 91–104.

Pickering, T., & Gorham, G. Learned heart-rate control by a patient with a ventricular parasystolic rhythm. *Lancet*, 1975, *1* (7901), 252–253.

Robinson, B. F. Relation of heart rate and systolic blood pressure to the onset of pain in angina pectoris. *Circulation*, 1967, *35*, 1073–1083.

Sirota, A. D., Schwartz, G. E., & Shapiro, D. Voluntary control of human heart rate: Effect on reaction to aversive stimulation. *Journal of Abnormal Psychology*, 1974, *83*, 261–267.

Sirota, A. D., Schwartz, G. E., & Shapiro, D. Voluntary control of human heart rate: Effect on reaction to aversive stimulation: A replication and extension. *Journal of Abnormal Psychology*, 1976, *85*, 473–477.

Smith, O., & Stebbins, W. Conditioned blood flow and heart rate in monkeys. *Journal of Comparative and Physiological Psychology*, 1965, *59*, 432–436.

Stephens, J. H., Harris, A. H., Brady, J. V., & Shaffer, J. W. Psychological and physiological variables associated with large magnitude voluntary heart-rate change. *Psychophysiology*, 1975, *12*, 381–387.

Steptoe, A. W. The regulation of blood pressure reactions to taxing conditions using pulse transit time feedback and relaxation. *Psychophysiology*, 1978, *15*, 429–438.

Victor, R., Mainardi, J. A., & Shapiro, D. Effects of biofeedback and voluntary control procedures on heart rate and perception of pain during the cold pressor test. *Psychosomatic Medicine*, 1978, *40*, 216–225.

# 10

## Behavior Patterns and Coronary Disease: A Critical Evaluation

DAVID S. KRANTZ
DAVID C. GLASS
MARC A. SCHAEFFER
JAMES E. DAVIA

## INTRODUCTION

Coronary heart disease (CHD), or ischemic heart disease, the major cause of death in this country, is a disorder thought to result from damage to the coronary arteries—a thickening of the arterial walls called atherosclerosis. The major clinical manifestations of the disease include myocardial infarction (death of heart tissue), angina pectoris (a syndrome of chest pain resulting from insufficient oxygen supply to heart muscle), and sudden death.

To understand the pathogenesis of these disorders, it is necessary to consider the interplay of hereditary factors, metabolic alterations, and

David S. Krantz. Department of Medical Psychology, Uniformed Services University School of Medicine, Bethesda, Maryland.

David C. Glass. Graduate Center, City University of New York, New York, New York.

Marc A. Schaeffer. Department of Medical Psychology, Uniformed Services University School of Medicine, Bethesda, Maryland.

James E. Davia. Walter Reed Army Medical Center and Department of Medicine, Uniformed Services University School of Medicine, Bethesda, Maryland.

the individual's life-style. An array of standard risk factors have been identified by epidemiological research (e.g., Brand, Rosenman, Sholtz, & Friedman, 1976; Kannel, McGee, & Gordon, 1976). The most widely accepted of these included age, hypertension, elevated low-density and low levels of high-density lipoproteins in the blood, cigarette smoking, family history of heart disease, and presence of diabetes mellitus. However, it has been asserted that the best combination of these risk factors still fails to identify most new CHD cases (Jenkins, 1971), and in recent years considerable evidence has implicated psychological and social factors in the pathogenesis of CHD (see Glass, 1977, and Jenkins, 1976, for reviews). Two categories of psychological variables have received the most support as coronary risk factors: psychological stress and certain personality characteristics or behavior patterns. The identification of these psychosocial risk factors highlights the role of life-style in the development of CHD and also directs attention from identification of static risk factors to the study of dynamic processes involving the interaction of the individual with his/her environment.

Psychological stress is often defined as an internal state that occurs when an individual confronts a threat to his/her physical or psychological well-being (Lazarus, 1966). Several classes of psychological stressors have been studied and found, with varying degrees of consistency, to be associated with coronary disease. Among these are chronic stressors such as job dissatisfactions, daily stress and tension, excessive work, and burdensome responsibility (Haynes, Feinleib, & Kannel, 1980; House, 1975; Jenkins, 1971, 1976). Acutely stressful life events beyond the individual's ability to control have also been linked to coronary disease (Glass, 1977; Parkes, Benjamin, & Fitzgerald, 1969; see Glass, 1977, and Jenkins, 1971, 1976, for reviews of the stress–CHD literature).

A second psychological factor which has important implications for CHD is the Type A or "coronary-prone" behavior pattern, a complex set of behaviors described by Friedman and Rosenman (e.g., 1959). Type A behavior is characterized by excessive competitive drive, impatience and hostility, and accelerated speech and motor movements. A contrasting Type B pattern is defined as the relative absence of these characteristics. No sharp division exists between the two behavior patterns; instead, the Type B person is a generally more relaxed and easygoing person who exhibits little aggressive drive and who is relatively devoid of time-urgent characteristics. It has been observed that the Type A pattern emerges in the presence of certain environmental challenges or stresses (Glass, 1977).

Encouraged by the development of the field of behavioral medicine, and also by a considerable body of data (including two large-scale prospective studies) documenting an association between Type A and coronary disease, research in this area has become increasingly popular among biomedical and behavioral researchers alike (see Dembroski, Weiss, Shields, Haynes, & Feinleib, 1978; Glass, 1977).

This chapter focuses on recent research developments on the Type A pattern. After a brief review of the evidence linking Pattern A to the occurrence of CHD, we consider its description and assessment, and address issues raised by the fact that Type A consists of a number of relatively independent dimensions of behavior. Following this, we discuss behavioral studies of situations which precipitate the Type A response, and biobehavioral mechanisms mediating associations between Type A and cardiovascular pathology. Our discussion concludes with a review of current psychophysiological research using patients with clinical coronary disease, and an outlook on directions for future investigation.

## TYPE A ASSOCIATIONS WITH CHD

People who are competitive, achievement oriented, time-urgent, and hostile have long been suspected of being at higher risk of clinical CHD (e.g., Osler, 1892). However, the major impetus for research validating this hypothesis comes from the work of cardiologists Friedman and Rosenman (1959), who described and defined the Type A pattern based on their observations of coronary patients. Since that time, several studies conducted by Rosenman, Friedman, Jenkins, and others have indicated that Type A individuals show a substantially higher incidence and prevalence of CHD than Type Bs. The most convincing evidence derives from the Western Collaborative Group Study (WCGS). This 8½-year prospective study (Rosenman, Brand, Jenkins, Friedman, Straus, & Wurm, 1975) demonstrated that men exhibiting Type A behavior at intake were more likely than Type B subjects to develop clinical CHD and were more likely to suffer a fatal heart attack. Type As were also more than twice as likely to suffer a recurrent heart attack during this interval. In the WCGS, the incidence of new (and recurrent) CHD increased in men exhibiting many of the standard risk factors, but step-wise regression analysis revealed that Pattern A was an independent risk factor associated with increased CHD. This latter point means that the predictive relationship of Pattern A cannot be accounted for entirely by the presence of other standard risk factors.

In an analysis of prospective data from the Framingham heart study, Haynes and her coworkers (Haynes, Feinleib, & Kannel, 1980) found that a questionnaire measure of Type A was related to incidence of CHD in women as well as men. Again, this finding was obtained even when standard risk factors were controlled. There does, however, tend to be a relationship between Pattern A and some of the standard risk factors. For example, some studies indicate that fully developed Type A subjects have significantly higher serum cholesterol levels than Type Bs, more rapid blood clotting times, and higher postprandial serum triglyceride levels (Rosenman & Friedman, 1974). There is little evidence, though, of a relationship between prevalence of hypertension and Pattern A (Shekelle, Schoenberger, & Stamler, 1976); neither is there a consistent relationship between Type A and basal blood pressure levels. We do, however, review extensive research indicating that Type As display greater *reactive* increases in blood pressure when confronted with challenging situations.

There is also an association between Pattern A and coronary atherosclerosis, although this relationship has been recently called into question (cf. Dimsdale, Hackett, Hutter, & Block, 1980). In an autopsy study, Friedman, Rosenman, Straus, Wurm, and Kositchek (1968) found evidence of greater coronary occlusion in men previously determined to be Type A, regardless of whether death was due to CHD or to other causes. More recent studies have examined the relationship between measures of Type A and extent of atherosclerosis demonstrated at coronary arteriography. This procedure, also called angiography, permits quantification of extent of coronary artery disease (CAD) in living patients. It involves passing a catheter through the peripheral vasculature into the heart, injecting a photosensitive dye, and filming coronary arterial anatomy. The evidence here is somewhat contradictory, but at least three studies (Blumenthal, Williams, Kong, Schanberg, & Thompson, 1978; Frank, Heller, Kornfeld, Sporn, & Weiss, 1978; Zyzanski, Jenkins, Ryan, Flessas, & Everist, 1976) concur in reporting positive associations between severity of coronary atherosclerosis and measures of Type A behavior. However, other investigations have not supported this finding (e.g., Dimsdale, Hackett, Hutter, Block, Catanzano, & White, 1979; Krantz, 1980). Finally, Krantz, Sanmarco, Selvester, and Matthews (1979) found evidence of a positive association between magnitude of Type A scores and progression of atherosclerosis. In this study of men who underwent repeat coronary angiograms over a 17-month period, extreme Type B subjects were unlikely to show significant increases in occlusion of coronary vessels.

## RESEARCH ON ASSESSMENT

### Measurement of Pattern A

Classification of subjects as Type A or Type B is based on a structured interview (SI) developed by Rosenman and Friedman (e.g., Rosenman & Friedman, 1974). In this interview, the subject is asked questions dealing with competitive drive, impatience, and daily irritations. These interviews are tape recorded for later assessment by trained raters. Research (Matthews, Krantz, Dembroski, & MacDougall, 1982; Scherwitz, Berton, & Leventhal, 1977; Schucker & Jacobs, 1977) has shown that speech characteristics (such as speed, explosiveness) and clinical ratings of tone and manner of response correlate more highly with overall Type A–Type B assessments in the interview than do purely content aspects of subjects' answers. Despite the fact that hostility is a defining characteristic of Type A, it may be underrepresented in the content of SI questions, showing itself in questions relating to irritation at being slowed down. Hostility must be inferred, instead, largely from the tone of answers. Interview ratings can be made on a four-point scale of intensity (extreme Type A, mild Type A, unclassifiable [X], Type B), but most research has relied on simple A-B dichotomy.

The other commonly used measure of Type A[1] is the Jenkins Activity Survey for Health Prediction, or JAS (Jenkins, Zyzanski, & Rosenman, 1971). This is a self-administered questionnaire which was developed to duplicate interview assessments. The JAS yields a continuous distribution of scores. Being a self-report measure, it relies on content and self-perceptions only, but the Type A scale can generally mimic dichotomous interview assessments in about 65–70% of cases (e.g., Jenkins *et al.*, 1971; MacDougall, Dembroski, & Musante, 1979). However, studies which have correlated continuous Type A JAS scores with the four-point inten-

---

1. A third, less frequently used measure of Type A is a scale developed by Haynes, Feinleib, Levine, Scotch, and Kannel (1978), which was validated in the Framingham heart study.

sity ratings made in the interview (Chesney, Black, Chadwick, & Rosenman, 1981; MacDougall *et al.*, 1979; Matthews *et al.*, 1982) show a disappointingly low degree of overlap between JAS and interview (correlations ranging between .25 and .40). This points to the fact that JAS and SI are measuring different components of Type A.

How are SI and JAS evaluated as coronary risk factors? In epidemiology, there are two measures of how precisely any test can correctly classify individuals who have a particular disease or risk characteristic; namely, sensitivity and specificity. Sensitivity indicates the percentage of diseased or "at-risk" individuals who will be correctly identified as being "at risk" by the test, whereas specificity indicates the percentage of nondiseased or "low-risk" individuals who will be designated "low risk" by the test (Peterson & Thomas, 1978). If we adopt prediction of coronary disease as the criterion, the sensitivity of measures of Type A appears to be adequate. Research consistently shows high percentages of Type As in populations with manifest heart disease and in individuals who later develop CHD. It is important to note, however, that a study comparing SI and JAS questionnaire as predictors of coronary disease in the WCGS (Brand, Rosenman, Jenkins, Sholtz, & Zyzanski, in press) found the interview to be a stronger predictor, and hence the more sensitive measure.

But the epidemiologic specificity of Type A behavior defined by interview leaves much to be desired.[2] While evidence indicates that the Type B pattern is related to low incidence of heart disease, large numbers of persons who suffer from heart disease are falsely being classified as "coronary prone" by interview. The largest currently available population sampling of the prevalence of Type A (defined by SI) comes from the WCGS, which was begun in 1960. This sampling of middle-class, middle-aged men was roughly evenly divided between As and Bs. However, more recent samples (both published and unpublished) of symptom-free men show a preponderance of Type As (as much as 65-70%) in populations similar to WCGS (Chesney *et al.*, 1981; Glass, unpublished data; Krantz, 1980) and even among college students (MacDougall *et al.*, 1979). At first glance, it seems that these difficulties might be overcome by shifting to the JAS. Recall, however, the JAS is often a weaker predictor of subsequent CHD (and also of certain physiological responses to be

---

2. In fairness to the predictive value of the A-B dichotomy, recall that no single standard risk factor is notably more successful in predicting cases of CHD (Kannel *et al.*, 1976).

described later). Shifting to this measure to correct the population prevalence problem of the SI technique may result, therefore, in sacrificing sensitivity for specificity.

## Toward Increased Specificity

Because Pattern A consists of several overlapping and somewhat independent dimensions of behavior, and because large percentages of individuals are classified as Type A who will not develop coronary disease, researchers have begun to look for ways of reducing the heterogeneity of the Type A group. This has resulted in an examination of separate components of the behavior pattern and also in attempts to move from the level of describing behavioral characteristics toward examining possible mediating physiological processes.

Research suggests that some aspects of the Type A pattern may be more important than others in contributing to CHD risk. Matthews, Glass, Rosenman, and Bortner (1977) conducted an item analysis of a subsample of interviews from the WCGS. They found that only some elements of the Type A pattern significantly predicted incidence of CHD. Attributes reflected in these items included competitive drive, impatience, vigorous voice stylistics, and potential for hostility. There is also suggestive evidence that different facets of the Type A pattern may be specifically associated with different clinical manifestations of coronary disease. In an item analysis of responses to the JAS in WCGS participants, Jenkins, Zyzanski, and Rosenman (1978) found that responses to the questionnaire items were characteristically different among those men who developed acute myocardial infarction (MI), angina pectoris, and clinically unrecognized (silent) MI. The conclusions of this study are in accord with other studies in the epidemiologic literature (dealing with standard and psychosocial risk factors) indicating that MI and angina pectoris might well have different physiological and psychosocial antecedents (e.g., Lebovitz, Shekelle, Ostfeld, & Paul, 1967; Medalie, Snyder, Groen, Newfeld, Goldbourt, & Riss, 1973). This finding is also consistent with data reported by Haynes (1980) indicating that the association between the Framingham Type A scale and later development of CHD was largely accounted for by cases of angina pectoris rather than MI. Preliminary data from an unpublished study of patients scheduled for cardiac catheterization (Krantz, 1980) indicated that many components of the Type A pattern were more strongly related to MI as a clinical end point than to extent of coronary atherosclerosis. Second, it was found that different Type A components seemed to relate to each of these two manifestations of CHD. For example, certain voice characteristics (e.g., response latency, rapid speech) were related to MI, whereas certain self-reports of behavior (e.g., resentment at being kept waiting) were related to extent of coronary atherosclerosis. Pending further replications of these findings, these data suggest that future research employing analyses of Type A components may improve the specificity of the link between psychological states and cardiovascular pathology.

It should also be noted that there is a literature documenting the association between heart disease incidence and a number of psychological characteristics (both trait and situational) themselves not a part of the Type A pattern as currently described and measured (see Jenkins, 1971, 1976, for reviews). Some examples of individual difference variables in this category are provided by associations between measures of anxiety[3] and incidence of angina pectoris, but not MI (Medalie et al., 1973; Zyzanski et al., 1976). In addition, Williams and colleagues (Williams, Haney, Lee, Kong, Blumenthal, & Whalen, 1980) have reported that both Type A behavior (defined by interview) and scores on an MMPI measure of interpersonal hostility were independently related to extent of coronary atherosclerosis. As previously mentioned, a variety of situational factors (e.g., stressful life events, job dissatisfaction) related to acute and chronic stress have also been related to CHD. These psychosocial risk factors for heart disease are not a necessary part of the Type A complex. Moreover, only certain aspects of Pattern A may be related to incidence of CHD. Therefore, it has been recommended that the terms "Type A" and "coronary-prone behavior" no longer be used interchangeably (Cooper, Detre, & Weiss, 1981).

Another way of approaching the specificity–sensitivity problem is to shift the emphasis of research so as to devote more attention to the smaller (cf. Chesney et al., 1981) group of subjects who are not classified as Type A by interview. These individuals seem to be relatively immune to developing CHD and its complications, and, as indicated, studies have consistently shown that Pattern B is associated with low incidence of coronary disease. In fact, the absence of disease in Type Bs is

---

3. Since several of these studies employ various measures of anxiety with questionable reliability and validity, this conclusion should be viewed as tentative (cf. Jenkins, 1971).

often more pronounced than the presence of disease in Type As. (That is, the "false-negative" rate for coronary risk is considerably less frequent than the "false-positive" rate.) Consider for example, two studies previously described which deal, respectively, with prevalence and progression of atherosclerosis in patients referred for cardiac catheterization. Blumenthal *et al.* (1978) found that fewer than 7% of patients with severe CAD were classified as Type Bs, and Krantz *et al.* (1979) found that roughly 11% of patients who evidenced progression of CAD were extreme Type Bs as defined by JAS. The point of this line of thought is that Pattern B seems to be a rather specific marker of the absence of pathology. However, because of its high prevalence in the general population, the counterpart Type A pattern is a poorer indicant of the presence of pathogenic processes. At present, precious little is known about Pattern B, which is defined as "the absence of Type A," and we may stand to learn much about the prevention of heart disease by directing more research toward understanding non-coronary-prone individuals.

There is one final issue related to the predictive ability of Type A for CHD which has only begun to receive consideration in the epidemiological literature. As we document in the next section of this chapter, Type A behavior in experimental settings emerges primarily in the presence of certain environmental challenges or stresses (Glass, 1977). If this is true, it follows that Type A behavior, when studied naturalistically, will interact with particular situational circumstances in the production of CHD. Despite ample evidence from laboratory studies (see following), at present there is little direct epidemiological evidence to support or refute this hypothesis. The WCGS, conducted largely on a population of white-collar middle-class men, did not report any data regarding the possible interactions between Type A and occupational or other environmentally challenging or stressful circumstances. Some support for an interaction comes from a retrospective study by Glass and coworkers (Glass, 1977) which found prevalence of CHD in men who evidence Type A behavior *and* also report higher occurrence of recent life events over which they have little control. An interaction between Type A and occupational type was demonstrated in the prospective data from the Framingham heart study (Haynes *et al.*, 1980), which reported an association between Type A and CHD among white-collar, but not blue-collar workers. If we assume that the life-styles and work demands on men in white-collar (but not blue-collar) occupations represent sufficient challenge to elicit Type A behavior, the interactional hypothesis receives some support from this study.

However, several retrospective studies did find a relationship between Type A and CHD in blue-collar populations (cf. Glass, 1977; Zyzanski, 1978), and the data are far from conclusive regarding possible interactions of Type A with occupational status in the development of CHD.

Answers to questions about the interaction of Type A with situational factors in the development of CHD require that research efforts be directed toward a delineation of the classes of environmental stimuli that elicit the primary facets of the behavior pattern. It is not enough to speak loosely about appropriately challenging and/or stressful events. These terms must be defined with precision and relevant parameters specified to determine, *a priori*, which types (and levels) of stress (or challenge) are sufficient to produce Type A behaviors and concomitant physiologic responses in both laboratory and field settings. In the following sections of this chapter, we review research bearing on these issues.

## BEHAVIORAL STUDIES OF TYPE A

It has been repeatedly emphasized in the literature (Friedman & Rosenman, 1959; Glass, 1977) that Type A behaviors emerge in the presence of certain challenges or stresses. Glass and his coworkers have demonstrated that given appropriate environmental elicitors, Type As display exaggerated achievement strivings and suppress subjective states (such as fatigue) that threaten their best efforts (Carver, Coleman, & Glass, 1976; Glass, 1977). Type As also become impatient with delays and perform poorly on tasks which require slow responding (Glass, Snyder, & Hollis, 1974). Type As are more aggressive than Bs when frustrated or provoked interpersonally (Carver & Glass, 1978). Matthews and her coworkers (Matthews & Brunson, 1979; Weidner & Matthews, 1978) have demonstrated that Type As focus attention on central tasks in achievement situations and often ignore peripheral cues that might deter performance. This attentional style is also related to a tendency to suppress the perception of symptoms which might interfere with performance (Weidner & Matthews, 1978).

### REACTIONS TO UNCONTROLLABLE EVENTS

It has been suggested (Glass, 1977) that the motivational basis of the foregoing Type A behaviors is an attempt to assert and maintain control over environmental challenges and demands. The concept of control (cf.

Seligman, 1975) is defined in terms of perceptions of contingencies. That is, if a person perceives that outcomes are contingent on his/her behavior, the outcome is defined as controllable. By contrast, if a person believes that his/her actions do not influence an outcome (for example, as in the case of failure), the outcome is uncontrollable. Type A subjects are engaged in a perpetual struggle to gain control, whereas Type B subjects are relatively free of such concerns and, therefore, show an absence of Pattern A behavioral traits. The accelerated pace and hard-driving, aggressive stance of the Type A individual can be seen as an attempt to avoid anxiety resulting from the threat of failure to cope with situations by quickly gaining mastery over them. On the other hand, if these efforts at control meet with repeated failure, Type As will give up responding and act helpless. Stated somewhat differently, initial exposure to a situation which threatens loss of control results in enhanced motivation to control on the part of As, whereas prolonged exposure without successful coping leads to a decrement in these behaviors. This pattern of responding has been described as initial "hyperresponsiveness" followed by subsequent "hyporesponsiveness." A series of experiments with healthy human subjects has provided support for these hypotheses (Brunson & Matthews, 1981; Glass, 1977).

Glass proposes that throughout life the Type A coping style is characterized by alternate periods of struggling to master potentially uncontrollable situations (hyperresponsiveness) and periods of resignation and giving up (hyporesponsiveness). More importantly, it is proposed that the cycle of enhanced coping and giving up is correlated with large fluctuations in sympathetic nervous system function (particularly epinephrine and norepinephrine excretion), which are thought to potentiate the development of CAD and its clinical complications (see the following section).

BIOBEHAVIORAL MECHANISMS

Most of the research already reviewed has been concerned with describing behavioral characteristics of so-called coronary-prone individuals. How might these behavior patterns be involved in the physiological mechanisms underlying CHD? The epidemiological evidence suggests that Type A behavior may either contribute to the atherosclerotic process itself or be involved in precipitating the clinical complications of CAD (Williams, 1978). Glass (1977) has hypothesized that an explanation of these mechanisms must take into account: (1) the role of environmental stress in eliciting the Type A response and (2) the psychophysiology of stress. We have already described behavioral research on Type A. Before considering psychophysiological research and behavioral–physiological interactions, an overview of the pathogenesis of CHD is in order.

## THE DISEASE PROCESS

It is believed that the initiating event in the atherosclerotic process involves injury to the inner wall of the coronary arteries called the endothelium of the intima (Gorlin, 1976). A change occurs in this lining wall of the artery, leading to a train of events which, according to current medical theory (Carruthers, 1969; Ross & Glomset, 1976), results in an atheromatous plaque. It is believed that this change can be produced by either physical or chemical injury because the spiral course of the coronary arteries around a constantly moving structure (the myocardium) introduces unique bends and bifurcations into the system. Bifurcations and other curves create points of differing "sheer stress" and turbulence of blood flow, which may be important in promoting endothelial injury and the impregnation of the intima with lipids and blood platelets (substances important in coagulation). It is via these processes that hypertension is thought to accelerate the atherosclerotic process. There are also numerous biochemical ways that intimal changes may be brought about. For example, there is evidence that certain lipids (very-low-density lipoproteins, or VLDL) are particularly toxic to the coronary arteries (Gorlin, 1976; Herd, 1978; Williams, 1978).

Once the arterial wall is injured, its permeability is thought to increase and there is an accumulation of smooth muscle cells, containing and surrounded by lipid and cholesterol deposits (the "fatty streak") (Gorlin, 1976; Ross & Glomset, 1976). Blood platelets, which are lipid rich, may actually enter the intima, and thus set the stage for a large lipid-filled lesion, the atheromatous plaque. The excess lipids and cholesterol accumulating at the base of the plaque interfere with blood supply needed by living cells within, thereby resulting in calcification. Blood platelets may also adhere to the surface of the plaque, causing its enlargement and setting the stage for clinical complications.

The clinical manifestations of coronary disease (angina pectoris, MI, sudden death) are thought by most cardiologists to be complications of atherosclerosis (Friedberg, 1966). Angina pectoris consists of chest pain arising from the inability of diseased coronaries to provide adequate blood flow to meet oxygen requirements of the myocardium. It may result from a variety of factors which either reduce oxygen delivery to the heart or increase demand for blood flow (Goldstein & Epstein, 1972). MI is often the result of a clot or a thrombus forming in a coronary artery, diminishing blood supply and killing heart tissue. MI may also occur without the specific production of thrombi (Eliot, 1979; Friedberg, 1966), but discussion of these processes as well as alternative views of MI is beyond the scope of this chapter. An acute MI may also involve a portion of the heart's conduction system. In such cases, cardiac arrhythmias or ventricular fibrillation may develop, leading to sudden death.

STRESS AND PATHOPHYSIOLOGY

The contributions of psychological factors (stress and the Type A behavior pattern) to coronary disease are probably mediated by activity of the sympathetic–adrenomedullary (SAM) system.[4] According to Herd (1978), for example, the physiological concomitants of increased SAM activity (increased blood pressure, heart rate, and myocardial oxygen consumption; elevated circulating levels of epinephrine, norepinephrine, and plasma concentrations of free fatty acids [FFA]; increased plasma renin activity) all have the potential to predispose to cardiovascular diseases and their clinical complications.

It appears that catecholamines (epinephrine and norepinephrine) may have a special significance in the development of coronary disease. These hormonal substances, released during stressful periods (Mason, 1972), are secreted from the adrenal medulla and, in the case of norepinephrine, also from sympathetic nerve endings. Catecholamines might induce acute hemodynamic effects related to coronary artery disease, including increases in heart rate and blood pressure, and release of FFA and other lipids in the blood. Carruthers (1969), for example, has proposed that stress of modern living results in release of catecholamines which mobilize FFA greatly in excess of metabolic requirements. Excess FFA is

4. The pituitary–adrenocortical axis may also be involved in the stress–CHD relationship. The corticosteroid cortisol increases free fatty acid release and generally leads to a rise to serum lipids (Netter, 1969).

then taken up directly by arterial walls or converted to triglycerides which later are deposited in arterial walls.

The catecholamines can also contribute to infarction by facilitating platelet aggregation (Mustard & Packham, 1969), potentiating bleeding in arterial atheromata by elevating blood pressure or by narrowing of capillaries nourishing blood vessels and associated coronary plaques (Januszewicz & Snajderman, 1972). Last, there is reason to believe that increased levels of catecholamines may predispose to ventricular arrhythmia and sudden death (Herd, 1978; Lown, Verrier, & Rabinowitz, 1977).

## Psychophysiological Correlates of Type A Behavior

Recent research indicates that Type A persons, compared to Type Bs, show evidence of elevated sympathetic nervous system arousal when confronted with situations that are appropriately stressful or challenging. Hemodynamic reactions and neurodendocrine responses have received the most attention.

### Cardiovascular Response

A series of studies indicate that while not differing in baseline levels, Type A individuals respond to a variety of laboratory challenges with greater elevations in blood pressure and heart rate (e.g., Dembroski, MacDougall, Shields, Petitto, & Lushene, 1978; Manuck, Craft, & Gold, 1978). This increased cardiovascular *reactivity* in Type A subjects has been reported in a variety of subject populations including male and female college students (Glass, Krakoff, Finkelman, Snow, Contrada, Kehoe, Mannucci, Isecke, Collins, Hilton, & Elting, 1980; MacDougall, Dembroski, & Krantz, 1981; Manuck & Garland, 1979), working-class adults (Glass, Krakoff, Contrada, Hilton, Kehoe, Mannucci, Collins, & Snow, 1980), and coronary patients (Dembroski, MacDougall, & Lushene, 1979; Krantz, Schaeffer, Davia, Dembroski, MacDougall, & Shaffer, 1981). Regarding the various measures of Type A behavior, it appears that across a variety of studies, the SI is a stronger predictor of cardiovascular response than is the JAS. (For a complete review of this research, see Dembroski, MacDougall, Herd, & Shields, in press.) Since these instruments capture different components of the Type A constellation of behaviors, it is reasonable to inquire how the various components relate to cardiovascular response. Dembroski, MacDougall, Shields, Petitto, and Lushene (1978) found that clinical ratings of style and manner of verbal response (such as rapid and accelerated speech, verbal competitiveness), and ratings of potential for hostility seem to show higher correlations with physiological reactivity than do self-reports of characteristics such as being competitive. This latter finding is particularly provocative. Many of the components found to be most highly related to physiological reactivity measures were those found to be predictive of later incidence of CHD in the Matthews *et al.* (1977) reanalysis of the WCGS data cited earlier in this chapter.

Neuroendocrine Response

Studies of neuroendocrine function also suggest excess sympathetic arousal in Type A subjects. Extreme Type As, for example, show more rapid blood clotting times and a smaller decrease in platelet aggregation in response to norepinephrine (e.g., Friedman & Rosenman, 1959; Simpson, Olewine, Jenkins, Ramsey, Zyzanski, Thomas, & Hames, 1974). Of greater significance, perhaps, are the findings that Type As show greater elevations of plasma levels of catecholamines during a harassing and stressful social competition (Friedman, Byers, Diamant, & Rosenman, 1975; Glass, Krakoff, Contrada, Hilton, Kehoe, Mannucci, Collins, & Snow, 1980). It should be emphasized that the enhanced neuroendocrine response of Type As occurs only under particular situational circumstances. For example, a study that is described later demonstrates that Type A subjects' greater catecholamine response in a competitive situation requires the additional instigation of harassment by a competitor (Glass, Krakoff, Contrada, Hilton, Kehoe, Mannucci, Collins, & Snow, 1980). Nevertheless, a major question in the field has been the potential mediation of the relation between Pattern A and coronary disease by the catecholamines, and we discuss this again at a later point in this chapter.

SITUATIONAL SPECIFICITY OF PHYSIOLOGICAL RESPONSE

Consistent with the definition of Type A behavior, and with the behavioral research already reviewed, A-B differences in physiological reactivity seem to emerge only under particular circumstances. A descriptive picture of the range of situations that elicit these differences is beginning to emerge, but there is no clear-cut consensus as to the conceptual similarities between a variety of these situations. Three studies by Goldband (1980) demonstrate that in order to elicit A-B differences, experimental tasks must be "relevant" to Type A characteristics. In accord with this formulation, experimental situations defined as competitive, time dependent, and potentially uncontrollable resulted in heightened cardiovascular response in Type A subjects, whereas the same tasks not so defined resulted in no A-B differences. In addition, two other psychological stressors not conceived to be "relevant" to Type A characteristics (a balloon bursting and cold-pressor stimulus) resulted in no physiological differences (Goldband, 1980).

Situations must also involve a certain degree of environmental challenge. Dembroski, MacDougall, Herd, and Shields (1979), for example, manipulated the instructions given to subjects exposed to cold-pressor and reaction time tests. "High-challenge" instructions were delivered in a crisp tone of voice and informed subjects of the difficulty of the task and the need for willpower, whereas "low-challenge" subjects were led to believe the task was routine. Results indicated only minimal A-B differences in the low-challenge condition and considerably larger and reliable differences in the high-challenge condition. Additionally, analyses of various Type A components (clinical ratings of voice stylistics and content of responses to questions) were coded in the structured interview and related to cardiovascular response. Paralleling a previous study (Dembroski, MacDougall, Shields, Petitto, & Lushene, 1978), clinical ratings of hostility and competitiveness were related to cardiovascular response, even in the low-challenge conditions. This result was interpreted by the authors to suggest that subjects exhibiting high hostility and competitiveness have lower thresholds for perceiving environmental challenge.

The situational specificity of Type A-Type B differences in psychophysiological response is further demonstrated by a study indicating that Type As showed more blood pressure reactivity than Bs when threatened with loss of self-esteem but not when threatened with shock (Pittner & Houston, 1980).

Differences in physiological response between Type A and Type B subjects have also been elicited by conditions of social competition, both actual (Friedman *et al.*, 1975; Glass, Krakoff, Contrada, Hilton, Kehoe, Mannucci, Collins, & Snow, 1980) and simulated (Van Egeren, 1979), as well as by conditions where cardiovascular measurements are taken during the course of the face-to-face interview (Dembroski, MacDougall, Herd, & Shields, 1979; Krantz *et al.*, 1981; MacDougall *et al.*, 1981). An early study (Friedman *et al.*, 1975) demonstrated that a stressful face-to-face competitive situation (which included moderate noise stress and verbal harassment from the experimenter) elicited greater plasma norepinephrine responses in Type A as compared to Type B men. Unfortunately, the particular technique used for drawing blood samples involved a repeated venipuncture procedure which in and of itself has been shown to elicit psychological stress and resultant elevated neuroendocrine response (Rose & Hurst, 1975).

A recent pair of studies by Glass, Krakoff, Contrada, Hilton, Kehoe, Mannucci, Collins, and Snow (1980) helps clarify the nature of the relationship between social competition and both cardiovascular and neuroendocrine responses in Type A and Type B subjects. In the first experiment, the relative effects of competition per se versus *hostile* competition were assessed. All subjects were led to believe they would compete with an opponent (who was actually an experimental confederate) on an electronic game called "Pong." The game was described as a test of coordination, and a gift certificate was offered to the winner of a nine-game tournament. A and B subjects were exposed to one of two experimental conditions. In the "no-harass" condition, the confederate remained silent and simply competed against the subject. (The confederate had been trained to a level of skill to win the gift certificate according to a pre-arranged schedule.) In the "harass" condition, the same procedure was followed with one variation: The confederate made a series of preprogrammed remarks designed to harass the subject. Throughout the task, blood pressure and heart rate (HR) were measured and blood samples were drawn from an in-dwelling catheter.

The results revealed no baseline differences, but harassment had an effect on systolic blood pressure (SBP) changes. Type As showed greater SBP increases, and an interaction between A-B and harass–no-harass conditions indicated that the harass-As showed higher SBP elevations than each of the other groups. Average HR elevations were also greatest for the harass-As. The catecholamine measures showed no baseline differences, but for plasma epinephrine, the increases for the harass-As were greater than for the other experimental groups. Changes in plasma norepinephrine were in a similar direction but not reliably different between groups.

This study indicates that relative to resting levels, face-to-face competition elicits similar increases in cardiovascular measures and plasma epinephrine in both Type A and B individuals. A hostile, harassing opponent heightens cardiovascular and neuroendocrine response over nonhostile competition in Type As but does not seem to affect Type Bs. In a subsequent follow-up study, subjects were tested *individually* and challenged to perform well on an individualized version of the "Pong" task. This time, Type As exhibited heightened cardiovascular and plasma epinephrine responses. Taken together, these studies suggest that nonhostile face-to-face competition elicits equal cardiovascular and neuroendocrine responses in As and Bs. Type As appear to be more reactive to solitary performance challenge and also to hostile competition.

### Other Individual Difference Variables

Several individual difference variables may interact with the A-B dichotomy in potentiating elevated physiological arousal of Type A subjects in particular situations. These individual difference variables probably alter the meaning and interpretation of a particular situation, and therefore confirm the notion that physiological reactivity is elicited by psychological, rather than purely physical, challenges. We have previously described particular Type A components, such as potential for hostility and certain speech characteristics (e.g., rapid and accelerated speech), which seem to be related to cardiovascular reactivity. In addition, there is a recent evidence of sex differences in the types of situations which elicit cardiovascular reactivity. For example, Manuck et al. (1978) found that JAS-defined Type A men (but not women) were more reactive during performance of a difficult cognitive task. MacDougall et al. (1981) found that Type A and B females showed no differences in physiological reactivity on a psychomotor performance task which previously yielded large A-B differences in males, but did differ in SBP elevations during interpersonal interactions with another female. The authors hypothesize that males and females differ in the type and range of situational events which lead to such responses (e.g., interpersonal confrontations are effective triggers for women).

Still another individual difference variable is self-involvement. Scherwitz, Berton, and Leventhal (1978) found no reactivity differences between As and Bs across a variety of experimental tasks. However, when subjects were subdivided on a dimension called "self-involvement"—measured by counting the rate of self-referencing personal pronouns (I, me, mine, etc.) used during the SI—it was found that self-involved Type As showed higher blood pressure levels and lower HR than low-self-involved Type As. By contrast, the Type B group had very few significant correlates of self-references. The self-involvement dimension is described by Scherwitz et al. (1978) as "the extent to which the subject is identifying with his attitudes, actions, feelings and imagery." In evaluating the Scherwitz et al. (1978) findings, it is not entirely clear whether this dimension can be best measured by number of personal pronouns used. Subsequent research, while confirming self-referencing as a variable related to cardiovascular responses, has produced results inconsistent with the notion that self-referencing potentiates the relationship between Type A behavior and physiological reactivity. For example, recent data (Glass, unpublished) suggest that number of self-references increases blood pressure reactivity of Type Bs (but not As) and also indicate that self-references are positively, rather than negatively, related to HR. These recent data suggest that rather than *interacting with* Type A, self-referencing *simulates* the action of Type A in terms of elevated cardiovascular response. Moreover, the significance of self-referencing for coronary disease risk is brought into question by another recent finding indicating that rate of self-referencing is *negatively* associated with prevalence of CAD in a cardiac catheterization sample, even after controlling for age and sex of patients (Krantz, 1980).

BIOBEHAVIORAL MODELS

Across a range of over a dozen studies conducted in several different laboratories, Type A subjects evidence increased hemodynamic and catecholamine response to situations which are appropriately "challenging" or stressful. From behavioral studies, we know also that given appropriate environmental elicitors, Type As display exaggerated achievement strivings, impatience, and aggressiveness; and suppress subjective states (such as fatigue) that threaten their best efforts (Glass, 1977). Several theoretical perspectives have been offered to define the motivational basis of Type A and to understand mechanisms whereby these behaviors are linked to CHD.

## Active Coping/Control Maintenance

Recall one approach toward integrating behavioral and biochemical processes which proposes that efforts to assert and maintain control (active coping) are accompanied by concomitant elevations in circulating catecholamines (Glass, 1977). As the realization develops that control has been lost, the person gives up and becomes behaviorally passive. During this period, catecholamine levels presumably decline, or at least the magnitude of elevation is lessened. According to this perspective, the behavioral sequence—efforts to exert control followed by giving up—occurs repeatedly over the course of a lifetime. The biochemical correlates of this sequence of coping and passivity may, according to this reasoning, play a role in the pathogenesis of coronary atherosclerosis.

The notion of efforts to control (or active coping) being accompanied by sympathetic activation resembles Obrist's (1976) hypothesis that sympathetic influences on the cardiovascular system are most pronounced when subjects are engaged in active coping behavior. A series of studies (Obrist, Gaebelein, Teller, Langer, Grignolo, Light, & McCubbin, 1978) offer support for this view and demonstrate, through the use of a pharmacological blocking agent, that these cardiovascular changes (increases in SBP, HR, and carotid $dP/dt$—a measure of left-ventricular performance) are $\beta$-adrenergically mediated. The behavioral evidence would suggest that Type A individuals exhibit a response style characterized by active coping under the very stimulus situations where this coping results in elevated cardiovascular and neuroendocrine hyperactivity. Therefore, an integration of the Glass (1977) and Obrist (1976) hypotheses may provide a useful model for specifying the mechanisms by which the behavior of Type As might be related to physiological reactivity.

## Attentional Processes

A second, albeit less fully developed, approach toward integrating bio-behavioral evidence on Type A places emphasis on physiological correlates of information processing and attention. Based on earlier work by the Laceys (e.g., Lacey & Lacey, 1970), Williams (1978) has proposed that sensory "intake" and "rejection" are accompanied by particular patterns of physiological response. According to this view, when a situation calls for shutting out or rejecting stimuli, the defense reaction is activated. This is characterized by emotional arousal, increased motor activity, and a cardiovascular response pattern characterized by increased cardiac output, with a shunting of this increased output away from the skin and viscera to the skeletal musculature. However, when vigilance and attentive observation to the environment are required, a different response pattern is elicited. This is characterized by decreased emotional expression and motor activity, decreased HR and cardiac output, and vasoconstriction in skeletal muscle, skin, and viscera (Williams, Bittker, Buschbaum, & Wynne, 1975).

Williams (1978) hypothesizes that Type A individuals may exhibit extreme (both in increase and decrease) hemodynamic and biochemical responses associated with these behavioral adjustments. There are currently very little physiological data bearing on this attentional hypothesis, but the behavioral research by Matthews and coworkers (e.g., Matthews & Brunson, 1979; Weidner & Matthews, 1978) is supportive of the notion that Type As focus their attention on central tasks and attend less to peripheral tasks. These findings on attentional differences did not find support in a recent study (Glass, Krakoff, Finkelman, Snow, Contrada, Kehoe, Mannucci, Isecke, Collins, Hilton, & Elting, 1980). In a dual task situation (a central task and peripheral task) which induced overload, there were no A-B differences in performance on either of the tasks, but the demands of the dual task did elicit greater blood pressure and plasma catecholamine responses in As. At present, much more research is necessary to support or refute the notion that physiological correlates of sensory intake and rejection are more pronounced in Type As.

## SYMPATHETIC ACTIVATION AND CHD: RESEARCH STRATEGIES AND EVIDENCE

Psychophysiological, biochemical, and behavioral studies reviewed in the previous sections suggest that the association between Pattern A and CHD may be mediated via the action of the SAM system. Although this assumption is biologically plausible (Herd, 1978), empirical evidence is needed linking these processes directly to various manifestations of coronary disease (see Goldband, Katkin, & Morell, 1979). It is tempting, for example, in the absence of hard data, to draw the (probably oversimplified) conclusion that each behavioral and/or physiological correlate of Type A behavior plays a role in the pathogenesis of all manifestations of coronary disease. However, we already know that certain components of Type A have stronger associations with CHD than others (e.g., Matthews *et al.*, 1977). Both on a psychological and physiological level, there is reason to believe that there are different mechanisms involved in the etiology and/or pathogenesis of angina pectoris, MI, and coronary atherosclerosis. For example, psychological evidence suggests that angina patients tend to be more anxious, dissatisfied, and more reactive to environmental stress than patients with MI (Jenkins, 1971, 1976; Medalie *et al.*, 1973). Physiologically, it is clear that all clinical manifestations of disease are often not present in the same individual. Given the same level of coronary atherosclerosis, some individuals suffer clinical symptomatology, whereas others do not.

Goldband, Katkin, and Morell (1979) have outlined a research strategy for determining biobehavioral mechanisms linking Type A to CHD. This strategy involves the *integration* of three basic phenomena: individual differences in overt behavior (Type A), individual differences in psychophysiological response, and incidence of new and recurrent CHD. Previous sections of this chapter describe research linking Type A to coronary disease and, second, to enhanced sympathetic nervous system activity. We have yet to discuss evidence of an association between the SAM system and coronary disease.

In previous sections of this chapter, we describe evidence that a variety of concomitants of SAM activity might play a role in the pathogenesis of ischemic heart disease and its clinical complications (see Glass, 1977; Herd, 1978). The two most frequently invoked mechanisms include (1) the chemical and physiological action of plasma catecholamines, and (2) pronounced hemodynamic reactivity. Given that these mechanisms are biologically plausible, several empirical approaches might be used to obtain evidence that either or both of these processes are, indeed, operative in the pathogenesis of ischemic heart disease.

One approach might be to examine cardiovascular and neuroendocrine reactivity to emotional stress in patients who have manifest coronary disease. Although studies of patients with disease are subject to several possible confounds (e.g., damage to heart tissue or other changes due to disease processes may alter or obscure responses), the association between Type A and both recurrence of MI and progression of atherosclerosis suggests that pathogenic mechanisms probably remain active after disease is manifest. Next, in conjunction with cross-sectional study, a more costly but also more definitive approach might be to establish a prospective association between aspects of SAM activity and subsequent incidence of

CHD end points. Finally, to establish causality and precise mechanisms, animal models would be useful. The following section reviews psychophysiological research concerning sympathetic activity and CHD.

## ASSOCIATIONS OF SAM ACTIVITY AND ISCHEMIC HEART DISEASE

In the only prospective study examining cardiovascular reactivity as a predictor of CHD incidence, Keys, Taylor, Blackburn, Brozek, Anderson, and Simonson (1971) reported that magnitude of diastolic blood pressure (DBP) response to cold pressor was a significant variable in predicting subsequent CHD. In fact, this response was a stronger predictor than many of the risk factors assessed in the study.

A variety of case-control studies have been conducted examining psychophysiological responses to emotional stress in cardiac patients. Several have noted pronounced ECG changes in patients during administration of challenging mental examinations (Schiffer, Hartley, Schulman, & Abelman, 1976; Taggert, Gibbons, & Somerville, 1969). Schiffer *et al.* (1976) also found that patients with angina pectoris and hypertension displayed higher mean and maximal HR and SBP during a challenging history quiz than a healthy control group, although increases over baseline were reliable only for SBP. An attempted replication of this study (Sime, Buell, & Eliot, 1980) reported that postinfarct patients with clinical symptoms (angina, hypertension, and ECG changes) showed significantly higher elevations in DBP and, unexpectedly, lower HR increases during a challenging quiz compared to a group of healthy control subjects and a group of asymptomatic postinfarct patients, who did not differ from the controls. A preliminary report of a follow-up study showed that those patients who tended to be more reactive on cardiovascular measures were more likely to suffer reinfarction (Sime, Buell, & Eliot, 1979); however, these data should be viewed as tentative because the sample size was very small. Voudakis (1971) also found that patients with arteriosclerosis (including peripheral vascular disease, cerebrovascular disease, and CHD) showed elevated SBP and pulse pressure response to a cold-pressor test. Elevated urinary excretion of catecholamine metabolites during emotional stress has also been demonstrated in patients with classical angina reactions compared to patients who reported to a cardiac clinic and were free of chest pain or had chest pain not ischemic in origin (Nestel, Verghese, & Lovell, 1967).

Dembroski, MacDougall, and Lushene (1979) compared Type A and Type B postinfarct patients and non-CHD controls in cardiovascular response to the Type A SI and a challenging history quiz. Type A, relative to Type B subjects, evidenced greater increases in both SBP and DBP during interview and quiz; and CHD cases, relative to controls, showed marginally higher SBP increases to the quiz but not during the interview. There were no HR effects. This study suggests that during a quiz which elicits cardiovascular reactivity in Type As, patients (even Type Bs), but not Type B controls, evidence elevated SBP response. Rosenman (1978) also reported that both coronary patients and Type A individuals without manifest CHD symptomatology respond to a competitive contest with greater elevations in plasma norepinephrine than Type B subjects.

In sum, a variety of studies demonstrate that patients with manifest CHD display evidence of heightened cardiovascular and/or neuroendocrine responses when confronted by challenging or stressful tasks. However, many of these studies do not distinguish between the various clinical manifestations of CHD, and others do not screen coronary cases for the presence of history of hypertension, the latter disorder often having been associated with differences in sympathetic nervous system activity (e.g., Julius & Esler, 1975). Most consistently, a finding of elevated reactivity has been demonstrated in patients who display overt symptomatology of ischemic heart disease or hypertension. Evidence for cardiovascular and/or sympathetic nervous system reactivity as a mechanism specifically linked to coronary atherosclerosis would be provided by research linking psychophysiological response to angiographic findings.

A recent study (Krantz et al., 1981) was conducted to test the notion that pronounced hemodynamic reactivity in Type A individuals might be one important factor in promoting the onset or progression of CAD. Patients scheduled for cardiac catheterization were subjected to the structured Type A interview and a history quiz while HR and blood pressure were monitored. Physiological changes were quantified for three portions of the interview and during the quiz. Blind to the psychophysiological testing, patients were categorized as having mild, moderate, or severe atherosclerosis based on results of subsequent cardiac catheterization. Analyses controlling for age and $\beta$-adrenergic blocking medications revealed some evidence of Type A-B differences in SBP, HR, and rate–pressure product during the interview, but not during the quiz. In terms of the relationship of hemodynamic variables to CAD, there was little systematic evidence that magnitude of response on any of the cardiovascular measures was positively related to severity of disease. Internal analyses of 24 nonmedicated patients and examination of data derived from cardiac catheterization were used to rule out the possible confounding effects of $\beta$-blocking drugs and myocardial damage.

Patients who undergo cardiac catheterization are, however, a select group of subjects and are not necessarily representative of the general population or of heart patients in general. Moreover, based on these data, no conclusions can be drawn about neuroendocrine responses, as no such measures were taken. Excessive output of plasma catecholamines and other chemical substances (e.g., FFA) which cause arterial endothelial injury remains an untested mechanism.

Although we do not consider the Krantz *et al.* (1981) study to be definitive, for reasons already presented, these data do not provide evidence that blood pressure and HR reactivity per se are predisposing mechanisms accounting for associations reported in some studies (e.g., Blumenthal *et al.*, 1978; Frank *et al.*, 1978) between Pattern A and initiation of promotion of the atherosclerotic process in coronary arteries. There is considerably more evidence that hemodynamic reactivity may be a physiological mechanism specifically linked to the development of clinical manifestations of CHD, such as MI or angina pectoris. For example, in the Krantz *et al.* (1981) study, Type A patients with a given level of CAD showed greater increases in rate–pressure product (a correlate of myocardial oxygen consumption) during a challenging interview. This is at least suggestive of a mechanism that might link Type A to ischemic symptoms. Indeed, recent research linking Type A behavior to increased reactivity during coronary artery bypass surgery and postoperative complications (Arabian, Krantz, & Davia, 1981; Kahn, Kornfeld, Frank, Heller, & Hoar, 1980) reinforces the assoiation between reactivity and *clinical* CHD outcomes.


CONCLUDING COMMENTS

Recent research has examined a number of mechanisms underlying the Type A–CHD relationship by studying both behavioral and physiological processes. This chapter has reviewed evidence in each of these two categories. A common theme that can be seen in many current investigations in the area is the notion of *specificity* on many levels of analysis. For example, specific components of the Type A construct seem to be most importantly linked to CHD risk, and there is preliminary evidence (at this point only suggestive) that particular behavioral and/or physiological characteristics may be selectively related to various clinical manifestations of CHD. In addition, physiological and behavioral reactivity in Type A individuals seems to emerge only under particular environmental circumstances.

Although we have focused on behavior–disease relationships, research on Pattern A may be useful not only for the information it reveals about mechanisms of CHD but also for the understanding it can provide of the behavior pattern itself and of basic biobehavioral mechanisms. However, Type A behavior remains largely a description of behaviors. Despite the fact that several investigators have offered theories of the psychological mechanisms underlying Type A behavior (Glass, 1977; Scherwitz et al., 1978), there is still no clear consensus as to the conceptual definition of Pattern A or the situations that promote this behavior. The eliciting situations for Type A behavior-associated physiological responses have been variously described as challenging (e.g., Dembroski, Weiss, Shields, Haynes, & Feinleib, 1978), threats to control over stressful events (Glass, 1977), and ego involving (Scherwitz et al., 1978). It remains difficult to predict a priori whether a particular situation fits into any of these conceptual or descriptive categories.

The lack of conceptual definition of Type A is particularly troublesome for research which deals with populations other than middle-aged, middle-class men, the group for which SI and JAS were validated. If one cannot define a "core" of Type A behavior that transcends the cultural environment, sex roles, and life-span development, then it is difficult to determine which definition(s) to use in studying these groups. Uncertainties about possible underlying mechanisms also translate into questions about which aspects of Type A behavior to try to change if intervention trials are undertaken.

A fundamental question is whether there is, in fact, a set of underlying psychological dimensions or constructs which form the basis of Type A, or is its association with coronary disease merely a reflection of behavioral arousal or physiological reactivity that can result from many causes? If enhanced sympathetic nervous system reactivity is the sine qua non of "coronary-prone behavior," one must still understand the kinds of situations which elicit the responses (or patterns of responses) which promote development of ischemic heart disease. Indeed, it is the biobehavioral approach, promising an integration of physiological and behavioral processes, which makes the Type A construct so appealing to psychological and biomedical researchers alike.

## ACKNOWLEDGMENTS

Research by the authors was supported by grants to David S. Krantz from the National Institutes of Health (HL-23674) and USUHS (CO-7201), and to David C. Glass from the National Institutes of Health (HL-2254).

## REFERENCES

Arabian, J. M., Krantz, D. S., & Davia, J. E. *Type A behavior, intra-operative blood pressure, and recovery from coronary bypass surgery.* Presentation to the annual meeting of the Society for Psychophysiological Research, Washington, D.C., October 1981.

Blumenthal, J. A., Williams, R., Kong, Y., Schanberg, S. M., & Thompson, L. W. Type A behavior and angiographically documented coronary disease. *Circulation*, 1978, *58*, 634–639.

Brand, R. J., Rosenman, R. H., Jenkins, C. D., Sholtz, R. I., & Zyzanski, S. J. Comparison of coronary heart disease prediction in the Western Collaborative Group Study using the structured interview and the Jenkins Activity Survey assessments of the coronary-prone Type A behavior pattern. *Journal of Chronic Diseases*, in press.

Brand, R. J., Rosenman, R. H., Sholtz, R. I., & Friedman, M. Multivariate prediction of coronary heart disease in the Western Collaborative Group Study compared to the findings of the Framingham Study. *Circulation*, 1976, *53*, 348–355.

Brunson, B. I., & Matthews, K. A. The Type A coronary-prone behavior pattern and reactions to uncontrollable stress: An analysis of performance strategies, affect, and attributions during failure. *Journal of Personality and Social Psychology*, 1981, *40*, 906–918.

Carruthers, M. A. Aggression and atheroma. *Lancet*, 1969, *2*, 1170.

Carver, C. S., Coleman, A. E., & Glass, D. C. The coronary-prone behavior pattern and suppression of fatigue on a treadmill test. *Journal of Personality and Social Psychology*, 1976, *33*, 460–466.

Carver, C. S., & Glass, D. C. Coronary-prone behavior pattern and interpersonal aggression. *Journal of Personality and Social Psychology*, 1978, *36*, 361–366.

Chesney, M. A., Black, G. W., Chadwick, J. H., & Rosenman, R. H. Psychological correlates of the coronary-prone behavior pattern. *Journal of Behavioral Medicine*, 1981.

Cooper, T., Detre, T., & Weiss, S. M. Coronary prone behavior and coronary heart disease: A critical review. *Circulation*, 1981, *63*, 1199–1215.

Dembroski, T. M., MacDougall, J. M., Herd, J. A., & Shields, J. L. Effects of level of challenge on pressor and heart rate responses in Type A and B subjects. *Journal of Applied Social Psychology*, 1979, *9*, 209–228.

Dembroski, T. M., MacDougall, J. M., Herd, J. A., & Shields, J. L. Perspectives on coronary-prone behavior. In D. S. Krantz, A. Baum, & J. E. Singer (Eds.), *Hand-*

*book of psychology and health* (Vol. 1: *Cardiovascular disorders*). Hillsdale, N.J.: Erlbaum, in press.

Dembroski, T. M., MacDougall, J. M., & Lushene, R. Interpersonal interaction and cardiovascular response in Type A subjects and coronary patients. *Journal of Human Stress*, 1979, *5*, 28–36.

Dembroski, T. M., MacDougall, J. M., Shields, J. L., Petitto, V., & Lushene, R. Components of the Type A coronary-prone behavior pattern and cardiovascular responses to psychomotor performance challenge. *Journal of Behavioral Medicine*, 1978, *1*, 159–176.

Dembroski, T. M., Weiss, S. M., Shields, J. L., Haynes, S. G., & Feinleib, M. (Eds.). *Coronary-prone behavior*. New York: Springer-Verlag, 1978.

Dimsdale, J. E., Hackett, T. P., Hutter, A. M., & Block, P. C. The risk of Type A mediated coronary disease in different populations. *Psychosomatic Medicine*, 1980, *42*, 55–62.

Dimsdale, J. E., Hackett, T. P., Hutter, A. M., Block, P. C., Catanzano, D. M., & White, P. J. Type A behavior and angiographic findings. *Journal of Psychosomatic Research*, 1979, *23*, 273–276.

Eliot, R. S. *Stress and the major cardiovascular diseases*. Mt. Kisco, N.Y.: Futura, 1979.

Frank, K. A., Heller, S. S., Kornfeld, D. S., Sporn, A., & Weiss, M. Type A behavior pattern and coronary angiographic findings. *Journal of the American Medical Association*, 1978, *240*, 761–763.

Friedberg, C. K. *Diseases of the heart* (3rd ed.). Philadelphia: W. B. Saunders, 1966.

Friedman, M., Byers, S. O., Diamant, J., & Rosenman, R. H. Plasma catecholamine response of coronary-prone subjects (Type A) to a specific challenge. *Metabolism*, 1975, *4*, 205–210.

Friedman, M., & Rosenman, R. H. Association of specific overt behavior pattern with increases in blood cholesterol, blood clotting time, incidence of arcus senilis and clinical coronary artery disease. *Journal of the American Medical Association*, 1959, *169*, 1286–1296.

Friedman, M., Rosenman, R. H., Straus, R., Wurm, M., & Kositchek, R. The relationship of behavior pattern A to the state of the coronary vasculature: A study of 51 autopsied subjects. *American Journal of Medicine*, 1968, *44*, 525–538.

Glass, D. C. *Behavior patterns, stress and coronary disease*. Hillsdale, N. J.: Erlbaum, 1977.

Glass, D. C., Krakoff, L. R., Contrada, R., Hilton, W. F., Kehoe, K., Mannucci, E. G., Collins, C., & Snow, B. Effect of harassment and competition upon cardiovascular and catecholamine responses in Type A and B individuals. *Psychophysiology*, 1980, *17*, 453–463.

Glass, D. C., Krakoff, L. R., Finkelman, J., Snow, B., Contrada, R., Kehoe, K., Mannucci, E. G., Isecke, W., Collins, C., Hilton, W. F., & Elting, E. Effect of task overload upon cardiovascular and plasma catecholamine responses in Type A and B individuals. *Basic and Applied Social Psychology*, 1980, *1*, 199–218.

Glass, D. C., Snyder, M. L., & Hollis, J. F. Time urgency and the Type A coronary-prone behavior pattern. *Journal of Applied Social Psychology*, 1974, *4*, 125–140.

Goldband, S. Stimulus specificity of physiological response to stress and the Type A coronary-prone personality. *Journal of Personality and Social Psychology*, 1980, *39*, 670–679.

Goldband, S., Katkin, E. S., & Morell, M. A. Personality and cardiovascular disorder: Steps toward demystification. In C. Spielberger & I. Sarason (Eds.), *Stress and anxiety*. Washington, D.C.: Hemisphere, 1979.

Goldstein, R. E., & Epstein, S. E. Medical management of patients with angina pectoris. *Progress in Cardiovascular Diseases*, 1972, *14*(4), 360–398.

Gorlin, R. *Coronary artery disease*. Philadelphia: W. B. Saunders, 1976.

Haynes, S. G. *The influence of personality and working status on coronary heart disease*. Presentation to the meeting of the Social Science Research Council Committee on Life Course Perspectives on Middle and Old Age: Stress, Disease, and Behavior, Stanford, Calif., May 5–6, 1980.

Haynes, S. G., Feinleib, M., & Kannel, W. B. Psychosocial factors and CHD incidence in Framingham: Results from an 8 year follow-up study. *American Journal of Epidemiology*, 1980, *108*, 229.

Haynes, S., Feinleib, M., Levine, S. Scotch, N., & Kannel, W. The relationship of psychosocial factors to coronary heart disease in the Framingham study: Prevalence of coronary heart disease. *American Journal of Epidemiology*, 1978, *107*, 384–402.

Herd, J. A. Physiological correlates of coronary prone behavior. In T. M. Dembroski, S. M. Weiss, J. L. Shields, S. G. Haynes, & M. Feinleib (Eds.), *Coronary-prone behavior*. New York: Springer-Verlag, 1978.

House, J. S. Occupational stress as a precursor to coronary disease. In W. D. Gentry & R. B. Williams, Jr. (Eds.), *Psychological aspects of myocardial infarction and coronary care*. St. Louis: C. V. Mosby, 1975.

Januszewicz, W., & Snajderman, M. Catecholamines and the cardiovascular system. *Acta Physiologica Polonica*, 1972, *23*, 585–595.

Jenkins, C. D. Psychologic and social precursors of coronary disease. *New England Journal of Medicine*, 1971, *284*, 244–255; 307–317.

Jenkins, C. D. Recent evidence supporting psychologic and social risk factors for coronary disease. *New England Journal of Medicine*, 1976, *294*, 987–994; 1022–1038.

Jenkins, C. D., Zyzanski, S. J., & Rosenman, R. H. Progress toward validation of a computer-scored test for the Type A coronary-prone behavior pattern. *Psychosomatic Medicine*, 1971, *33*, 193–202.

Jenkins, C. D., Zyzanski, S. J., & Rosenman, R. H. Coronary-prone behavior: One pattern or several? *Psychosomatic Medicine*, 1978, *40*, 25–43.

Julius, S., & Esler, M. Autonomic nervous cardiovascular regulation in borderline hypertension. *American Journal of Cardiology*, 1975, *36*, 685–696.

Kahn, J. P., Kornfeld, D. S., Frank, K. A., Heller, S. S., & Hoar, P. F. Type A behavior and blood pressure during coronary artery bypass surgery. *Psychosomatic Medicine*, 1980, *42*, 407–414.

Kannel, W. B., McGee, D., & Gordon, T. A general cardiovascular risk profile: The Framingham Study. *American Journal of Cardiology*, 1976, *38*, 46–51.

Keys, A., Taylor, H. L., Blackburn, H., Brozek, J., Anderson, J. T., & Simonson, E. Mortality and coronary heart disease among men studied for 23 years. *Archives of Internal Medicine*, 1971, *128*, 201–214.

Krantz, D. S. *Behavior patterns and coronary disease: Some research issues*. Presentation to the meeting of the Social Science Research Council Committee on Life Course Perspectives on Middle and Old Age: Stress, Disease, and Behavior, Stanford, Calif., May 5–6, 1980.

Krantz, D. S., Sanmarco, M. E., Selvester, R. H., & Matthews, K. A. Psychological correlates of progression of atherosclerosis in men. *Psychosomatic Medicine*, 1979, *41*, 467–475.

Krantz, D. S., Schaeffer, M. A., Davia, J. E., Dembroski, T. M., MacDougall, J. M., & Shaffer, R. T. Extent of coronary atherosclerosis, Type A behavior, and cardiovascular response to social interaction. *Psychophysiology*, 1981, *18*, 654–664.

Lacey, J. I., & Lacey, B. C. Some autonomic–central nervous sytem interrelationships. In H. Black (Ed.), *Physiological correlates of emotion.* New York: Academic Press, 1970.

Lazarus, R. S. *Psychological stress and the coping process.* New York: McGraw-Hill, 1966.

Lebovitz, B. Z., Shekelle, R. B., Ostfeld, A. M., & Paul, O. Prospective and retrospective psychological studies of coronary heart disease. *Psychosomatic Medicine,* 1967, *29,* 265–272.

Lown, B., Verrier, R. L., & Rabinowitz, S. Neural and psychologic mechanisms and the problem of sudden cardiac death. *American Journal of Cardiology,* 1977, *39,* 890–902.

MacDougall, J. M., Dembroski, T. M., & Krantz, D. S. Effects of types of challenge on pressor and heart rate responses in Type A and B women. *Psychophysiology,* 1981, *18,* 1–9.

MacDougall, J. M., Dembroski, T. M., & Musante, L. The structured interview and questionnaire methods of assessing coronary-prone behavior in male and female college students. *Journal of Behavioral Medicine,* 1979, *2,* 71–83.

Manuck, S. B., Craft, S. A., & Gold, K. J. Coronary-prone behavior pattern and cardiovascular response. *Psychophysiology,* 1978, *15,* 403–411.

Manuck, S. B., & Garland, F. N. Coronary-prone behavior pattern, task incentive and cardiovascular response. *Psychophysiology,* 1979, *16,* 136–142.

Mason, J. W. Organization of psychoendocrine mechanisms: A review and reconsideration of research. In N. S. Greenfield & R. A. Sternbach (Eds.), *Handbook of psychophysiology.* New York: Holt, Rinehart, & Winston, 1972.

Matthews, K. A., & Brunson, B. I. The attentional style of Type A coronary-prone individuals: Implications for symptom reporting. *Journal of Personality and Social Psychology,* 1979, *37,* 2081–2090.

Matthews, K. A., Glass, D. C., Rosenman, R. H., & Bortner, R. W. Competitive drive, pattern A, and coronary heart disease: A further analysis of some data from the Western Collaborative Group Study. *Journal of Chronic Diseases,* 1977, *30,* 489–498.

Matthews, K. A., Krantz, D. S., Dembroski, T. M., & MacDougall, J. M. The unique and common variance in the structured interview and Jenkins Activity Survey estimates of Type A behavior. *Journal of Personality and Social Psychology,* 1982, *42,* 303–313.

Medalie, J. H., Snyder, M., Groen, J. J., Newfeld, H. N., Goldbourt, V., & Riss, E. Angina pectoris among 10,000 men. *American Journal of Medicine,* 1973, *55,* 583–594.

Mustard, J. F., & Packham, M. A. Platelet function and myocardial infarction. In S. Bondurant (Ed.), *Research on acute myocardial infarction.* New York: American Heart Association, 1969.

Nestel, P. J., Verghese, A., & Lovell, R. R. Catecholamine secretion and sympathetic nervous system responses to emotion in men with and without angina pectoris. *American Heart Journal,* 1967, *73,* 227–234.

Netter, F. H. *The Ciba collection of medical illustrations* (Vol. 5: *Heart*). Summit, N.J.: Ciba Publications Department, 1969.

Obrist, P. A. The cardiovascular–behavioral interaction—As it appears today. *Psychophysiology,* 1976, *13,* 95–107.

Obrist, P. A., Gaebelein, C. J., Teller, E. S., Langer, A. W., Grignolo, A., Light, K. C., & McCubbin, J. A. Relationship among heart rate, carotid dP/dt, and blood pressure in humans as a function of the type of stress. *Psychophysiology,* 1978, *15,* 102–115.

Osler, W. *Lectures on angina pectoris and allied states.* New York: Appleton, 1892.

Parkes, C. M., Benjamin, B., & Fitzgerald, R. G. Broken heart: A statistical study of increased mortality among widowers. *British Medical Journal*, 1969, *1*, 740–743.

Peterson, D. R., & Thomas, D. B. *Fundamentals of epidemiology: An instruction manual.* Lexington, Mass.: D. C. Heath, 1978.

Pittner, N. S., & Houston, B. K. Response to stress, cognitive coping strategies, and the Type A behavior pattern. *Journal of Personality and Social Psychology*, 1980, *39*, 147–157.

Rose, R. M., & Hurst, M. W. Plasma cortisol and growth hormone responses to intravenous catheterization. *Journal of Human Stress*, 1975, *1*, 22–36.

Rosenman, R. H. The role of the Type A behavior pattern in ischemic heart disease: Modification of its effects by beta-blocking agents. *British Journal of Clinical Practice*, 1978, *32* (Suppl. 1), 58–65.

Rosenman, R. H., Brand, R. J., Jenkins, C. D., Friedman, M., Straus, R., & Wurm, M. Coronary heart disease in the Western Collaborative Study: Final follow-up experience of 8½ years. *Journal of the American Medical Association*, 1975, *223*, 872–877.

Rosenman, R. H., & Friedman, M. Neurogenic factors in pathogenesis of coronary heart disease. *Medical Clinics of North America*, 1974, *58*, 269–279.

Ross, R., & Glomset, J. A. The pathogenesis of atherosclerosis. *New England Journal of Medicine*, 1976, *295*, 369–377; 420–425.

Scherwitz, L., Berton, K., & Leventhal, H. Type A assessment and interaction in the behavior pattern interview. *Psychosomatic Medicine*, 1977, *39*, 229–240.

Scherwitz, L., Berton, K., & Leventhal, H. Type A behavior, self-involvement, and cardiovascular response. *Psychosomatic Medicine*, 1978, *40*, 593–609.

Schiffer, F., Hartley, L. H., Schulman, C. L., & Abelman, W. H. The quiz electrocardiogram: A new diagnostic and research technique for evaluating the relation between emotional stress and ischemic heart disease. *American Journal of Cardiology*, 1976, *37*, 41–47.

Schucker, B., & Jacobs, D. R. Assessment of behavioral risks for coronary disease by voice characteristics. *Psychosomatic Medicine*, 1977, *39*, 219–228.

Seligman, M. *Helplessness.* San Francisco: Freeman, 1975.

Shekelle, R. B., Schoenberger, J. A., & Stamler, J. Correlates of the JAS Type A behavior pattern score. *Journal of Chronic Diseases*, 1976, *29*, 381–394.

Sime, W. E., Buell, J. C., & Eliot, R. S. Psychophysiological (emotional) stress testing: A potential means of detecting the early reinfarction victim. *Circulation*, 1979, *59 & 60* (Suppl. 2), II-56. (Abstract)

Sime, W. E., Buell, J. C., & Eliot, R. S. Cardiovascular responses to emotional stress (quiz interview) in post-infarct cardiac patients and matched control subjects. *Journal of Human Stress*, 1980, *6*(3), 39–46.

Simpson, M. T., Olewine, D. A., Jenkins, C. D., Ramsey, F. H., Zyzanski, S. J., Thomas, G., & Hames, C. G. Exercise-induced catecholamines and platelet aggregation in the coronary-prone behavior pattern. *Psychosomatic Medicine*, 1974, *36*, 476–487.

Taggert, P., Gibbons, D., & Somerville, W. Some effects of motor car driving on the normal and abnormal heart. *British Medical Journal*, 1969, *4*, 130.

Van Egeren, L. F. Social interactions, communications, and the coronary-prone behavior pattern: A psychophysiological study. *Psychosomatic Medicine*, 1979, *41*, 2–18.

Voudakis, I. A. Exaggerated cold-pressor response in patients with arteriosclerotic heart disease. *Angiology*, 1971, *22*, 57–62.

Weidner, G., & Matthews, K. A. Reported physical symptoms elicited by unpredictable events and the Type A coronary-prone behavior pattern. *Journal of Personality and Social Psychology*, 1978, *36*, 213–220.

Williams, R. B. Psychophysiological processes, the coronary-prone behavior pattern, and coronary heart disease. In T. M. Dembroski, S. M. Weiss, J. L. Shields, S. G. Haynes, & M. Feinleib (Eds.), *Coronary-prone behavior*. New York: Springer-Verlag, 1978.

Williams, R. B., Bittker, T. E., Buschbaum, M. S., & Wynne, L. C. Cardiovascular and neurophysiologic correlates of sensory intake and rejection. *Psychophysiology*, 1975, *12*, 427–438.

Williams, R. B., Haney, T. L., Lee, K. L., Kong, Y., Blumenthal, J. A., & Whalen, R. E. Type A behavior, hostility, and coronary atherosclerosis. *Psychosomatic Medicine*, 1980, *42*, 539–550.

Zyzanski, S. J. Coronary-prone behavior pattern and coronary heart disease: Epidemiologic evidence. In T. M. Dembroski, S. M. Weiss, J. L. Shields, S. G. Haynes, & M. Feinleib (Eds.), *Coronary-prone behavior*. New York: Springer-Verlag, 1978.

Zyzanski, S. J., Jenkins, C. D., Ryan, T. J., Flessas, A., & Everist, M. Psychological correlates of coronary angiographic findings. *Archives of Internal Medicine*, 1976, *136*, 1234–1237.

# 11

## Cardiovascular Psychophysiology: A Systems Perspective

GARY E. SCHWARTZ

## INTRODUCTION

As the preceding chapters in this volume illustrate, research in cardiovascular psychophysiology is inherently complex. It is complex not only because the cardiovascular system is a very complex structure having multiple, interrelated functions, but also because the cardiovascular system is intimately connected, both structurally and functionally, with virtually every other organ system in the body. It turns out that these properties make the cardiovascular system a model system for conducting psychophysiological research in general. No function of an organism can be carried out independently of some adjustment somewhere in the cardiovascular system. Every class of behavior must directly and/or indirectly involve some adjustment in relevant components of the cardiovascular system.

Unfortunately, despite the fact that the cardiovascular system is ideally suited for examining behavior from a systems perspective, to date

Gary E. Schwartz. Department of Psychology, Yale University, New Haven, Connecticut.

most theory and research in cardiovascular psychophysiology have not adopted this general perspective. Most researchers in cardiovascular psychophysiology, regardless of their specific disciplinary training (be it in psychology, physiology, or medicine), have not received formal training in the concepts and methods of systems "thinking" (see Weinberg, 1975). The present author is no exception, having only recently acquired training in the concepts and mathematics of systems theory (see DeRosnay, 1979; Jones, 1973; Miller, 1978).

The thesis of this chapter is that systems theory can make important and unique contributions to improving research in cardiovascular psychophysiology. These improvements can come not only in conceptualizing and analyzing cardiovascular activity but in linking this activity to the "behavior" of organisms (broadly defined). The purpose of this chapter is to provide a brief introduction to systems theory and to give a few examples of how systems theory can be applied to common problems in psychophysiology. The chapter is designed to be illustrative rather than comprehensive, with the hope of stimulating the reader's further interest in the general topic.

This chapter is primarily theoretical and does not review a particular body of empirical research. The chapter includes some general discussions of philosophy of science as it applies to current research. The reader should, therefore, be prepared for the fact that the discussion that follows is not typically included in the standard psychophysiology text. However, as I hope will become clear as the chapter unfolds, the conceptual issues addressed in this chapter have direct relevance for theory and research in cardiovascular psychophysiology, and deserve to be aired, especially in the present volume. Toward this end, the chapter includes a general structure for organizing physical, biological, psychological, and social data in cardiovascular psychophysiology, and makes some general suggestions for advancing the mathematical description of cardiovascular functioning over time.

## WHAT IS SYSTEMS THINKING?

Systems thinking—or more appropriately, general systems thinking (Weinberg, 1975)—involves a particular orientation or perception of nature. This perception is guided by certain principles, one of which is that the orientation should be potentially applicable to any system, regardless of its specific nature, level, or degree of complexity. The principles, therefore, are truly general—they can, for example, be applied equally well to the fluid, chemical, humoral, neural, vascular, muscular, or integrative levels of analysis of cardiovascular structure and functioning. The book by Weinberg (1975) is an excellent introduction to general systems thinking and is highly recommended.

It is impossible to summarize the Weinberg volume in a few pages and do it justice. However, the general flavor of systems thinking can be readily appreciated by considering the research of Harris, Fontana, and Dowds (1977). Harris *et al.* operationalized the philosophical writings of Pepper (1942). Pepper has proposed that there are four main philosophical (conceptual) systems or "world hypotheses," that is, coherent sets of assumptions about the world. These four cognitive systems are formism, mechanism, organicism, and contextualism.

Briefly, "formistic thinking" is the simplest, and most immediate, way of conceptualizing nature. It involves the relatively quick placement of a single instance into a general category. Events are seen as discrete and limited. Consequently, events can be placed in specific categories and be labeled as such. For example, we can have specific categories for apples versus pears. If we see a round, greenish object, depending upon the shape, we may classify the object as a green apple *or* a green pear. Note that the round object cannot be both—it must be one or the other. A higher-level example of categorization is that the apple and pear can both be classified as fruit, whereas another green object, such as a green pepper, would be classified as a vegetable. However, once again, if something is a fruit, it cannot be a vegetable, and vice versa.

Labeling and categorization are examples of formistic thinking. Although the labeling process is necessary and can be quite complex (e.g., consider the field of zoology, which is a highly complex field of classifying organisms), it is nonetheless the simplest of cognitive styles or conceptual systems. Note that the very process of describing world hypotheses as consisting of four separate categories is itself an example of formistic thinking! Similarly, the process of labeling the heart and not the lungs, kidney, or brain as part of the cardiovascular system (since the latter are typically considered to be solely part of the respiratory, urinary, and central nervous systems, respectively) is also an example of simple formistic thinking. According to the research of Harris *et al.* (1977), there are certain people who tend to view the world *primarily* from the perspective of formistic thinking, and they may be highly motivated to do so. Such individuals are prone to classify people (or nations, or things, etc.) as either "good" *or* "bad," either "in" *or* "out," and so forth, and, therefore, tend to hold a "prejudiced" and restricted view of the world.

The next level of cognitive processing, the second category in Pepper's (1942) structure, is "mechanistic thinking." Mechanistic thinking takes formistic categories and looks for direct cause–effect relationships between them. In simple mechanistic thinking, each behavior or event has a discrete and particular existence in space and time, and each event may have a single direct effect on certain other events. Higher-level mechanistic thinking examines *chains* of cause–effect relationships, where Category A (a cause) influences B (an effect), and then B (now a cause) influences C (an effect). Cause–effect relationships occur in fixed times (e.g., they cannot go backward), and it is presumed that every effect has a specific, and single, cause (a final common pathway).

Mechanistic thinking is, of course, a fundamental aspect of basic science. Mechanistic thinking represents an advance over formistic thinking in that causal links between categories are pursued. Mechanistic thinking has led to many of the major discoveries in classical physics and chemistry, and has become a world view for many scientists, including physiologists and psychologists. According to research by Harris *et al.* (1977), there are certain people who tend to view the world *primarily* from the perspective of mechanistic thinking, who are apparently highly motivated to do so, and who are prone to see *all* events as having single causes. For example, they will tend to view a person's behavior as being caused by a specific, single event, as well as the behavior of a biological system (e.g., a disease is caused solely by a single germ) or a social system (e.g., a nation goes to war for a single reason).

Mechanistic thinking, like formistic thinking, is quite useful. However, modern physical and biological scientists have recently been forced to the conclusion that mechanistic thinking is oversimplified and ultimately incorrect (von Bertalanffy, 1968). Although cause–effect relationships do hold, they hold *only under certain conditions*. If certain conditions are changed, the cause–effect relationship will change accordingly. The cause–effect relationship can disappear or radically change (even to the point of producing opposite or counterintuitive effects). If the relationship between any two categories or events is *always* determined to various degrees by other categories or events (directly or indirectly), it becomes difficult to justify viewing a single event as being a single cause having a single effect. All events are, therefore, seen as multidetermined, having multiple causes. A full description of the characteristics (behavior) of a general category (event), regardless of its level (be it physical, chemical, physiological, psychological, social, and so forth), therefore, requires the specification of unique *combinations* or *patterns* of events (causes).

This is the essence of Pepper's (1942) third category of world hypotheses, what he calls "organistic thinking." Organistic thinking presumes that component parts of systems interact in unique ways, producing higher-level characteristics that are determined by the complex interactions of the various components. An organistic thinker would never conclude that increased vagal tone, for example, "causes" heart rate slowing without also emphasizing that this relationship occurs *only under certain circumstances* (e.g., when the sinoatrial node is appropriately connected to the atriaventricular node—for if these connections are impaired, for whatever reason, increased vagal firing can sometimes lead to ventricular tachycardia!). Heart rate slowing is an "emergent" property in the sense that it emerges out of an *interaction* of multiple factors (i.e., a pattern of factors), and this interaction is orderly and relatively fixed. In other words, specific patterns of processes determine what the relative effects of increased vagal tone will have on the heart.

According to Harris *et al.* (1977), there are people who tend to view the world *primarily* from the perspective of organistic thinking, who appear to be highly motivated to do so, and who are prone to see all events as having multiple causes and reflecting a developmental process. For instance, they tend to seek complex solutions to seemingly simple problems. Sometimes organistic thinkers will miss specific ("simple") relationships (implied in mechanistic conceptions) because they overattend to the complexities. Such is the risk of adopting an organistic perspective.

The last level of cognitive processing, in Pepper's (1942) framework, is "contextualism," or "relational thinking." For the prototypical contextual thinker there are no absolute truths or standards. Rather, events or elements take their meaning from the contexts in which they are embedded. These contexts are not fixed but are variable and subject to manipulation and reconstruction. Moreover, a single element can exist as part of more than one context at the same time. According to Harris *et al.* (1977), there are people who are prone to view the world *primarily* from a perspective of contextual thinking, who appear to be highly motivated to do so, and who tend to see all events as being relative. Their thinking is very fluid and sometimes difficult to pin down, for what is true today in one context may be questionable tomorrow in another.

Although this last category of thinking may at first glance sound "unscientific," it need not be. In fact, many physical phenomena discovered at subatomic levels have properties that *require* contextual thinking to comprehend them (e.g., consider Heisenberg's uncertainty principle or Einstein's theory of relativity). Contextual thinking, in less extreme forms, can be profitably applied to the psychophysiological systems such as the cardiovascular system.

Consider homeostasis, a process emerging out of the interaction of central–peripheral (brain–bódy) components, operating in a negative feedback, self-regulatory fashion (Wiener, 1948). From the perspective (context) of the neurologist, the brain (by neural and humoral links) controls the heart and vasculatory system. From the perspective (context) of the cardiovascular physiologist, the heart and vasculature (by various feedback links) control the brain. Each of these specialists sees only a partial picture of the self-regulatory process (their perception is context limited).

Systems theory, on the other hand, proposes that self-regulation emerges out of the *interaction* of the central–peripheral components. *Each* component controls (regulates/constrains) the *other*, and only out of this set of interdependencies does homeostatic stabilization emerge. If the linkages between the components are altered in certain ways (delaying the information, distorting or attenuating the information, or, in extreme cases, disconnecting the information linking the components), the self-regulation process will be distorted accordingly. I have referred to this general process of distortion as "disregulation." In general systems terms, disregulation is a prerequisite for the promotion of disorder and, ultimately, disease (Schwartz, 1977, 1978, 1979).

Ideally, a comprehensive researcher, from a general systems perspective, should be skilled in all four (formistic, mechanistic, organistic, and contextual) styles of thinking. The challenge facing researchers is to *integrate* these different styles so as to enrich the process of theory construction, research design, data analysis, interpretation, and synthesis. The issue of synthesis (of integrating various levels of analysis) is a major challenge facing cardiovascular psychophysiologists, especially in the broad context of behavioral medicine (Schwartz, 1982). The remainder of this chapter describes and operationalizes a few of the major concepts in systems theory, and illustrates how they can be applied to some common issues in cardiovascular psychophysiology.

## DO ALL SYSTEMS "BEHAVE"?

Systems theorists seek general principles that can potentially be applied to any system. The ability to distinguish when a term is used in a general sense versus use in a context-specific sense takes practice. As a result, this distinction is often confused in scientific literature.

Consider the term "behavior." As shown in Table 11-1, the term "behavior" has been used in four different ways, with the first definition being the most specific and narrow and the last definition being the most general and broad. The first definition uses the term to refer only to overt actions of organisms that can be measured "directly." Hence, to the naked eye, opening and closing one's jaw is "behavior"; whereas the muscular activity that pulls on the bone and enables the jaw to move is not "behavior," nor is the verbal thought preceding the overt verbal behavior. To behaviorists such as Skinner (1953), "behavioral" science refers to a subset of the science of psychology, though strict "behaviorists" would like to see all of psychology adopt their particular perspective.

TABLE 11-1. Four Definitions of "Behavior," Using Behavioral Medicine as an Example, Moving Up Levels of Complexity (in Systems Terms)

1. Behavior from the perspective of behaviorists and behavior therapists. "Behavior" here refers to one subarea in the discipline of psychology, emphasizing learning and the strict measurement of observable events. "Behavioral medicine" here refers to the application of behavior therapy per se (learning theory) to medicine.

2. Behavior from the perspective of general psychology. "Behavior" here refers to the study of behavior of organisms, broadly defined, and encompasses the entire discipline of psychology. Here psychology is "the" behavioral science. "Behavioral medicine" here refers to the application of all subareas of the discipline of psychology to medicine.

3. Behavior from the perspective of the arts and sciences. "Behavior" here refers to the study of behavior of organisms, very broadly defined, and encompasses not only the discipline of psychology but the disciplines of anthropology, sociology, political science, and so forth. "Behavioral medicine" here refers to the application of all behavioral sciences (psychology being only one such science) to medicine. This is the definition of "behavioral science" used at the Yale Conference on Behavioral Medicine (Schwartz & Weiss, 1978).

4. Behavior from the perspective of systems theory. "Behavior" here refers to the study of behavior of systems, not just organisms. All scientific disciplines, including physics, chemistry, and biology, as well as the "behavioral sciences" mentioned in Definition 3, would be reclassified here as "behavioral sciences." "Behavioral medicine" here refers to the application of systems theory, and the integration of all scientific disciplines, to medicine (Schwartz, 1979).

*Note.* From "Integrating Psychobiology and Behavior Therapy: A Systems Perspective," by G. E. Schwartz. In G. T. Wilson and C. M. Franks (Eds.), *Contemporary Behavior Therapy: Conceptual and Empirical Foundations.* New York: Guilford Press, 1982.

However, the term "behavior" can be, and often is, used more broadly, as indicated in Definitions 2 and 3. Definition 2 broadens the term to refer to the functioning of organisms, whether the behavior can be directly observed or is inferred (e.g., through self-reports). Here behavioral science refers to the whole of psychology as a science. Definition 3 broadens the term to include other social sciences such as anthropology and sociology. This definition of "behavior" is the one that was adopted at the Yale Conference on Behavioral Medicine (Schwartz & Weiss, 1978). The Yale Conference viewed medical and health psychology, medical sociology, medical anthropology, and so forth, as all reflecting the "behavioral" side of behavioral medicine.

However, it is the last definition of "behavior" that is the most general and is the one adopted by general systems theorists. Simply stated, all systems have certain properties, all systems react to specific stimulation from their environments, and they also can all produce specific actions. The general definition of "behavior," according to Webster, involves "action and reaction." Subatomic particles, atoms, chemicals, cells, organisms, groups, organizations, and so forth, all have properties (actions and reactions) as systems which can be detected and quantified. Therefore, all systems "behave."

To a systems scientist, the scientific method requires that the functioning of a given system be measurable. However, the systems scientist makes a special effort to distinguish between observation and inference. For example, subatomic physics attempts to study the behavior of subatomic particles in bubble chambers. However, these physicists do not "directly" measure the behavior of these particles, but rather detect the paths these particles take from the trails they leave as they interact with each other and *infer* their behavior from these indirect measurements.

Obviously, certain behaviors of certain systems can potentially be more "directly" measured than others. For example, with indwelling catheters it is possible for a cardiovascular physiologist to measure "directly" the pressure in an artery. I put the term "directly" in quotes, however, to emphasize what we often forget; namely, that what the physiologist *actually sees* in this example is not *the* pressure per se but rather the movement of a pen leaving a trail of ink on paper, or light leaving a trail on an oscilloscope screen. The physiologist *infers* the concept of pressure by *observing* the "behavior" of the pen leaving ink on paper or light leaving a path on the screen (the path is produced as a side effect of electrons striking the chemicals on the face of the cathode ray tube).

The general systems meaning of the term "behavior" is not often used by psychologists and physiologists. To help distinguish between Definition 4 and Definition 2 (from Table 11-1), in the following discussion I use capital letters to refer to the BEHAVIOR of systems and use small letters to refer to the overt (or inferred) psychological behavior of organisms (see Schwartz, 1982). I have adopted the same procedure with other terms to distinguish between general use and context-specific use.

The systems scientist, therefore, recognizes that, ultimately, all scientific disciplines involve the study of the BEHAVIOR of systems, and all scientists ultimately infer this BEHAVIOR from measurements that are, ultimately, to various degress, indirect. From this perspective, physics is not a "harder" science than physiology, which in turn is not a "harder" science than psychology. In fact, as various writers have noted (see especially DeRosnay, 1979, or Zukav, 1979), the ratio of inference to observation is probably highest today in physics, the "hardest" of the sciences.

I might also note that it is curious how the most general meaning of the term BEHAVIOR (BEHAVIOR of systems) parallels the most specific meaning of the term behavior (overt behavior of organisms). Like the strict behavioral scientist, the systems theorist attempts to distinguish inference from observation (see Schwartz, 1982). However, the important difference between the two is not that one is broad and the other is narrow, but rather that one acknowledges the need for inference and does so carefully, while the other operates under the myth that it does not require inference (when, in fact, it does—operant conditioning implies that learning exists, and that memories are presumably stored inside the organism, which is an inferred process).

## BEHAVIOR AND LEVELS IN SYSTEMS

Why devote so much space to a discussion of the general term BEHAVIOR in a book on cardiovascular psychophysiology? The reasons are many. Of primary concern is the fact that cardiovascular psychophysiologists attempt to study processes that cut across various levels in systems. As shown in Table 11-2 (from Schwartz, 1982), systems vary

TABLE 11-2. Levels of Complexity in Systems and Associated Academic Disciplines

According to systems theory, in order to understand the behavior of an open system at any one level, it is essential to have some training in the academic disciplines below that level, plus have some training at least in the relevant discipline at the next highest level as well.

| Level and complexity of the system | Academic field associated with the level of the system |
| --- | --- |
| beyond earth | astronomy |
| supranational | ecology |
| national | government, political science, economics |
| organizations | organizational science |
| groups | sociology |
| organism | psychology, ethology, zoology |
| organs | organ physiology (e.g., neurology, cardiology) |
| cells | cellular biology |
| biochemicals | biochemistry |
| chemicals | chemistry, physical chemistry |
| atoms | physics |
| subatomic particles | subatomic physics |
| abstract systems | mathematics |

Note. From "Integrating Psychobiology and Behavior Therapy: A Systems Perspective," by G. E. Schwartz. In G. T. Wilson and C. M. Franks (Eds.), Contemporary Behavior Therapy: Conceptual and Empirical Foundations. New York: Guilford Press, 1982.

in complexity, and different scientific disciplines have evolved to study the BEHAVIOR of systems at different levels of complexity. A basic tenet of systems thinking, as discussed in the previous section (recall organistic thinking), is that multiple processes interact, and that new properties (BEHAVIORS) emerge from the interactions of the components. In other words, although the concept of emergent property is a general concept that cuts across all levels of systems, unique BEHAVIORS specific to each system emerge at each level of complexity.

It is essential, therefore, that researchers who study processes that cut across multiple levels should organize their data in a systematic fashion. However, since general systems theory is currently not widely adopted, there is no commonly held set of principles for organizing and describing the BEHAVIORS that are measured at each level. The lack of a general structure leads to confusion and inaccuracies in interpreting data and describing results.

## LEVELS IN SYSTEMS AS APPLIED TO THE
## CARDIOVASCULAR SYSTEM

Consider current psychophysiological research on Type A behavior and cardiovascular functioning (e.g., Glass, Krakoff, Contrada, Hilton, Kehoe, Mannucci, Collins, Snow, & Elting, 1981; Krantz, Glass, Schaeffer, & Davia, Chapter 10, this volume), and consider what are the various "dependent measures" (BEHAVIORS) commonly made. In a given study, one might use: (1) self-report scales tapping a subject's memory of his/her behavior, (2) a structured interview in which the researcher focuses on "nonverbal" behaviors such as loudness of speech and angry facial expressions as more "direct" measures of Type A, (3) physiological measures such as blood pressure and heart rate, and (4) endocrine measures such as circulating epinephrine and norepinephrine. In common language, Measure 1 (self-report) is not labeled as behavior, whereas Measure 2 (the nonverbal, overt responses in the interview) is. Measures 3 and 4 are also not labeled as behavior but represent physiology and endocrinology, respectively.

However, in systems language, all of these measures are BEHAVIORS, though they tap processes occurring at different levels in a very complex system (the human being). The relationship between these various BEHAVIORS must be specified in some organized way in order to correctly interpret their interrelationships. In other words, a structure is needed so that the levels of inference connecting one set of BEHAVIORS with another can be made explicit.

Figure 11-1 presents a highly simplified but nonetheless useful first approximation for conceptualizing levels of cardiovascular processes ultimately controlling blood pressure in systems terms. Briefly, blood pressure (for simplicity, called Level 1) is a composite of the patterns of determining hemodynamic factors (Level 2), each of which in turn is generated by a pattern of peripheral organ activity (Level 3). The Level 3 effector BEHAVIOR is determined by patterns of peripheral neural and humoral mechanisms (Level 4), which are ultimately expressions of (are regulated by) patterns of central neurogenic processes (Level 5) (higher levels, e.g., social, are not shown in this figure). The development of actual anatomical alterations or organ pathology in cardiovascular diseases (a Level 3 effect) is believed to be in part a direct consequence of sustained high blood pressure (Level 1), shown by Feedback Loop A. Feedback Loop B shows

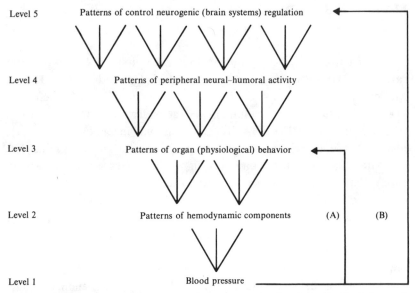

Level 5      Patterns of control neurogenic (brain systems) regulation

Level 4      Patterns of peripheral neural–humoral activity

Level 3      Patterns of organ (physiological) behavior

Level 2      Patterns of hemodynamic components     (A)     (B)

Level 1      Blood pressure

FIG. 11-1. Behavioral regulation of blood pressure: levels of analysis. Feedback Loops A and B represent internal (organ physiology and pathophysiology) and external ("biofeedback") effects of blood pressure. From "Behavioral Medicine Approaches to Hypertension," by G. E. Schwartz, A. P. Shapiro, D. P. Redmond, D. C. E. Ferguson, D. R. Ragland, and S. M. Weiss, *Journal of Behavioral Medicine*, 1979, *2*, 311–363. Reprinted by permission.

how biofeedback for blood pressure (Level 1) enters the CNS (Level 5). Other feedback loops, as well as various interactions within sublevels, are not indicated for the sake of simplicity.

The interactions among Levels 3, 2, and 1 have been traditionally the province of cardiovascular physiologists. By "mechanisms of blood pressure regulation" (Level 1) is meant the particular pattern of hemodynamic factors (Level 2) generating the pressure in a given instance (blood pressure as a Level 1 BEHAVIOR emerges out of the interaction of the Level 2 BEHAVIORS of hemodynamic factors). The pattern of effector organ BEHAVIORS (Level 3) in turn regulates the pattern of hemodynamic factors (Level 2). Among the interactions (not shown) within Level 3 are those termed "autoregulatory." For example, intrinsic mechanisms within the heart directly influence both heart rate and the force of contraction. These provide important Level-3-to-Level-2 feedback relationships, contributing stability and "fine tuning" of blood pressure (Level 1). Likewise, autoregulatory Level 3 mechanisms within the kidney and peripheral vasculature contribute to regulation of local perfusion and may play a role in cardiovascular pathology.

Guyton, Coleman, and Granger (1972) have provided a comprehensive flow chart for such Level 3 mechanisms. However, their discussion of Level 4 control of the Level 3 mechanisms is less complete, and treatment of the complex patterns of CNS subsystems (Level 5) regulating Level 4 is at best cursory. Omission of Level 4 and Level 5 mechanisms from detailed consideration is the traditional paradigmatic orientation of internal medicine and physiology, and partly reflects the limitation of techniques (including pharmacological, biomedical, and surgical) for measuring Level 4 and Level 5 BEHAVIORS. Nevertheless, it is precisely these considerations which provide the biological links connecting environmental factors to cardiovascular regulation and, ultimately, blood pressure (Level 1).

The brain is shown as the "highest" level (Level 5) because it is the most complex and integrative of organs; it interconnects and coordinates all the various sensory, motor, and autonomic organs (all Level 3 BEHAVIORS). In addition, it is physically the farthest removed and thus the least "direct" in the control of blood pressure (Level 1). However, this view is not meant to imply that the brain is the "primary" determinant of blood pressure regulation or that it operates independently of the lower levels. On the contrary, complex control loops from the lower to higher levels influence the behavior of the brain itself. For example, it is known that the brain (Level 5) can, via the sympathetic nervous system (Level 4), regulate the release of renin from the kidney (Level 3); in turn, angiotension in the blood stream (Level 1) can feed back and influence brain function. Similarly, renal modulation of sodium and water excretion ultimately influences the brain, while the brain affects both their intake and elimination. A complete systems description of the regulation of blood pressure, then, would involve descriptions *at all of these levels*, including their interrelationships.

A more complete description of cardiovascular regulation, using a five-level structure (Schwartz *et al.*, 1979), is provided in Table 11-3. This table extends the preceding discussion, illustrating the complex patterns of processes that can occur at a given level and the various interactions that are possible as one crosses levels.

TABLE 11-3. Cardiovascular Regulation in Systems Terms

Levels of integration (from Figure 11-1): Function is tissue perfusion via capillary pressure.

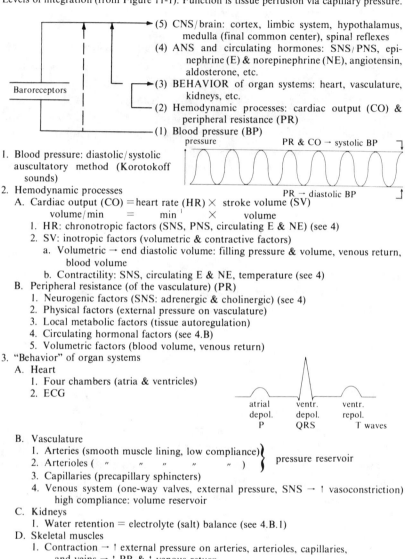

(5) CNS/brain: cortex, limbic system, hypothalamus, medulla (final common center), spinal reflexes

(4) ANS and circulating hormones: SNS/PNS, epinephrine (E) & norepinephrine (NE), angiotensin, aldosterone, etc.

Baroreceptors

(3) BEHAVIOR of organ systems: heart, vasculature, kidneys, etc.

(2) Hemodynamic processes: cardiac output (CO) & peripheral resistance (PR)

(1) Blood pressure (BP)

pressure        PR & CO → systolic BP

PR → diastolic BP

1. Blood pressure: diastolic/systolic auscultatory method (Korotokoff sounds)
2. Hemodynamic processes
   A. Cardiac output (CO) = heart rate (HR) × stroke volume (SV)
      volume/min = min$^{-1}$ × volume
      1. HR: chronotropic factors (SNS, PNS, circulating E & NE) (see 4)
      2. SV: inotropic factors (volumetric & contractive factors)
         a. Volumetric → end diastolic volume: filling pressure & volume, venous return, blood volume
         b. Contractility: SNS, circulating E & NE, temperature (see 4)
   B. Peripheral resistance (of the vasculature) (PR)
      1. Neurogenic factors (SNS: adrenergic & cholinergic) (see 4)
      2. Physical factors (external pressure on vasculature)
      3. Local metabolic factors (tissue autoregulation)
      4. Circulating hormonal factors (see 4.B)
      5. Volumetric factors (blood volume, venous return)
3. "Behavior" of organ systems
   A. Heart
      1. Four chambers (atria & ventricles)
      2. ECG

      atrial       ventr.      ventr.
      depol.       depol.      repol.
      P            QRS         T waves

   B. Vasculature
      1. Arteries (smooth muscle lining, low compliance)⎱
      2. Arterioles ( ″      ″    ″    ″      ″ ) ⎰ pressure reservoir
      3. Capillaries (precapillary sphincters)
      4. Venous system (one-way valves, external pressure, SNS → ↑ vasoconstriction) high compliance: volume reservoir
   C. Kidneys
      1. Water retention = electrolyte (salt) balance (see 4.B.1)
   D. Skeletal muscles
      1. Contraction → ↑ external pressure on arteries, arterioles, capillaries, and veins → ↑ PR & ↑ venous return
      2. Isotonic rhythm → ↑ blood flow
      3. Isometric contraction → sustained vasoconstriction → ↑ PR
   E. Respiration of lungs
      1. Rhythmic change in thoracic pressure → ↑ venous return
                                                 sinus arrhythmia (stretch receptors in lungs, etc.)
                                                    inspiration → ↑ HR
                                                    expiration → ↓ HR

    2. Dive reflex (see chemoreceptor reflex)
    3. Hyperventilation, hypoventilation
    4. Valsalva maneuver
  F. Adrenal glands
    1. Medulla → E & NE (see 4.B.2)
    2. Cortex → aldosterone (see 4.B.1)
4. Autonomic nervous system and circulating hormones
  A. Autonomic nervous system (ANS) (neurogenic control mediator)
    1. Parasympathetic nervous system (PNS): cholinergic (Ach is neurotransmitter)
      a. Vagus nerve: vagal tone controls resting HR (SA & AV nodes) (also to atrial muscle tissue)
        ↑ vagal tone → ↓ HR
        ↓   "   " → ↑ HR
    2. Sympathetic nervous system (SNS): adrenergic/NE = transmitter (except in sympathetic vasodilator system)
      a. SNS nerves to cardiac pacemakers (SA node & AV node)
      b. SNS nerves to ventricular muscle tissue (inotropic/SV effects) ($\beta$-receptors)
                 ↑ HR
        ↑ SNS ⟨
                 ↑ SV
      c. SNS adrenergic vasoconstrictor system (all arteries & arterioles) (separately to venous system) (vasodilatation in coronary arteries)
        (controls tone at rest)
        ↑ SNS → ↑ vasoconstriction → ↑ PR
                ($\alpha$-receptors)
      d. SNS cholinergic vasodilator system (muscle arteries & arterioles)
        ↑ SNS → ↑ vasodilatation → ↓ PR
  B. Circulating hormones
    1. Pituitary/adrenal/kidney system

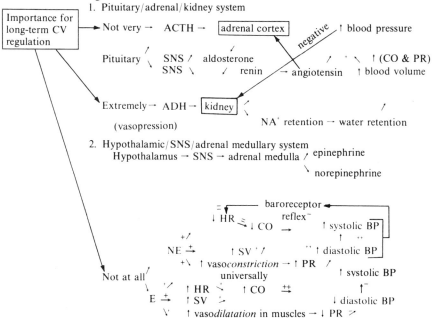

    2. Hypothalamic/SNS/adrenal medullary system

(continued)

TABLE 11-3. (*continued*)

3. Vasodilators: prostaglandins, kinins, local metabolites
5. Central nervous system (brain & spinal cord)
  A. Spinal reflexes
  B. Medulla (three centers)
    1. Cardioinhibitory → ↑ vagus → ↓ HR

    2. Vasodepressor → ↓SNS ⟨ ↓ HR ⎫ ↓ BP
                            ↓ vasoconstriction → ↓ PR ⎭

    3. Vasopressor → ↑ SNS ⟨ ↑ HR- ⎫ ↑ BP
                           ↑ vasoconstriction → ↑ PR ⎭
  C. Hypothalamus
    1. Sympathetic "defense center"
    2. Parasympathetic "relaxation response (trophotropic) center"
  D. Limbic system ("emotional brain")
    1. Amygdala: "sham rage"
  E. Cerebral cortex
Baroreceptor reflex: ↑ aortic/carotid pressure → ↓ HR (via cardioinhibitory & vasodepressor
                                                  centers)
                              ↓ PR (↓ vasoconstriction)
  pressure receptors in aorta and carotid arteries (tonically active)
  short-term (2-day) effects, hence receptor/reflex becomes "reset" in hypertension
Chemoreceptor reflex: ↑ $P_{CO_2}$ or ↓$P_{O_2}$ or ↓ pH → ↑ vasopressor center activity

        if apnea: "dive reflex" (↑ vasoconstriction → ↑ PR → bradycardia)

        if respiration normal: ↑ PR/$\dot{V}_E$, ↑ HR,↑BP       ↓ HR

        opposite effects of central vasoconstriction and local vasodilatation

*Note.* Prepared by Stephen Warrenburg for a psychophysiology course taught at Yale University that used a systems perspective.

Returning to Type A behavior and cardiovascular responding, it becomes clear that Measure 1, the self-report data, represents Level 5 information produced by the subject via cortical mechanisms involved in self-reflective cognitive processing. Note that the subject is asked to rate his/her behavior and intentions in terms of his/her memory. The subject's memory may be incomplete and/or distorted; plus, the subject may choose to answer the questions in a less honest, more socially desirable fashion.

Measure 2, the interview, also represents Level 5 information, but this information is inferred by an outside observer by measuring parameters such as loudness of voice. Note that loudness of voice is a Level 1 BEHAVIOR, just like blood pressure. Loudness of voice is determined by patterns of sounds interacting in the mouth and sinuses (Level 2), which are generated by complex patterns of organ BEHAVIOR (Level 3 vocal, respiratory, and facial organ behavior), which in turn are generated by complex patterns of neural control (Level 4) and ultimately mediated by the brain (Level 5). However, the loudness of the voice per se, especially if it is occurring spontaneously (as opposed to being consciously self-regulated by the subject), may be mediated more directly by subcortical, limbic processes. Similarly, one can think of spontaneous facial expressions of emotions as being "windows into the hypothalamus," bridging Level-1-to-Level-5 processes again (what one sees overtly in facial expression are patterns of skin movement—Level 1, which psychologists and laymen label as "behavior").

Note that Measure 3, the cardiovascular measures, is actually a combination of Levels 3 and 1. Heart rate is a Level 3 parameter vis-à-vis its relationship to blood pressure, whereas blood pressure is a Level 1 parameter. Actually, splitting mean pressure into systolic and diastolic pressure provides a closer link between Levels 1 and 2, and, therefore, between Levels 2 and 3. As we will see later, interpreting *patterns* of Level 1 and 3 measures helps to organize and differentiate between different psychobiological states.

Finally, Measure 4, the endocrine measures, concerns Level 4 BEHAVIORS. Epinephrine and norepinephrine each have multiple effects on patterns of Level 3 processes, and these patterns of effects are not identical. Norepinephrine tends to have more of a vasoconstrictive effect, whereas epinephrine has more of a contractility and heart rate effect. Thus, patterns of epinephrine and norepinephrine can lead to complex patterns of organ BEHAVIOR.

## CAN SYSTEMS "DISSOCIATE"?

Organizing the measures in this fashion is useful because it helps organize one's thinking on a variety of topics, including the degree to which it is possible (and valuable) to discover *dissociations* among the different dependent variables within and across levels, and the extent to which one can ideally select other dependent variables to help link the various levels of processes.

Let us consider the question of dissociation more closely. DISSOCIATION can be thought of as a general systems concept in the same way that BEHAVIOR can be thought of as a general systems concept. "Dissociation" to a psychologist might imply a personality disorder (e.g., the multiple personality syndrome), whereas DISSOCIATION to a systems theorist simply means lack of ASSOCIATION. Different measures (i.e., BEHAVIORS) can be ASSOCIATED or DISSOCIATED to various degrees. Note that DISSOCIATIONS can occur both within levels and across levels. When psychologists speak about dissociations between autonomic measures, they are referring to DISSOCIATIONS within a level (e.g., Level 3); whereas when they speak of dissociations between self-report, behavioral, and physiological measures (e.g., Lang, 1977), they are referring to DISSOCIATIONS across various levels. Theoretically, the more distant two measures are in terms of levels, the greater the potential for their DISSOCIATION.

The relative lack of correlation typically reported in the literature across different physiological responses (measured at Levels 3, 2, and 1) partly reflects the capacity of different response systems to DISSOCIATE or ASSOCIATE under different environmental conditions. The confusing array of findings in the literature might be clarified if a systems perspective was adopted for conceptualizing how different responses within and across levels can be ASSOCIATED.

## IS THERE SUCH A THING AS A "SINGLE" CARDIOVASCULAR MEASURE? A RESPONSE IS NOT A RESPONSE IS NOT A RESPONSE

A fundamental systems principle implied in Figure 11-1 and in our prior discussion of organistic thinking is that no *single* measure (BEHAVIOR) is ultimately a *single* measure of anything. That is an illusion. Every response is multiply determined to various degrees by parameters interacting within and across levels. For example, consider blood pressure. Blood pressure (Level 1) can increase as a function of increased cardiac output or increased peripheral resistance (Level 2). Many different patterns of cardiac output and peripheral resistance can all lead to the same mean blood pressure increase. Therefore, a blood pressure increase is not a blood pressure increase is not a blood pressure increase.

If two subjects show the same mean increase in blood pressure (Level 1) to a given external stimulus, this does not necessarily mean that the subjects have responded by the same mechanisms (by the same pattern of Level 2 processes, and hence patterns of processes in Levels 3-5). Or, if a given subject responds to two different situations with the same mean increase in blood pressure, this does not necessarily mean that the subject responded to both situations with the same pattern of Level 2 processes and above. Note that I use the term "pattern" here to denote the fact that combinations of higher-level processes (BEHAVIORS) can mediate similar outcomes at lower levels (BEHAVIORS).

This same principle applies to BEHAVIORS at all levels. If one were to measure cardiac output (at Level 2), one would quickly determine that cardiac output can increase due to an increase in heart rate or an increase in stroke volume. Again, many different combinations of heart rate and stroke volume can lead to the same increase in cardiac output. Hence, cardiac output is not cardiac output is not cardiac output.

Moving up levels does not eliminate this problem. The general principle continues to apply. Consider heart rate (Level 3). Heart rate can increase due to increased sympathetic tone, decreased parasympathetic tone, or increased circulating epinephrine, to list but a few possible Level 4 mechanisms. A given heart rate increase can occur as a result of numerous combinations/patterns of these Level 4 processes. Therefore, a heart rate increase is not a heart rate increase is not a heart rate increase.

Once this principle is deeply understood, one will never be content to measure a single parameter in isolation again! Rather, one will seek not only to measure patterns of processes occurring at different levels but also to describe statistically how the measured BEHAVIORS are organized under different conditions.

Consider, for example, recent research from our laboratory on patterning of heart rate, systolic blood pressure, and diastolic blood pressure, in different emotional states (Schwartz, Weinberger, & Singer, 1981). Briefly, 36 subjects imagined walking up and down a step, and then actually walked up and down a step, simultaneously expressing one of six different emotions nonverbally. The emotional conditions were happiness, sadness, anger, fear, control, and relaxation. Systolic and diastolic blood pressure, and heart rate, were measured intermittently during baseline periods, after the imagery period, and after the approximately 1-min exercise period.

Subjects rated their own emotions during the imagery and exercise periods. In addition, the experimenter rated their nonverbal behavior for overt evidence of their emotional responding during the imagery and exercise periods. Thus, similar to the Type A example mentioned previously, we had three categories of measures (1, 2, 3—we lacked the 4th, neuroendocrine measure, as mentioned in the Type A example).

The cardiovascular measures were examined for configurations/ patterns, using various multivariate statistics. Importantly, data differentiating the different emotional states emerged not only in terms of the patterns of *mean* changes in the cardiovascular parameters (e.g., fear was accompanied by increases in systolic blood pressure and heart rate but not diastolic blood pressure, whereas anger was accompanied by increases in all three parameters) but more importantly in their *interrelationships* as a function of different emotional conditions. For example, during exercise, changes in systolic and diastolic pressure were dissociated (became uncorrelated) for all the emotions except sadness, suggesting that "sadness produced a psychobiological state which was incompatible with the normal adjustments of exercise" (Schwartz *et al.*, 1981). Or, discriminate analyses revealed for the first linear combination a positive discriminate weight for happiness (.36) and a negative discriminate weight for sadness (−.35), whereas the second linear combination revealed a negative discriminate weight for happiness (−.31) and a positive discriminate weight for sadness (.75), indicating that the cardiovascular adjustments were organized differently for happiness and sadness.

The interrelationships between the two "psychological" measures (self-report and observer ratings) and the three cardiovascular parameters were also investigated. Importantly, the cardiovascular changes were more reliably associated with the *observer*'s ratings of the subject's *overt* behavior than with the subject's *self-ratings*. As described in Schwartz (1981), this finding makes good sense in systems terms, since the cardiovascular and somatic BEHAVIORS (the latter inferred by the observer ratings) are more closely linked (anatomically in the CNS, Level 5; and proximally, Level 3) than are the subject's perceptions of his/her emotions with either of the Level 3 or 1 BEHAVIORS.

Systems theory provides the conceptual structure for stimulating novel ways of describing interrelationships among different BEHAVIORS measured within and across levels. In fact, as described in the next section, not only does system theory encourage the use of pattern recognition statistics, but it also stimulates the use of more dynamic, time-oriented statistics to assess changes in patterns of responses over time.

However, I do not mean to imply that what is needed is simply the attaching of more electrodes and the production of more computer printout. Rather, what I am suggesting is that modern systems theory can be used to help integrate our approach to the design, analysis, and interpretation of multilevel experiments, thereby helping to guide our choice of measures and the types of analyses most appropriate for describing the systems' functioning.

## WHAT IS CONTROL THEORY? AN ANALYSIS OF
## REGULATION AND DISREGULATION

An important subset of general systems theory is referred to as "control theory" (or cybernetics; Wiener, 1948). Control theory is concerned with the mechanisms by which systems regulate themselves, drawing on dynamic processes of feedback that change the BEHAVIOR of a system over time. As Jones (1973) describes in his superb book titled *Principles of Biological Regulation: An Introduction to Feedback Systems*, systems such as the cardiovascular system are never static nor are they "closed." Rather they are "open" and constantly adjusting to stimuli or demands imposed upon them. If the feedback processes are connected and are functioning appropriate to the system, the BEHAVIOR of the system will not be random but will show an orderly pattern of change over time.

Figure 11-2 is taken from Carver and Scheier's (1981) recent book titled *Attention and Self-Regulation*, which is an excellent introduction to control theory as applied to psychology. This figure nicely illustrates how negative and positive feedback can differentially alter the BEHAVIOR of a system to a load/stress/demand placed upon it. The figure illustrates that if the feedback is negative, and it is not excessive, the negative feedback will serve to restore the system back to some prior value or "reference value." This is the essence of Cannon's concept of homeostasis. However, if the negative feedback is excessive, it can act as positive feedback, which will drive the system's behavior to extremes.

The mathematics of control theory are quite complex and are beyond the scope of this chapter (see Jones, 1973, for an excellent overview of control theory; also see the volume by Basar, 1976, who provides a nice introduction to a biophysical and physiological systems analysis of broad relevance to psychophysiology). However, the reader should quickly grasp a few key properties that illustrate the importance of this general perspective for studying cardiovascular psychophysiology.

For example, note that the cardiovascular responses to moderate-intensity psychological stimuli in normal, healthy individuals look quite similar to Panel (b) of Figure 11-2. Beat-by-beat changes in heart rate to moderate-intensity psychological stimuli often show a repeatable pattern of relative decreases and increases in rate. This temporal pattern of response is highly suggestive of a mildly overcompensating negative feedback system.

Theoretically, by specifying more precisely—that is, by quantifying

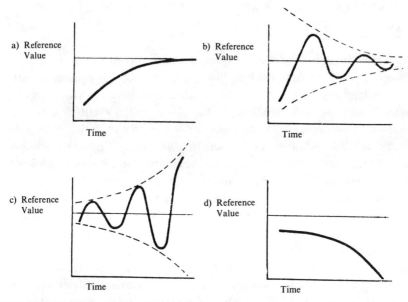

FIG. 11-2. Responses of four feedback systems to an initial deviation: (a) a smoothly functioning negative feedback loop, (b) a negative feedback loop with slight overcompensation, (c) a negative feedback loop with sufficient overcompensation that positive feedback occurs, and (d) a positive feedback loop. From *Attention and Self-Regulation: A Control-Theory Approach to Human Behavior*, by C. S. Carver and M. F. Scheier. New York: Springer-Verlag, 1981. Reprinted by permission.

the ordering, timing, and peaking of the total response (both the reaction and recovery process)—it becomes possible to better describe the underlying mechanisms that are called into play as they are expressed in the cardiovascular system. By manipulating various properties of the external stimulus, plus the subjects' interpretation of the stimulus, it becomes possible to infer: (1) whether the reference value has been altered, (2) whether the signal has been amplified (or dampened) by the subject on the input side, and/or (3) whether the feedback has been amplified (or dampened) on the output/recovery side.

It should be immediately apparent that by specifying input/output functions more precisely, as they deviate from normal patterns, it becomes possible to specify more precisely the mechanisms contributing to individual differences in response and recovery. The recovery process is especially interesting in this regard, because it reflects the extent to which the normal negative feedback, homeostatic processes are operating effectively. It is possible, in fact, to have patterns, or combinations, of input (e.g., peak) and output (e.g., time to recovery) BEHAVIORS that will reflect disruptions in patterns of input and output functioning.

For example, two subjects can have similar peak amplitude responses to a given stimulus, yet recover at markedly different rates and with different degrees of under- or overcompensation. Theoretically, these differences in recovery will be reflecting differences in the generation and processing of negative feedback. Conversely, two subjects can have similar recovery times, yet show markedly different peak amplitude responses to a given stimulus. Theoretically, these differences in peak response will be reflecting differences in the input processing of the stimuli.

Note that if a subject's negative feedback was markedly attenuated or, in extreme cases, was disconnected, not only would his/her recovery be markedly disordered if not eliminated entirely, but the lack of feedback would have the additional effect of allowing the initial response to rise more to begin with! In other words, if two subjects differ in their initial peak response to a stimulus, it is possible that increased response may be a byproduct of a disregulated negative feedback process (Schwartz, 1979). In this case of disregulation, one would theoretically observe that the timing of the peak would be delayed as well, since the feedback normally restraining the peak would be eliminated. Conversely, the time to reach a given value might actually be increasing, again for the same reason. Thus, if two subjects show a heightened peak response, the heightened peak may be due to different mechanisms. By measuring time to peak, and recovery from the peak, it becomes possible to better specify why the peak is peaking as it does. Thus, it follows from systems theory that a peak response is not a peak response is not a peak response.

The solution to the problem of distinguishing between different mechanisms contributing to under- or overresponding, or under- or over-recovery, is to measure patterns of information *temporally* as well as across different physiological responses. An elegant approach to the study of cardiovascular self-regulation and disregulation would be to measure various parameters in terms of *levels* (both within the cardiovascular system and possibly across relevant physiological systems) and then examine their *temporal* response and recovery patterns to different stimuli. Using systems and control theory as a guide, it should be possible to better organize the resulting information, draw predictions about possible outcomes, specify the patterns of information statistically, and interpret the results.

The reader should also note that negative and positive feedback processes are actually both "self-regulating" processes in the sense that the system BEHAVES in a manner governed by the components as they control each other in a feedback loop fashion. Positive feedback does not lead to "disordered" BEHAVIOR—it leads to ordered BEHAVIOR of a given type, one that is as self-regulatory as BEHAVIOR generated by negative feedback. If negative or positive feedback is delayed, distorted, or, in extreme cases, disconnected, the system will show a relative decrease in self-regulated BEHAVIOR (as governed by the particular feedback process), which will be expressed as disordered functioning. I use the term "disregulation" to refer to this general process (Schwartz, 1977, 1978, 1979).

"Disregulation" is a general concept and actually should be capitalized, as should the term "regulation." Since REGULATION can occur at any level, DISREGULATION can also occur in any feedback process at any level. Hence, DISREGULATION can occur at the periphery (Levels 3–1 in Figure 11-1) or can occur more centrally (within the CNS, Level 5 itself). The resulting DISORDERED BEHAVIOR can be measured at various levels, depending upon the level of the initial DISREGULATION. In certain cases, DISREGULATION at one level may lead to REGULATION at another level. However, space precludes a detailed discussion of REGULATION and DISREGULATION in complex systems and their quantification mathematically. Nonetheless, the reader should see the potential for organizing different biological, psychological, and social sources of information in terms of levels and in terms of their dynamic degrees of REGULATION and DISREGULATION expressed over time.

## SUMMARY AND CONCLUSIONS

The goal of this chapter has been to present some basic concepts of systems theory and to illustrate how these concepts might be applied to future research in cardiovascular psychophysiology. Clearly, the intent of this chapter has not been to focus on specific data per se. Rather, the goal has been to describe a general orientation that has broad implications for organizing data, collecting information, describing results mathematically, and interpreting interrelationships. Systems theory is, of course, no stranger to physiology (e.g., von Bertalanffy, 1968). However, systems theory is not typically applied in a *general* sense to organizing information that cuts across various levels of complexity (recall Table 11-2).

Cardiovascular psychophysiology, and especially cardiovascular social psychophysiology, cuts across so many levels as to make the task of interpreting the data almost impossible without some general organizing structure. The comprehensive researcher must be able to think formistically, mechanistically, organistically, and contextually; and have some familiarity with concepts in physics and electronics, chemistry, physiology, psychology, and even sociology (e.g., consider how social class and ethnic background influence cardiovascular responding to certain classes of psychosocial stimulation)! The emergence of behavioral medicine, broadly defined, illustrates this growing movement toward synthesis, with an accompanying paradigmatic shift toward multivariate, multilevel thinking (Schwartz, 1982).

Clearly, some general structure is needed for organizing this information, for specifying when levels are crossed and how various parameters relate to each other within and across different levels. Systems theory provides such a general structure. In addition, systems theory helps formulate general principles and techniques for describing the BEHAVIOR of any system over time, especially self-regulating BEHAVIOR. Thus, accompanying the organizational structure of systems theory is a mathematical structure for approaching the analysis of patterns of information over time.

The intent of systems theory, however, is not to lead researchers to become loose in their thinking, nor is it antagonistic to scientific specialization per se. On the contrary, the goal of systems theory is to help *structure* one's thinking so as to better integrate one's specialized training and knowledge with the larger body of skills and information that must be integrated in order to do research that cuts across physical, biological, psychological, and social levels of functioning. Whether research in cardiovascular psychophysiology will become more advanced in terms of organization, methodology, and integration as a function of developments in systems theory remains an empirical question.

## REFERENCES

Basar, E. *Biophysical and physiological systems analysis.* Reading, Mass.: Addison-Wesley, 1976.

Carver, C. S., & Scheier, M. F. *Attention and self-regulation: A control-theory approach to human behavior.* New York: Springer-Verlag, 1981.

deRosnay, J. *The macroscope.* New York: Harper & Row, 1979.

Glass, D. C., Krakoff, L. R., Contrada, R., Hilton, W. F., Kehoe, K., Mannucci, E. G., Collins, C., Snow, B., & Elting, E. Effect of harassment and competition upon cardiovascular and plasma catecholamine responses in Type A and Type B Individuals. *Psychophysiology*, 1981, *17*, 453–463.

Guyton, A. C., Coleman, T. G., & Granger, H. J. Circulation: Overall regulation. *Annual Review of Physiology*, 1972, *34*, 13–46.

Harris, M., Fontana, A. F., & Dowds, B. N. The world hypotheses scale: Rationale, reliability and validity. *Journal of Personality Assessment*, 1977, *41*, 337–347.

Jones, R. W. *Principles of biological regulation: An introduction to feedback systems.* New York: Academic Press, 1973.

Lang, P. J. Anxiety: Toward a psychophysiological definition. In H. S. Akiskal & W. L. Webb (Eds.), *Psychiatric diagnosis: Exploration of biological predictors.* New York: Spectrum, 1977.

Miller, J. G. *Living systems.* New York: McGraw-Hill, 1978.

Pepper, S. C. *World hypotheses.* Berkeley: University of California Press, 1942.

Schwartz, G. E. Psychosomatic disorders and biofeedback: A psychobiological model of disregulation. In J. D. Maser &ᵗ°M. E. P. Seligman (Eds.), *Psychopathology: Experimental models.* San Francisco: W. H. Freeman, 1977.

Schwartz, G. E. Psychobiological foundations of psychotherapy and behavior change. In S. L. Garfield & A. E. Bergin (Eds.), *Handbook of psychotherapy and behavior change* (2nd ed.). New York: Wiley, 1978.

Schwartz, G. E. Disregulation and systems theory: A biobehavioral framework for biofeedback and behavioral medicine. In N. Birbaumer & H. D. Kimmel (Eds.), *Biofeedback and self-regulation.* Hillsdale, N.J.: Erlbaum, 1979.

Schwartz, G. E. Psychophysiological patterning and emotion revisited: A systems perspective. In C. Izard (Ed.), *Measuring emotions in infants and children.* Cambridge: Cambridge University Press, 1981.

Schwartz, G. E. Integrating psychobiology and behavior therapy: A systems perspective. In G. T. Wilson & C. M. Franks (Eds.), *Contemporary behavior therapy: Conceptual and empirical foundations.* New York: Guilford Press, 1982.

Schwartz, G. E., Shapiro, A. P., Redmond, D. P., Ferguson, D. C. E., Ragland, D. R., & Weiss, S. M. Behavioral medicine approaches to hypertension: An integrative analysis of theory and research. *Journal of Behavioral Medicine*, 1979, *2*, 311–363.

Schwartz, G. E., Weinberger, D. A., & Singer, J. A. Cardiovascular differentiation of happiness, sadness, anger, and fear following imagery and exercise. *Psychosomatic Medicine*, 1981, *43*, 343–364.

Schwartz, G. E., & Weiss, S. M. *Proceedings of the Yale Conference on Behavioral Medicine* (DHEW Publication No. [NIH] 78-1424). Washington, D.C.: Department of Health, Education, and Welfare, 1978.

Skinner, B. F. *Science and human behavior.* New York: Macmillan, 1953.

von Bertalanffy, L. *General systems theory.* New York: Braziller, 1968.

Weinberg, G. M. *An introduction to general systems thinking.* New York: Wiley, 1975.

Wiener, N. *Cybernetics or control and communication in the animal and machine.* Cambridge, Mass.: MIT Press, 1948.

Zukav, G. *The dancing Wu Li masters.* New York: Morrow, 1979.

# Author Index

Starr, I., 38, 39, 90*n.*
Stebbins, W. C., 270, 295*n.*, 297, 314*n.*
Steele, J. M., 54, 90*n.*
Stegall, H. F., 59, 90*n.*
Stein, L., 97, 126*n.*
Stephens, J. H., 312, 314*n.*
Steptoe, A. W., 46, 63–65, 85*n.*, 90*n.*, 299, 314*n.*
Sterman, M. B., 243, 260*n.*, 261*n.*
Stern, J. A., 105, 106, 124*n.*, 146, 148*n.*
Stern, M., 54, 57, 89*n.*
Stern, R. M., 71, 90*n.*, 153, 168, 187*n.*
Sternbach, R. A., 2, 3*n.*, 50, 90*n.*, 130, 149*n.*, 279, 295*n.*
Stewart, G. N., 68, 90*n.*
Stone, T. W., 192, 220*n.*
Strange, P. W., 71, 90*n.*
Straus, R., 317, 318, 342*n.*, 345*n.*
Stringfellow, J. C., 29, 86*n.*
Strongman, K. T., 154, 187*n.*
Sturmfels, L., 105, 124*n.*
Surwit, R. S., 67, 90*n.*
Sutterer, J. R., 11, 18*n.*, 32, 36, 88*n.*, 98, 101, 113, 114, 119, 125*n.*, 225, 263*n.*, 267, 273, 283, 295*n.*
Svensson, T. H., 191, 222*n.*
Swammerdam, 67
Swaney, K., 283, 292*n.*
Swanson, J., 214
Szpiler, J. A., 100, 126*n.*

Taggert, P., 337, 345*n.*
Tahmoush, A. J., 76, 87*n.*, 90*n.*
Talbot, S. A., 81, 82, 90*n.*
Tam, R. M. K., 236, 260*n.*
Tang, P. C., 239, 264*n.*
Taubman, F., 38, 84*n.*
Tavel, M. E., 63, 64, 90*n.*
Taves, P. A., 158, 160, 161, 184*n.*
Taylor, H. L., 337, 343*n.*
Taylor, K., 28, 90*n.*
Teller E. S., 104, 125*n.*, 268, 294*n.*, 334, 344*n.*
Terry, B. S., 235, 261*n.*
Tesser, A., 168, 187*n.*
Thackray, R. I., 50, 61, 88*n.*, 90*n.*
Thauer, R., 32, 91*n.*
Thomas, D. B., 320, 345*n.*
Thomas, G., 329, 345*n.*
Thompson, H. B., 1, 3*n.*, 7, 18*n.*
Thompson, L. W., 198, 209, 222*n.*, 318, 341*n.*
Thoren, P., 191, 222*n.*
Thorne, P. R., 29, 91*n.*
Thurstone, L. L., 154, 187*n.*
Tiniter, C. M., 54, 83*n.*

Tosheff, J. G., 275, 291*n.*
Tournade, A., 190, 222*n.*
Trap-Jensen, J., 306, 313*n.*
Traube, 232
Treolar, A. E., 51, 91*n.*
Triandis, H. C., 154, 187*n.*
Troyer, W. G., 176, 186*n.*
Turpin, G., 223, 263*n.*
Tursky, B., 1, 19–82, 19, 20, 24, 25, 26, 29–31, 46, 50, 52, 54, 55, 57–59, 61, 67, 76, 77, 81, 83*n.*, 84*n.*, 86*n.*, 88*n.*, 91*n.*, 130, 149*n.*, 173, 176*n.*, 187*n.*, 200, 222*n.*
Twentyman, C. T., 31, 87*n.*
Tyler, S. W., 176*n.*, 188*n.*
Tyrer, P., 128, 132, 150*n.*
Tzankoff, S. P., 300

Uviller, E. T., 132, 149*n.*, 153, 186*n.*
Uzmann, J. W., 61, 91*n.*

Valimaki, I., 239, 261*n.*
Valins, S., 133, 150*n.*, 152, 167, 188*n.*
Vallbona, C., 236, 239, 252, 262*n.*, 264*n.*
Van Bergen, F. H., 51, 91*n.*
Vandenberg, J., 75, 84*n.*
VanDercar, D. H., 26, 89*n.*
Van Egeren, L. F., 93, 126*n.*, 330, 345*n.*
Van Gelder, D., 10, 18*n.*
VanderHoeven, G. M. A., 63, 64, 91*n.*
Van Toller, C., 156, 188*n.*
Vendrik, A. J. H., 78, 79, 83*n.*
Verghese, A., 337, 344*n.*
Verrier, R., 255, 260*n.*, 262*n.*, 328, 344*n.*
Victor, R., 134–137, 140, 143, 144, 150*n.*, 299, 314*n.*
Vigier, D., 192, 220*n.*
Vinci, Leonardo da, 5
Volpitto, P. P., 65, 89*n.*
von Bertalanffy, L., 350, 370, 372*n.*
Voudakis, I. A., 337, 345*n.*

Walker, B. B., 2, 25, 83*n.*, 152, 183*n.*, 189–219, 196, 203, 204, 220*n.*, 222*n.*
Wallach, J. H., 240, 261*n.*
Walter, D. O., 243, 260*n.*, 261*n.*
Walter, G. F., 30, 91*n.*, 253, 263*n.*
Weatherhead, D. S., 51, 91*n.*
Webb, G. N., 34, 88*n.*
Webb, R. A., 11, 18*n.*, 32, 88*n.*, 99, 126*n.*, 225, 263*n.*, 267, 273, 294*n.*
Weber, F., 76, 90*n.*
Webster, J. G., 34, 47, 66, 70, 73, 74, 76, 91*n.*
Wechsler, A., 175*n.*, 184*n.*

# Subject Index

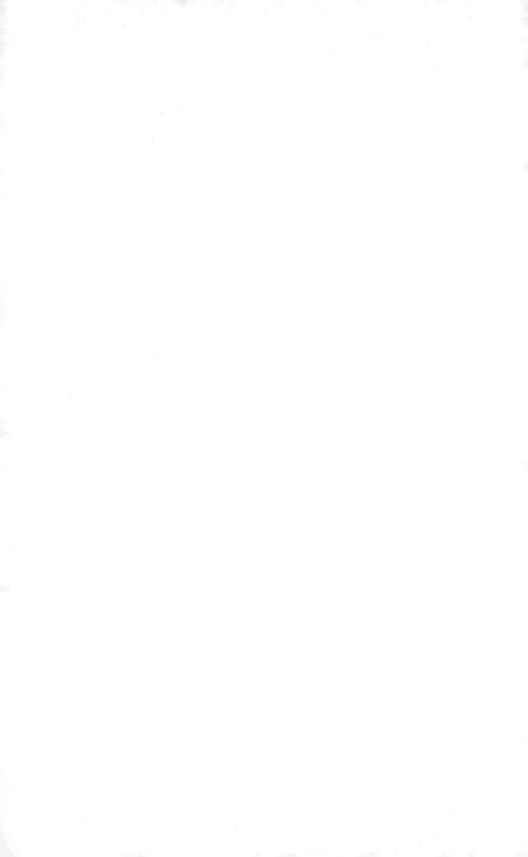